Disruptive Behavior Disorders: Symptoms, Evaluation and Treatment

Disruptive Behavior Disorders: Symptoms, Evaluation and Treatment

Editors

Annarita Milone
Gianluca Sesso

MDPI • Basel • Beijing • Wuhan • Barcelona • Belgrade • Manchester • Tokyo • Cluj • Tianjin

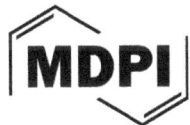

Editors
Annarita Milone
Department of Child Psychiatry
and Psychopharmacology
IRCCS Stella Maris Foundation
Pisa
Italy

Gianluca Sesso
Department of Clinical and
Experimental Medicine
University of Pisa
Pisa
Italy

Editorial Office
MDPI
St. Alban-Anlage 66
4052 Basel, Switzerland

This is a reprint of articles from the Special Issue published online in the open access journal *Brain Sciences* (ISSN 2076-3425) (available at: www.mdpi.com/journal/brainsci/special_issues/ Disruptive_Behavior_Disorders_Symptoms_Evaluation_Treatment).

For citation purposes, cite each article independently as indicated on the article page online and as indicated below:

LastName, A.A.; LastName, B.B.; LastName, C.C. Article Title. *Journal Name* **Year**, *Volume Number*, Page Range.

ISBN 978-3-0365-3628-6 (Hbk)
ISBN 978-3-0365-3627-9 (PDF)

Cover image courtesy of Erika Riciniello

© 2022 by the authors. Articles in this book are Open Access and distributed under the Creative Commons Attribution (CC BY) license, which allows users to download, copy and build upon published articles, as long as the author and publisher are properly credited, which ensures maximum dissemination and a wider impact of our publications.
The book as a whole is distributed by MDPI under the terms and conditions of the Creative Commons license CC BY-NC-ND.

Contents

Preface to "Disruptive Behavior Disorders: Symptoms, Evaluation and Treatment" vii

Annarita Milone and Gianluca Sesso
Disruptive Behavior Disorders: Symptoms, Evaluation and Treatment
Reprinted from: *Brain Sci.* **2022**, *12*, 225, doi:10.3390/brainsci12020225 1

Claudia A. Robles-Haydar, Marina B. Martínez-González, Yuliana A. Flórez-Niño, Luz M. Ibáñez-Navarro and José J. Amar-Amar
Personal and Environmental Predictors of Aggression in Adolescence
Reprinted from: *Brain Sci.* **2021**, *11*, 933, doi:10.3390/brainsci11070933 7

Marina B. Martínez-González, Yamile Turizo-Palencia, Claudia Arenas-Rivera, Mónica Acuña-Rodríguez, Yeferson Gómez-López and Vicente J. Clemente-Suárez
Gender, Anxiety, and Legitimation of Violence in Adolescents Facing Simulated Physical Aggression at School
Reprinted from: *Brain Sci.* **2021**, *11*, 458, doi:10.3390/brainsci11040458 23

Gennaro Catone, Luisa Almerico, Anna Pezzella, Maria Pia Riccio, Carmela Bravaccio and Pia Bernardo et al.
The Relation of Callous–Unemotional Traits and Bullying in Early Adolescence Is Independent from Sex and Age and Moderated by Conduct Problems
Reprinted from: *Brain Sci.* **2021**, *11*, 1059, doi:10.3390/brainsci11081059 33

Laura López-Romero, Olalla Cutrín, Lorena Maneiro, Beatriz Domínguez-Álvarez and Estrella Romero
Psychopathic Traits in Childhood: Insights from Parental Warmth and Fearless Temperament via Conscience Development
Reprinted from: *Brain Sci.* **2021**, *11*, 923, doi:10.3390/brainsci11070923 47

Martina Smorti, Emanuela Inguaggiato, Lara Vezzosi and Annarita Milone
Parenting and Sibling Relationships in Family with Disruptive Behavior Disorders. Are Non-Clinical Siblings More Vulnerable for Emotional and Behavioral Problems?
Reprinted from: *Brain Sci.* **2021**, *11*, 1308, doi:10.3390/brainsci11101308 63

Eleonora Marzilli, Luca Cerniglia and Silvia Cimino
Antisocial Personality Problems in Emerging Adulthood: The Role of Family Functioning, Impulsivity, and Empathy
Reprinted from: *Brain Sci.* **2021**, *11*, 687, doi:10.3390/brainsci11060687 79

Pamela Fantozzi, Gianluca Sesso, Pietro Muratori, Annarita Milone and Gabriele Masi
Biological Bases of Empathy and Social Cognition in Patients with Attention-Deficit/Hyperactivity Disorder: A Focus on Treatment with Psychostimulants
Reprinted from: *Brain Sci.* **2021**, *11*, 1399, doi:10.3390/brainsci11111399 95

Carla Balia, Sara Carucci, Annarita Milone, Roberta Romaniello, Elena Valente and Federica Donno et al.
Neuropsychological Characterization of Aggressive Behavior in Children and Adolescents with CD/ODD and Effects of Single Doses of Medications: The Protocol of the Matrics_WP6-1 Study
Reprinted from: *Brain Sci.* **2021**, *11*, 1639, doi:10.3390/brainsci11121639 115

John E. Lochman, Caroline L. Boxmeyer, Chuong Bui, Estephan Hakim, Shannon Jones and Francesca Kassing et al.
Substance Use Outcomes from Two Formats of a Cognitive-Behavioral Intervention for Aggressive Children: Moderating Roles of Inhibitory Control and Intervention Engagement
Reprinted from: *Brain Sci.* **2021**, *11*, 950, doi:10.3390/brainsci11070950 . . . . **135**

Caroline L. Boxmeyer, Shari Miller, Devon E. Romero, Nicole P. Powell, Shannon Jones and Lixin Qu et al.
Mindful Coping Power: Comparative Effects on Children's Reactive Aggression and Self-Regulation
Reprinted from: *Brain Sci.* **2021**, *11*, 1119, doi:10.3390/brainsci11091119 . . . . **153**

Gabriele Masi, Ilaria Lupetti, Giulia D'Acunto, Annarita Milone, Deborah Fabiani and Ursula Madonia et al.
A Comparison between Severe Suicidality and Nonsuicidal Self-Injury Behaviors in Bipolar Adolescents Referred to a Psychiatric Emergency Unit
Reprinted from: *Brain Sci.* **2021**, *11*, 790, doi:10.3390/brainsci11060790 . . . . **173**

Carlo Buonanno, Enrico Iuliano, Giuseppe Grossi, Francesco Mancini, Emiliana Stendardo and Fabrizia Tudisco et al.
Forgiveness in the Modulation of Responsibility in a Sample of Italian Adolescents with a Tendency towards Conduct or Obsessive–Compulsive Problems
Reprinted from: *Brain Sci.* **2021**, *11*, 1333, doi:10.3390/brainsci11101333 . . . . **187**

Preface to "Disruptive Behavior Disorders: Symptoms, Evaluation and Treatment"

The principal aims of this Special Issue were to address three core features of the clinical management of Disruptive Behavior Disorders (DBD), namely, its clinical presentations and epidemiologic correlates, the multidimensional assessment of callous–unemotional traits, empathic faults and emotional dysregulation, and the available treatment options. In this Special Issue, twelve relevant contributions, which provide novel insights for the assessment and treatment of DBD in clinical practice, have been collected by the editors, Dr Annarita Milone and Dr Gianluca Sesso. The editors would like to thank colleagues and friends worldwide who fruitfully contributed to this Special Issue and helped them make it a concrete achievement. They also thank the colleagues of the Department of Child Psychiatry and Psychopharmacology of the IRCCS Stella Maris Foundation and especially Dr Gabriele Masi, the Head of the Department, for supporting the research in the field of Disruptive Behavior Disorders.

Annarita Milone and Gianluca Sesso
Editors

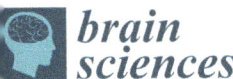

Editorial

Disruptive Behavior Disorders: Symptoms, Evaluation and Treatment

Annarita Milone [1,*] and Gianluca Sesso [1,2]

1. Department of Developmental Neuroscience, IRCCS Stella Maris Foundation, 56128 Pisa, Italy; gsesso@fsm.unipi.it
2. Department of Clinical and Experimental Medicine, University of Pisa, 56128 Pisa, Italy
* Correspondence: annarita.milone@fsm.unipi.it

Citation: Milone, A.; Sesso, G. Disruptive Behavior Disorders: Symptoms, Evaluation and Treatment. *Brain Sci.* **2022**, *12*, 225. https://doi.org/10.3390/brainsci12020225

Received: 28 January 2022
Accepted: 28 January 2022
Published: 7 February 2022

Publisher's Note: MDPI stays neutral with regard to jurisdictional claims in published maps and institutional affiliations.

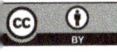

Copyright: © 2022 by the authors. Licensee MDPI, Basel, Switzerland. This article is an open access article distributed under the terms and conditions of the Creative Commons Attribution (CC BY) license (https://creativecommons.org/licenses/by/4.0/).

1. Introduction

Disruptive behavior disorders (DBD) refer to a group of conditions that typically share difficulties in modulating aggressive conducts, self-control, and impulses, with resulting behaviors that constitute a threat to others' safety and to social norms. Problematic issues with self-control associated with these disorders are commonly first observed in childhood, but may often persist into adolescence and adulthood, or pose a developmental risk for subsequent negative outcomes. The clinical management of DBD in childhood and adolescence has seen great advances in recent years, and research has also focused on identifying early signs, predictors, and risk factors, which may help clinicians to disentangle and subtype the heterogeneous manifestations of BDB. This has allowed significant progress to be made in defining specific developmental trajectories, targeted prevention programs, and timely treatment strategies.

The principal aims of this Special Issue were thus to address three core features of DBD clinical management, namely, its clinical presentations and epidemiologic correlates, including predictors of aggressiveness, gender-specific manifestations, and the role of familiar factors; the multidimensional assessment of callous–unemotional traits, empathic faults, executive dysfunctions, and emotional dysregulation; and the available treatment options, which comprise rehabilitative and pharmacological interventions. In this Special Issue, twelve relevant contributions, including ten original articles, one systematic review, and one study protocol, which provide novel insights for the assessment and treatment of DBD in clinical practice, are reported here (see Table A1).

2. Personality Traits and Socio-Environmental Factors as Correlates of Aggressiveness

The study by Robles-Haydar and colleagues [1] primarily aimed to identify the correlates of aggression in non-referred adolescents, hypothesizing a major contribution for moral disengagement in the development of antisocial tendencies. This study examined a set of clinically relevant sociodemographic, personal, and familiar variables, using structural equation models to determine causal relationships. While values of conformity and transcendence seem to inhibit aggressive behaviors, openness, moral disengagement and leadership are among its main predictors, a causal role for gender was also detected. Personality traits and environmental risk factors have been confirmed as well-known essential contributors involved in the development of antisocial conducts in adolescents. These results provide crucial cues, with major relevance in defining primary aims of therapeutic interventions and the prevention of DBD in childhood and adolescence.

Among the predictors of aggressiveness, gender and anxiety were also assessed in a study conducted on 1147 adolescents by Martínez-González and coworkers [2]. In this study, participants watched animated situations of simulated physical aggression against peers and filled out a questionnaire to assess the legitimation of violent behaviors and anxiety levels. While gender was not associated with the behaviors chosen to solve the situation, those adolescents who applied diffusion of responsibility and dehumanization to justify their behavior also showed higher levels of anxiety. Similarly, girls who expected legitimation from their peers presented higher anxiety as well. These results are essential to develop individual and groups of adolescents' educational programs that improve the awareness of aggressive behaviors' consequences, modify the way to manage interpersonal conflicts, and change gender-based stereotypes.

Similar findings were also reported by Catone and collaborators [3] in the Bullying and Youth Mental Health Naples study on cyberbullying behaviors in early adolescence. The aim of the study was to replicate and extend previous findings in a large Italian sample. Conduct problems, callous unemotional traits, traditional bullying and cyberbullying behaviors were assessed by self-rated measures. A significant and specific association between callous unemotional traits and traditional bullying was confirmed, and findings were extended to cyberbullying. This relationship was moderated by conduct problems, while it is independent from gender and age. In particular, males, older adolescents, and those with high scores on conduct problems or CU traits had higher scores on measures of traditional and cyberbullying perpetration. The results of this work can allow one to build psychological and social models of bullying, capable of having a greater impact on prevention and intervention programs.

3. Child Temperament, Parenting Style and Family Functioning

Other risk factors for the development of persistent patterns of conduct problems in youths, along with callous unemotional traits, include early parenting style and child temperament. Previous evidence has shown how low parental warmth and fearlessness predict later psychopathic traits in children at increased risk of psychosocial maladjustment. The two-year follow-up study conducted by López-Romero and colleagues [4] on a very large cohort of preschoolers aged 3 to 6 years aimed to disentangle how these factors interact with each other to predict the later occurrence of psychopathic traits. Direct effects from fearlessness to interpersonal and behavioral psychopathic traits were identified, as well as a negative effect of parental warmth, fearless temperament, and their interaction on the development of individual conscience, which in turn mediated the indirect effect of these variables on psychopathic traits. Overall, this study contributed to better understanding the development of child moral adjustment and providing additional insights into effective preventive strategies that may help one to restrain potentially high-risk profiles in early childhood.

Although parenting style is a key factor in the emergence of conduct problems, research has neglected, so far, the impact of harsh parenting on the siblings of children with DBD. The study performed by Smorti and collaborators [5] indeed aimed to assess parenting styles and siblings' relationships in sibling dyads of families composed of a DBD child and a non-clinical sibling, and compare them with control families composed of two non-clinical siblings. Sixty-one families were thus recruited and grouped accordingly. Findings indicated differential parenting styles with higher negative parenting toward the DBD child than the sibling, while no difference emerged in sibling relationships within sibling dyads. Externalizing and internalizing problems were also higher in DBD children and their siblings compared to control, confirming psychopathology vulnerability in siblings of children with DBD. Hence, based on these results, the authors of the paper suggested prevention strategies via the inclusion of siblings evaluation in the clinical assessment in DBD children families, and the involvement of parents in multimodal treatments to promote positive parenting, which could have positive effects not only on DBD children, but also for their siblings, in preventing internalizing and externalizing problems.

To further explore the role of family functioning in shaping impulsivity and empathetic abilities in adolescents, the study by Marzilli and coworkers [6] assessed the complex interplay between these variables and the development of antisocial personality traits during emerging adulthood. The study was conducted on a community sample of 350 emerging adults, and found predictive effects of parental control, impulsivity, and empathetic concern in antisocial personality problems. Moreover, motor impulsivity and empathetic concern mediated the relationship between parental control and antisocial personality traits. These results highlight the importance of considering the complex relationship between family functioning, empathy, and impulsivity when evaluating antisocial conducts in youths, and suggest a major protective role, both directly and indirectly, of parental control over behavioral problems. This is crucial for planning more targeted and effective intervention programs that involve parents to ensure the success of prevention goals, but also focus on the promotion of self-control and empathic abilities.

4. Pharmacological Interventions for DBD and Comorbid Conditions

Many DBD patients exhibit an impulsive type of aggressiveness beyond their antisocial behaviors, which is often related to the underlying presence of comorbid ADHD, as one of the most frequently observed in clinical settings. Indeed, in the systematic review conducted by Fantozzi and colleagues [7], the interest was focused on investigating the effects of targeted pharmacological treatments for ADHD on empathic competences, social skills, and aggressiveness in youths. Treatment options included methylphenidate and other stimulant and non-stimulant medications. Thirteen studies were finally included in the review, and data retrieved from individual studies were collected. Ten out of them assessed changes in empathy and the theory of mind, and reported significant improvements in youths treated with either stimulants or nonstimulant drugs. Similarly, seven studies evaluated changes in emotion recognition, though fewer consistent findings were reported. Nonetheless, despite the great heterogeneity in the methodology of the included studies, this systematic review provided evidence for a beneficial effect of medications for ADHD, not only on its core features, but also on cardinal symptoms and drawbacks of DBD.

Though DBD is among the most common reasons for referral to youth mental health services, the efficacy of therapeutic interventions in clinical practice still remains somewhat unclear. To define more appropriate targets for novel pharmacological treatments for DBD, Balia and collaborators [8], together with the European Commission within the Seventh Framework Program, here proposed the protocol for a multicenter case-control study which will be followed by a single-blind, placebo-controlled, cross-over, randomized acute single-dose medication challenge. This study is part of a larger program aimed to identify the neural, genetic, and molecular underpinnings of aggression and antisocial behaviors in preclinical models and clinical samples, known as the Multidisciplinary Approaches to Translational Research in Conduct Syndromes (MATRICS) project. Aggressive children and adolescents with DBD are here compared to age-matched typically developing controls on a neuropsychological battery, while selected autonomic measures are simultaneously recorded. The acute response to methylphenidate/atomoxetine, risperidone/aripiprazole, or placebo is also examined.

5. Evidence-Based Psychotherapy Approach: The Coping Power Program

Along with pharmacological treatments, evidence-based psychotherapy-oriented interventions are among the cornerstones of the preventive approach for youths with DBD. Among these latter, Coping Power programs have previously shown evidence of clinical effectiveness on children with DBD in reducing the risk of subsequent substance use. In the six-year follow-up study performed by Prof John E. Lochman [9], founder of the Coping Power program and one of the major leading experts in the field of psychoeducational and psychotherapeutic interventions for DBD, a sample of 360 children were randomly assigned to receive either the group or individual program of the Coping Power intervention. The authors observed lower increases in substance use risk for children with low inhibitory control, receiving individual intervention, and for children with higher inhibitory control receiving group intervention. In other words, the level of inhibitory control in aggressive children may help clinicians to tailor specific types of interventions to prevent the risk of later substance use.

Other formats of the Coping Power intervention program have been conceptualized. The study by Boxmeyer and colleagues [10] was indeed aimed to assess the efficacy of a novel adaptation of the program, known as Mindful Coping Power, on reactive aggression and self-regulation. In a cohort of 102 children, this novel version produced significantly greater improvement in the self-rated measures of emotional, behavioral, and cognitive dysregulation than the classic program; moderate effects were also observed in inhibitory control and breath awareness, as well as in parent-rated measures of attention and social skills, though with milder effects on externalizing problems and reactive aggression. Thus, enhancing effects on more internal embodied experiences are observed with the Mindful Coping Power.

6. Developmental Outcomes and Comorbidities of DBD

Among the severest clinical outcomes of DBD and emotional dysregulation, bipolar disorders with suicidality are often encountered in the developmental trajectory of these adolescents, and often represent a major challenging comorbidity, which is a relevant target for therapeutic purposes. The study by Masi and coworkers [11] aimed to compare suicidality and non-suicidal self-injury (NSSI) in 95 referred bipolar adolescents. The authors found that both were associated with female gender, borderline personality disorder, and symptoms of anxiety and depression; while NSSI was specifically associated with somatic problems, severe suicidal ideation, and attempts were mostly related with adverse life events, bullying, social problems, and feelings of rejection. Thus, both shared and differential features of suicidal ideation and NSSI in adolescence may represent possible targets for early interventions.

Although obsessive compulsive disorder (OCD) and DBD usually exhibit non-overlapping symptoms, they might be theoretically viewed as different developmental outcomes that are derived from a common matrix. On one hand, individuals with OCD show high levels of sense of responsibility and guilt, while, on the other hand, DBD patients lack guilt and are often guided by anti-social purposes. The study by Buonanno and collaborators [12] specifically aimed to investigate the role of forgiveness in responsibility and guilt, and its putative influence by tendencies towards OCD and DBD. Findings with 231 adolescents showed that self-forgiveness predicted high levels of sense of responsibility, while guilt was predicted by both self- and situation-forgiveness. Moreover, the effects of OCD but not DBD symptoms on responsibility and guilt were mediated by self- and situation-forgiveness.

7. Conclusions

Overall, the twelve contributions included in this Special Issue provided novel and fruitful insights from major experts in the field (see Table A1). Indeed, though an increasingly greater amount of studies covering the areas of interest of the present Special Issue has appeared in the literature from all over the world in the past two decades, especially dealing with the heterogeneity of clinical presentations of DBD, their etiopathogenetic factors, and their assessment and treatment options, there are still many questions to be answered. The articles here presented provide novel and helpful elements both for the identification of brand new areas of research, and the development of more effective assessment procedures and treatment strategies in clinical practice. Thus, we would like to express our deepest gratitude to all authors who contributed to this Special Issue "Disruptive Behavior Disorders: Symptoms, Evaluation and Treatment", and the reviewers, for their dedicated time and help in improving the quality of published manuscripts.

Author Contributions: A.M. and G.S. conceptualized the Special Issue and wrote the Editorial. All authors have read and agreed to the published version of the manuscript.

Funding: This work has been partially supported by grant from the IRCCS Stella Maris Foundation (RC 2763762, "Treatment of Aggressiveness in Disruptive Behavior Disorders") and the 5x1000 voluntary contributions, Italian Ministry of Health.

Acknowledgments: We thank colleagues and friends worldwide who fruitfully contributed to this Special Issue and helped us make it a concrete achievement. We also thank the colleagues of Department of Child Psychiatry and Psychopharmacology of IRCCS Stella Maris Foundation and especially Gabriele Masi, the Head of our Department, for supporting our research in the field of Disruptive Behavior Disorders.

Conflicts of Interest: The authors declare no conflict of interest.

Appendix A

Table A1. Summary of the included studies.

Ref	Authors	Country	Institution	Type
[1]	Robles-Haydar CA, Martínez-González MB, Flórez-Niño YA, Ibáñez-Navarro LM, Amar-Amar JJ.	Colombia	Universidad de la Costa, Universidad del Corte	Article
[2]	Martínez-González MB, Turizo-Palencia Y, Arenas-Rivera C, Acuña-Rodríguez M, Gómez-López Y, Clemente-Suárez VJ.	Colombia, Spain	Universidad de la Costa, Universidad Europea de Madrid	Article
[3]	Catone G, Almerico L, Pezzella A, Riccio MP, Bravaccio C, Bernardo P, Muratori P, Pascotto A, Pisano S, Senese VP.	Italy	Suor Orsola Benincasa University, University of Campania "Luigi Vanvitelli", Federico II University, Santobono-Pausilipon Children Hospital, IRCCS Stella Maris Foundation	Article
[4]	López-Romero L, Cutrín O, Maneiro L, Domínguez-Álvarez B, Romero E.	Spain, Netherlands	Universidade de Santiago de Compostela, Leiden University	Article
[5]	Smorti M, Inguaggiato E, Vezzosi L, Milone A.	Italy	University of Pisa, IRCCS Stella Maris Foundation	Article
[6]	Marzilli E, Cerniglia L, Cimino S.	Italy	University of Rome "La Sapienza", International Telematic University Uninettuno	Article
[7]	Fantozzi P, Sesso G, Muratori P, Milone A, Masi G.	Italy	IRCCS Stella Maris Foundation, University of Pisa	Systematic Review
[8]	Balia C, Carucci S, Milone A, Romaniello R, Valente E, Donno F, Montesanto A, Brovedani P, Masi G, Glennon JC, Coghill D, Zuddas A, The Matrics Consortium.	Italy, Ireland, Netherlands, Australia	University of Cagliari, "Cao" Pediatric Hospital, ARNAS "Brotzu" Hospital Trust, IRCCS Stella Maris Foundation, University College Dublin, Radboud University, University of Dundee, Murdoch Children's Research Institute of Melbourne, University of Melbourne	Study Protocol
[9]	Lochman JE, Boxmeyer CL, Bui C, Hakim E, Jones S, Kassing F, McDonald K, Powell N, Qu L, Dishion T.	USA	University of Alabama, Arizona State University	Article
[10]	Boxmeyer CL, Miller S, Romero DE, Powell NP, Jones S, Qu L, Tueller S, Lochman JE.	USA	University of Alabama, University of Texas at San Antonio	Article
[11]	Masi G, Lupetti I, D'Acunto G, Milone A, Fabiani D, Madonia U, Berloffa S, Lenzi F, Mucci M.	Italy	IRCCS Stella Maris Foundation	Article
[12]	Buonanno C, Iuliano E, Grossi G, Mancini F, Stendardo E, Tudisco F, Pizzini B.	Italy	School of Cognitive Psychotherapy, InMovement Center, University of Rome "Guglielmo Marconi", University of Campania "Luigi Vanvitelli"	Article

References

1. Robles-Haydar, C.A.; Martínez-González, M.B.; Flórez-Niño, Y.A.; Ibáñez-Navarro, L.M.; Amar-Amar, J.J. Personal and environmental predictors of aggression in adolescence. *Brain Sci.* **2021**, *11*, 933. [CrossRef] [PubMed]
2. Martínez-González, M.B.; Turizo-Palencia, Y.; Arenas-Rivera, C.; Acuña-Rodríguez, M.; Gómez-López, Y.; Clemente-Suárez, V.J. Gender, anxiety, and legitimation of violence in adolescents facing simulated physical aggression at school. *Brain Sci.* **2021**, *11*, 458. [CrossRef] [PubMed]
3. Catone, G.; Almerico, L.; Pezzella, A.; Riccio, M.P.; Bravaccio, C.; Bernardo, P.; Muratori, P.; Pascotto, A.; Pisano, S.; Senese, V.P. The relation of callous–unemotional traits and bullying in early adolescence is independent from sex and age and moderated by conduct problems. *Brain Sci.* **2021**, *11*, 1059. [CrossRef] [PubMed]
4. López-Romero, L.; Cutrín, O.; Maneiro, L.; Domínguez-álvarez, B.; Romero, E. Psychopathic traits in childhood: Insights from parental warmth and fearless temperament via conscience development. *Brain Sci.* **2021**, *11*, 923. [CrossRef]
5. Smorti, M.; Inguaggiato, E.; Vezzosi, L.; Milone, A. Parenting and sibling relationships in family with disruptive behavior disorders. Are non-clinical siblings more vulnerable for emotional and behavioral problems? *Brain Sci.* **2021**, *11*, 1308. [CrossRef]
6. Marzilli, E.; Cerniglia, L.; Cimino, S. Antisocial personality problems in emerging adulthood: The role of family functioning, impulsivity, and empathy. *Brain Sci.* **2021**, *11*, 687. [CrossRef]
7. Fantozzi, P.; Sesso, G.; Muratori, P.; Milone, A.; Masi, G. Biological bases of empathy and social cognition in patients with attention-deficit/hyperactivity disorder: A focus on treatment with psychostimulants. *Brain Sci.* **2021**, *11*, 1399. [CrossRef] [PubMed]
8. Balia, C.; Carucci, S.; Milone, A.; Romaniello, R.; Valente, E.; Donno, F.; Montesanto, A.; Brovedani, P.; Masi, G.; Glennon, J.C.; et al. Neuropsychological characterization of aggressive behavior in children and adolescents with CD/ODD and effects of single doses of medications: The protocol of the matrics_WP6-1 study. *Brain Sci.* **2021**, *11*, 1639. [CrossRef] [PubMed]
9. Lochman, J.E.; Boxmeyer, C.L.; Bui, C.; Hakim, E.; Jones, S.; Kassing, F.; McDonald, K.; Powell, N.; Qu, L.; Dishion, T. Substance use outcomes from two formats of a cognitive-behavioral intervention for aggressive children: Moderating roles of inhibitory control and intervention engagement. *Brain Sci.* **2021**, *11*, 950. [CrossRef]
10. Boxmeyer, C.L.; Miller, S.; Romero, D.E.; Powell, N.P.; Jones, S.; Qu, L.; Tueller, S.; Lochman, J.E. Mindful coping power: Comparative effects on children's reactive aggression and self-regulation. *Brain Sci.* **2021**, *11*, 1119. [CrossRef] [PubMed]
11. Masi, G.; Lupetti, I.; D'Acunto, G.; Milone, A.; Fabiani, D.; Madonia, U.; Berloffa, S.; Lenzi, F.; Mucci, M. A comparison between severe suicidality and nonsuicidal self-injury behaviors in bipolar adolescents referred to a psychiatric emergency unit. *Brain Sci.* **2021**, *11*, 790. [CrossRef] [PubMed]
12. Buonanno, C.; Iuliano, E.; Grossi, G.; Mancini, F.; Stendardo, E.; Tudisco, F.; Pizzini, B. Forgiveness in the modulation of responsibility in a sample of italian adolescents with a tendency towards conduct or obsessive–compulsive problems. *Brain Sci.* **2021**, *11*, 1333. [CrossRef] [PubMed]

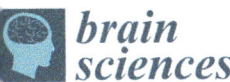

Article

Personal and Environmental Predictors of Aggression in Adolescence

Claudia A. Robles-Haydar [1], Marina B. Martínez-González [1,*], Yuliana A. Flórez-Niño [1], Luz M. Ibáñez-Navarro [1] and José J. Amar-Amar [2]

[1] Department of Social Science, Universidad de la Costa, Barranquilla 080001, Colombia; crobles@cuc.edu.co (C.A.R.-H.); yflorez1@cuc.edu.co (Y.A.F.-N.); libanez@cuc.edu.co (L.M.I.-N.)
[2] Department of Psychology, Universidad del Norte, Barranquilla 080003, Colombia; jamar@uninorte.edu.co
* Correspondence: mmartine21@cuc.edu.co

Abstract: This study aims to find causal factors of aggression in a group of Latino adolescents to achieve a greater understanding of human nature, taking into account personal and contextual variables. The fundamental hypothesis is that moral disengagement, personality traits, self-esteem, values, parenting, sex, and socioeconomic situation can function as possible casual factors of aggression in adolescents. The study examined the variables using the structural equations model (SEM) to determine causal factors of aggression in a sample of 827 adolescents (54% men and 46% women) between 11 and 16 years of age. According to the scientific literature review, sociodemographic, personal, and familiar variables were included in the causal model. The influence of the variables occurred in two ways: one that inhibits aggression and the other that reinforces it. The results are discussed based on identifying protective and risk factors against aggression: biological sex and values of conformity and transcendence as aggression's inhibitors and, on the other hand, openness, moral disengagement, and leadership values as the most important predictors of aggression.

Keywords: big five personality traits model; childrearing; disruptive behavior; moral disengagement; mother rejection; structural equation modeling; values

Citation: Robles-Haydar, C.A.; Martínez-González, M.B.; Flórez-Niño, Y.A.; Ibáñez-Navarro, L.M.; Amar-Amar, J.J. Personal and Environmental Predictors of Aggression in Adolescence. *Brain Sci.* **2021**, *11*, 933. https://doi.org/10.3390/brainsci11070933

Academic Editors: Annarita Milone and Gianluca Sesso

Received: 17 May 2021
Accepted: 5 July 2021
Published: 15 July 2021

Publisher's Note: MDPI stays neutral with regard to jurisdictional claims in published maps and institutional affiliations.

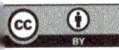

Copyright: © 2021 by the authors. Licensee MDPI, Basel, Switzerland. This article is an open access article distributed under the terms and conditions of the Creative Commons Attribution (CC BY) license (https://creativecommons.org/licenses/by/4.0/).

1. Introduction

Aggression is considered a behavior whose objective is to cause harm to another person [1]. The physical forms of aggression are motor behaviors that cause bodily harm, and the verbal forms can be direct and indirect, such as offensive comments, rumors, and nagging [2]. During adolescence, more intense relationships with aggression have been found, and it is in adolescence where criminal trajectories usually begin, and defiant and antisocial behaviors can be generated [3].

Sex represents a sociodemographic variable frequently associated with aggression, and there is some consensus stating that it is higher in men than in women [4,5]. The reasons for these differences are not entirely clear [6]. However, much has been said about evolutionary inheritance, the biological aspects of sexual differences, and care or socialization practices around the dimensions of masculinity and femininity [7]. In addition, some studies agree that children and young people from violent communities show more significant risks of developing criminal or antisocial behaviors than those in an enriched environment [8–10].

On the other hand, values are defined as subjective and emotional beliefs, and motivational constructs, representing what is important in people's lives. They guide the choice and evaluation of behaviors and events, essential in recognizing the motivations that underlie decision-making and reflection on human behavior [11,12]. This variable has been frequently related to moral judgment and prosocial behavior [13]. Values can be classified as those that regulate the expression of personal characteristics (self-direction, hedonism, achievement, power, stimulation) versus values that regulate relationships with others or those that are oriented to transcendence (universalism, benevolence, tradition, conformity, and security) [14]. There is evidence that values such as benevolence, universalism, and security positively affect personal development, while values such as power and achievement could be related to some difficulties such as depression, stress, and aggression [15–17].

Personality is understood as the individual and lasting attributes and inclinations that transmit a sense of identity, integrity, and singularity [18]. According to the Big Five theory, personality traits as kindness, tenacity or awareness, and emotional stability have predictive power on aggressive and antisocial behaviors [19]. Therefore, these behaviors would be modulated by a constellation of low scores in the traits of kindness, tenacity, and emotional stability [18,19].

Another critical aspect to understand the causes of aggression could be self-esteem. Low self-esteem predicts significant psychological imbalances, including aggression and violence [20,21]. However, there is also evidence to support the opposite: some research indicates that violent behavior is mainly related to high self-esteem [22,23]. Furthermore, the most violent criminals and the most hostile nations in the world are characterized by their high levels of self-esteem [22]. In this sense, both high and low self-esteem are probably related to aggression [24].

The relation of childrearing with aggression is taken into account. Support and affection refer to the warmth in parent–child interactions. These are observed in acceptance and tenderness, physical proximity, containment, and negative pole due to rejection [25,26]. The understanding of rejection is related to negative feelings such as anxiety, insecurity, low self-esteem, dependence, and destructive emotions such as anger and emotional insensitivity in children and adults [26]. The dimension of control implies authority and different disciplinary strategies to guide children's behavior [27]. There are findings on the adverse effects of physical punishment and its relationships with anxiety and aggression in children and adolescents [28–30]. Likewise, studies on the effects of inductive discipline, where the parental figure guides the child in reflecting on the repercussions that actions have for others, show positive relationships with prosocial behavior and the internalization of the norm [8,31].

Moral disengagement (MD) has been studied as a predictor of aggression and crime [32,33], bullying [34–36] and cyberbullying [37], aggression in young people [4,38–40], intimate partner violence [41,42], and terrorism, among others [43–45]. Moral disengagement is conceptually defined as the psychological process through which self-reactions are disconnected from inhuman behavior [46], allowing inhuman behaviors to be carried out with little or no self-reproach [47]. MD is present in all people as a propensity to evoke restructuring cognitions of harmful behaviors, making the subject perform actions that are harmful to others with little anguish and guilt [48,49].

The present study aims to provide an integrative view of the multi-causal relationships that affect aggression in Latino adolescents where behavior, environment, and personal factors operate interactively to elucidate the causes of human behavior. We expect to contribute to the prevention and mitigation of the negative consequences of aggression and attempt to achieve a greater understanding of human nature and its potentialities. The fundamental hypothesis is that moral disconnection, personality traits, self-esteem, values, rearing, sex, and socioeconomic situation are possible causes of aggression in adolescents. In this sense, it can be hypothesized that the most critical factors for the prediction of aggression are as follows: the personality trait of emotional instability, moral disconnection, self-improvement values (power and achievement), paternal and maternal rejection, discipline based on punishment, belonging to the male sex, and living in a low socioeconomic level. Likewise, those variables that decrease aggressive behaviors are as follows: personality traits of conscience and kindness, self-transcendence values (universalism and benevolence), inductive discipline, and belonging to the female sex. Self-esteem is expected to influence aggression.

2. Materials and Methods

The participants were contacted from four schools in Barranquilla (Colombia) with different socioeconomic conditions. The determination of socioeconomic conditions was obtained according to the classification of the National Statistical System (DANE), which classifies residential properties for the allocation of subsidies and differential charges for home public services in Colombia.

The institutional authorities and teachers sent the information to parents, promoted students' participation in the research, and obtained informed consent documents.

The following inclusion and exclusion criteria were maintained for the sample.

Inclusion criteria:

- Be between the ages of 11 and 16.
- Consent to participation in the study (parents and adolescents).

Exclusion criteria:

- Reside in towns outside the Barranquilla city.
- Cognitive conditions or language difficulties that affect the correct completion of the questionnaire.

The procedure was approved by the Universidad del Norte ethical committee (approval code 146) and conducted following the Helsinki Declaration (revised in Brazil, 2013). The participants completed the questionnaires in their classrooms for 100 and 180 min. During the session, they were accompanied by a psychologist and a teacher. The data were collected anonymously.

2.1. Participants

A total of 827 volunteer adolescents participated in this research. Owing to the characteristics of the population and the difficulties in accessing schools, the sampling was non-probabilistic. See Table 1 for sociodemographic information of the participants.

Table 1. Sociodemographic characteristics of the participants.

Variable	Description	Percent
Biological sex	Men	54%
	Woman	46%
Socioeconomic level	High	14.50%
	Medium	48%
	Low	37.60%

The adolescents were men (54%) and women (46%) with a mean age of 13.6 years (SD = 2) from different socioeconomic levels of the city. A higher proportion were participants from a medium socioeconomic level (47.9%), followed by those from a low level (37.6%), and a lesser proportion from a high socioeconomic level (14.5%).

2.2. Measurements

The Moral Disengagement Scale [50] is a 32-item questionnaire to measures children's proneness to moral disengagement. The scale allows a score per dimension according to the eight mechanisms of MD and a global score of DM. The scale is Likert-type and is rated in a range of five points: (1) not at all agree to (5) totally agree. The 32-item version is one of the most used in cross-cultural research. Likewise, its reliability levels have been greater than 0.82 [51–54]. In the present sample, a McDonald's Omega of 0.94 was obtained.

The Big Five Questionnaire short version [55] is a reduced version of the Big Five Questionnaire for Children BFQ-C [56]. It consists of 30 items and contains five subscales for each personality trait. Each subscale includes six items, rated on a five-point Likert scale: from 1 (almost never) to 5 (almost always). The reliability levels oscillate between 0.75 to 0.82, showing a good internal consistency [55]. In the present study, the results for

McDonald's Omega in each of the factors were above 0.7, which is considered good, except in factor 5 (openness), where the values were 0.65, indicating acceptable reliability.

The Rosenberg Self-Esteem Scale is one of the most used instruments evaluating this construct. It measures a single global dimension of self-esteem through 10 items on a Likert scale, whose alternatives range from 1 point (strongly disagree) to 4 points (strongly agree). The scale has been used in more than 53 countries and has adequate psychometric properties, with reliability levels greater than 0.70 [57,58]. In the present sample, a good level of reliability was obtained ($\Omega = 0.88$).

The Portrait Values Questionnaire (PVQ) is a questionnaire developed by Schwartz [11] to measure ten universal values: self-direction, stimulation, hedonism, achievement, power, security, conformity, tradition, benevolence, and universalism in the adolescent population. The questionnaire consists of 40 items presenting a description of the wishes or aspirations of a hypothetical person, those that implicitly affirm a value, for example, "Having new ideas and being creative is important for him/her. He/she likes to do things originally" (Self-direction) [12]. The scale is Likert-type with six response alternatives, where 1 point is equivalent to the highest perception of similarity with the character (he/she looks a lot like me) and 6 points to the greatest perception of disparity (he/she does not look like me at all), so the score is inverted [16]. Regarding the overall internal consistency of the sample, a McDonald's Omega of 0.96 was obtained.

Child–Parental Acceptance–Rejection Questionnaire (PARQ-C) measures young people's perceptions about parental upbringing [59]. It has two identical versions, one for each parent, with 29 items grouped into five subscales: warmth/affection, hostility/aggression, indifference/neglect, undifferentiated rejection, and control. It is a Likert-type scale, with response alternatives ranging from 1 (almost never) to 4 (every day). It allows obtaining scores for each subscale and grouping the scores in a single bipolar dimension of perceived acceptance–rejection [60]. The instrument has been used in more than 500 studies, with excellent psychometric properties [39,60]. The Spanish adaptation's reliability values oscillate between 0.71 and 0.92 for the father version and between 0.72 and 0.85 for the mother version [60]. Therefore, both versions of the PARQ-C have a good and excellent internal consistency ($\Omega = 0.90$ for the mother and $\Omega = 0.93$ for the father) in this study.

Discipline Interview Children and Adolescents' version measures how frequently parents use different disciplinary strategies in raising their children [61]. It has 18 items and four subscales: positive discipline, physical discipline, verbal discipline, and induction of guilt. The scale is Likert-type with response alternatives ranging from 1 (never) to 5 (almost every day). Their reliability levels range between 0.51 and 0.72 for each of the subscales [28,62]. Regarding the global internal consistency of the sample, the results were $\Omega = 0.93$ for the maternal version and $\Omega = 0.94$ for the paternal version.

Physical and Verbal Aggression Scale AFV measures aggressiveness in children and adolescents through two subscales: physical and verbal aggression, including a global aggression score [63]. The questionnaire consists of 20 items, five of which correspond to control statements not scored in the final grade. Thus, the physical aggression subscale has eight items, and the verbal aggression subscale has seven. The response alternatives are from 1 point (almost never) to 5 points (very often). The Hispanic version presents adequate internal consistency, with test reliability coefficients 0.84 and re-test 0.70 [64]. In addition, an excellent level of reliability was obtained in the present research, with a McDonald's Omega of 0.93.

Finally, we used a sociodemographic questionnaire developed for this study, including age, gender, family structure, and socioeconomic level.

2.3. Statistical Analysis

We carried out an exploratory data analysis using regression, case suppression, and frequency analysis using SPSS 22. Next, an analysis of structural equations was carried out through the AMOS v16 program. From the model, the path coefficients or Beta (β) coefficients were analyzed, for 99% [*] and 95% [**] confidence; significance values lower than 0.05 were considered relevant. Thus, the direction effects were established, either excitatory (positive sign) or inhibitory (negative sign), and their nature, direct on the variables of interest, or that their effect was mediated, through others or another variable of the model [65].

Subsequently, the indirect effects on the endogenous variable of aggression were determined. For this, the Beta (β) pathway coefficients were multiplied, from the first variable, through the intermediate variable, to the final one, obtaining the total effect or total Beta (βtotal). Then, all the inhibitory effects were added. We carried out the same procedure for the excitatory effects, allowing us to identify the direction of the most significant explanatory power of the model. Finally, the quality indicator of the model transformed into the determination coefficient R^2 was determined, as well as the Mardia coefficient and the adjustment indicators: [χ^2], [Sig], RMSEA, ECVI, NCP, CFI, NNFI, NFI, PNFI, and [GL], testing a single model for the variables.

3. Results

The following variables were included in the proposed model: sex, socioeconomic level, personality traits (energy, openness, agreeableness, conscientiousness, emotional instability), maternal discipline (positive discipline, punishment, negative discipline, verbal discipline) and paternal discipline (positive discipline, punishment, physical discipline, verbal discipline, guilt induction), and maternal affection (affection, aggression/rejection, control, indifference, trust/friendship) and paternal (affection, aggression/rejection, control)—all exogenous variables. At the next level, endogenous variables were introduced: values (openness to life, leadership, conservation/conformity, transcendence, and power), self-esteem, moral disengagement, and finally aggression.

The assumption of multivariate normality was verified, evaluated from the Mardia kurtosis coefficient (Ku). The standard error (δ) is higher than the criterion of 1.96 (δKu = 93.659), which indicates the absence of multivariate normality. It implies using unweighted least squares (ULS) to interpret the structural equation adjustment indicators. Among the adjustment indicators, we took those whose values do not depend on the comparison between models, as showed in Table 2.

Table 2. Structural equation model fit indicators.

Fit Indicators	[χ^2]	χ^2	p-Value χ^2	RMSEA	p-Value RMSEA	NCP	ECVI	NNFI	NFI	CFI	PNFI
Aggression prediction model	3381.24	3.04	0	0.05	0.586	2270.24	5.687	0.728	0.76	0.76	0.511

The adjustment indicators were interpreted following the scale established by Hair [66] as follows:

RMSEA (root mean square error of approximation) (between 0.05 and 0.08): it is at a suitable value of 0.05.

Significance of RMSEA or p-value of RMSEA (>0.05): the model value was 0.58. So, it was not fulfilled.

NNFI (non-normed fit index) (≈1): these values should tend to 1, so the value of 0.73 that the model produced is considered an acceptable measure.

NFI (normed fit index) (≈1): a value of 0.76 is considered an acceptable measure by the model.

CFI (comparative fit index) (≈1): the value of 0.76 is considered acceptable.

Although there is an adequate adjustment in the model's variables, it does not explain the total variability of the endogenous variable: aggression.

That is why the results indicate an adequate adjustment in the model's variables with a good, but not excellent value of the multivariate correlation coefficient (R = 0.43). The significant (β) links were analyzed to explain the causal effects of the independent variables. This is to understand the links and later reflect on which variables should be incorporated in future studies, as well as to contribute to increasing the explanatory capacity of the model.

Some of the variables evidenced an inhibitory and direct effect on aggression (Figure 1). For the biological sex (β = −0.15), women were less likely to manifest aggressive behaviors than men. The transcendence values (β = 0.11) and conservation/conformity (β = 0.08) were higher in adolescents with lower levels of aggression.

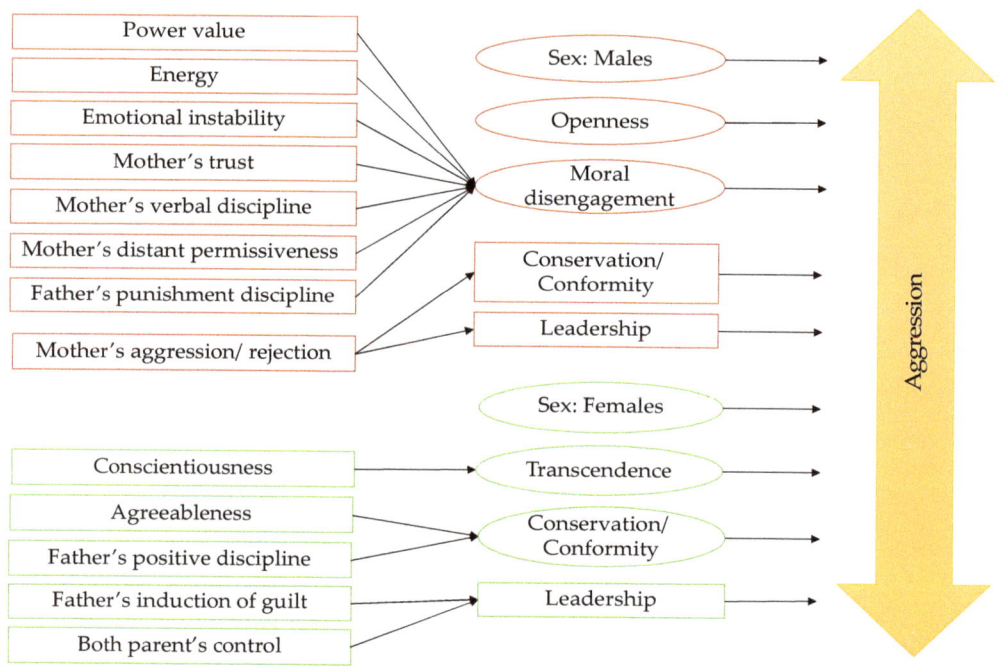

Figure 1. Model to explain aggression in Latin adolescents. The shape used within the path graph represents the variable's nature if it directly influences aggression (oval shape) or an indirect influence (rectangle). The red color represents the stimulating route of aggression, and the green represents the inhibitory.

Other inhibitory variables that indirectly affected aggression were the personality traits of conscientiousness (βtotal = −0.03) and agreeableness (βtotal = −0.01). The path from conscientiousness stimulates the value of transcendence (β = −0.25), decreasing aggression (β = 0.11). The route from agreeableness to aggression passes through the value of conservation/conformity (β = −0.19), and from there, it reduces aggression (β = 0.08). Thus, at higher levels of conscientiousness and agreeableness, aggression is lowered.

Continuing with the inhibitory route, the induction of guilt (βtotal = −0.01) as paternal childrearing affects the leadership value, and from there, it inhibits aggression (β = −0.07). Positive discipline used by the father (βtotal = −0.01) affects the conservation/conformity value (β = −0.10), and from there, it affects aggression (β = 0.08). Therefore, the greater the fathers' use of guilt and induction, the lower their children's aggressiveness.

Paternal affection was also highlighted in its control dimension (β = −0.01), affecting leadership value (β = 0.09), and from there, decreasing aggression (β = −0.07). Likewise, maternal control (β = −0.0001) passing through leadership value (β = −0.08) affects aggression (β = −0.07), demonstrating the importance of monitoring and limits imposed by the parents on mitigating the aggression.

On the other hand, some variables evidenced a direct and stimulating influence on aggression. The personality trait of openness (β = 0.12) was higher in adolescents with higher levels of aggression. The moral disengagement (β = 0.09) and the leadership value (β = −0.07) showed that those adolescents who seek to maintain a dominant position within the group tend to be more aggressive.

Other variables showed the same stimulating effect on aggression but indirect. The mother's affection expressed as aggression/rejection (βtotal = 0.02) passes through the leadership value (β = −0.11) and from there to aggression (β = −0.07). In the same way, mother's aggression/rejection passes through the conservation value (β = 0.13), increasing aggression (β = 0.08). In this way, the greater the maternal aggression/rejection, the greater the identification of young people with the leadership value and less the identification with the value of conservation/conformity, establishing that, at greater maternal rejection, higher levels of aggression are present in adolescents.

The rest of the variables exciting aggression indirectly are those whose route of influence goes through moral disengagement. The distant maternal permissiveness (βtotal = 0.01) and maternal trust (βtotal = 0.01) increase the levels of aggression. Maternal verbal discipline (βtotal = 0.01) and punishment-based discipline from the father (βtotal = 0.0001) are associated with aggressive behaviors in young people. The value of power (βtotal = −0.01) shows that, the greater the pursuit of material success and popularity in adolescents, the higher the levels of aggression. Likewise, the traits of emotional instability (βtotal = 0.01) and energy (βtotal = 0.01) show that, the more emotionally unstable and energetic young people are, the more aggressive they will tend to be.

Finally, variables as socioeconomic level and self-esteem had no significant effect on aggression.

4. Discussion

The present work aimed to know the influence of personal and environmental factors on aggression in adolescents. According to the model obtained, we found two ways of influencing aggression: one that inhibits it and another that reinforces it.

As protective factors, the most significant effects were found for sex, the values of transcendence and conformity, as well as the personal trait of conscientiousness. The following factors were found to have lesser effects: the personal trait of agreeableness and aspects of parenting as maternal and paternal control, induction of guilt, and positive discipline applied by the father.

Regarding risk factors, those variables with the most relevant effect were the openness personality trait, moral disengagement, and leadership value. The rest of the variables that reinforce aggression have moral disengagement as a mediator. Then, this variable directly affects aggression and moderates other routes of influence as emotional instability, energy, and power value, as well as maternal breeding factors such as distant permissiveness, trust/friendship, verbal discipline, and rejection.

The literature showed that women present less orientation to aggression than men in all cultures, regarding the inhibitory pathway. These differences in aggressive behavior have been attributed to higher levels of testosterone in males [67]. However, other studies have shown that men and women behave more aggressively when they believe they have higher testosterone levels, regardless of whether they have them or not [68]. Social constructions around masculinity highlight strength, virility, and arrogance in men, stimulating relations of power and submission so that the prevailing masculinity model and its heteronormative framework could constitute an adequate explanation for this phenomenon [4,31].

Personal values such as transcendence and conformity are inhibiting factors of aggression. The first motivates altruism by concern for others and the search for social justice [11,16,69], and the second inhibits actions that can cause harm to others, showing more obedience in individuals who show high levels of conformity [70,71]. It is necessary to mention that conformity also represents the effort to accomplish the norm and moderate actions to maintain the group's functioning [12]. The interest for not violating social norms or expectations is a kind of subordination to others' impositions that could be related to avoiding aggressive actions at least in conventional contexts in which the rules are created to protect life and humankind.

Similarly, traits of conscientiousness indirectly reduce aggression. For example, adolescents with high levels of consciousness are trustworthy and self-regulating [63,72]. Likewise, agreeableness indirectly decreases aggression as it stimulates prosocial behaviors by maintaining a positive and empathetic vision of human nature [73].

The effects of parenting are minor around the inhibition of aggression. However, control strategies with norms established and behavior monitoring constitute essential aspects in preventing disruptive behaviors [8]. Positive discipline refers to the use of induction and positive reinforcement to control children's behavior. Our findings exhibit that occurs when the father uses inductive discipline, calls to reason, and reflection on the consequences of the actions, which have been linked to prosocial behavior and empathy in children [8,9]. On the other hand, guilt induction is the disciplinary technique that promotes shame in children for their bad behavior [28] and has been related to psychological control and conditional love [74,75]. However, the role of guilt in maintaining interpersonal relationships is undeniable as it increases anxiety when harming others and promotes the search for reparation [76]. Guilt is an aspect promoted in all cultures because of its influence on internalizing the norm and regulating behavior [28]. This paradoxical result on the effects of guilt induction as a disciplinary technique may depend significantly on how the parent implements it. In this sense, one of the most important aspects is where the focus of criticism is placed, that is, if the parents decide to criticize the child's behavior instead of his personality, or if they highlight the negative consequences of the wrongdoing for the victim or the negative feelings that they are experiencing [77].

This disciplinary technique can be effective in preventing aggression, at least in a positive discipline context. However, the fact that it stands out in the paternal bond may be because of the traditional roles in the parenting of Latin American families, where the father is the one who mainly imposes the norm and discipline in the home.

These results are in line with previous research, where aggressive behavior is explained by the combination of attributes that allows the person to exercise adequate control over their impulses, which endow them with empathy and concern for the welfare of others [46,73]. It is not enough to possess the capacities to self-regulate, but rather one must have the motivation and desire to put them into practice [46].

Regarding the combination of variables that stimulate aggressive behavior, the openness trait was the one that had the highest incidence and a direct influence on aggression. Young people with a moderate-disruptive behavior had scores above the average in the openness trait [78]. People characterized by this trait are open to novelty, questioning authority, and social conventions [79], which could lead them to enroll in risky behaviors, especially if they are outspoken, energetic, and emotionally unstable.

Another significant predictor of aggression was moral disengagement, coinciding with previous studies [4,9,38,80,81]. Most acts of human cruelty are the product of a deliberative conscience, in which the person engages in aggressive or malicious behaviors, justifying their actions to reduce feelings of guilt and self-concept [32,49,82].

Finally, and as the last variable whose influence directly affects aggression, is the value of leadership, defined as the importance that people give to having a dominant position within the group, making decisions, and telling others what to do. In this study, maternal aggression increased this value, while the induction of guilt by the father decreased it. In this case, leadership refers to a restrictive aspect of the freedoms of others and the search for control [83]. Autocratic leadership has related to hostile behavior [84].

Among the variables that indirectly incited aggression were significant aspects such as permissiveness, trust, and mother rejection. In correspondence with other variables of the family relationship and the adolescent's personality characteristics, permissive parenting would produce negative results in development and social performance [85].

A second aspect of the affective relationship with the mother is the trust/friendship dimension. This result reveals a more horizontal relationship, which could reduce the mother's chances of establishing herself as an authority capable of redirecting adolescent maladaptive behaviors [86]. It is not an inherently negative relationship, although it can become permissive, lacking affection or hostile context as maternal rejection was also evident. Maternal rejection implies feelings of anger, detachment, or resentment towards the child, involving behaviors that intentionally harm them, such as sarcasm, threats, hurtful gestures, slapping, or pinching. In general, rejection has been one of the most studied and documented aspects in research on the influence of parenting on child and adolescent adjustment, with one of its main consequences being feelings of hostility and problems in handling anger and aggression [59].

Most of the studies that have dealt with parenting have been configured around the maternal figure [85]. Few studies have sought to establish differences between the influence of the father and the mother in parenting [87]. Some of these have revealed that maternal rejection would have worse consequences on children's psychological adjustment and would be involved with greater internalizing and externalizing behavioral manifestations in children and young people [27]. The mother is usually configured as the principal caregiver and giver of affection and tenderness [88]. In this sense, aggression from the mother could have a more harmful effect because she is the figure in charge of giving affection and because of cultural expectations that the children would have about the mother [88]. In the case of discipline, the influence of both parental figures appears, including verbal discipline from the mother and punishment from the father—not physical, but symbolic. Verbal discipline is based on shouting, threats, and insults to control children's behavior, which is why it has been connected to aggressive behavior in children and young people [89,90]. Likewise, the mother's verbal discipline was related to the prediction of aggression, and the physical dimensions that did not appear may be because of some limitations in the use of instruments, which make it difficult to establish the limit between discipline and physical abuse [91].

Another critical aspect of the indirect influence on aggression is the value of power relative to ambition and materialism. Power refers to searching for a dominant position within the group and is integrated into the self-improvement dimension, in which personal interests are pursued instead of group interests [12]. In this work, the power dimension includes aspects related to the search for personal success and the desire to obtain lots of money, be admired, and impress others. It is known that the persecution of this type of value motivates selfish behaviors [16,69].

Some authors have found how money and its pursuit have been associated with criminal acts [92], behavioral problems, low social productivity, and in general psychological maladjustment, warning about the devastating consequences that a materialistic view of the world can generate [93,94]. Likewise, people who aspire excessively to the goals of fame and fortune tend to be more narcissistic and Machiavellian [95].

The value of power must be analyzed concerning the amalgam of factors where adolescents' personality is integrated. Thus, traits as the emotional instability make one prone to the experimentation of negative emotions such as sadness, fear, and anger, with little tolerance to stress and difficulties for self-regulation [96]. In this sense, people with difficulties controlling their negative emotionality would be more likely to act on it [38,97]. In the case of energy, this trait is characterized by the search for social stimulation and dominance and has been linked to high extraversion and high neuroticism with antisocial results [98]. Extraverted people would experience greater difficulties in inhibiting their aggressive impulses; at the same time, their permanent need for stimulation would put them in search of novel and intense situations [98].

Neither self-esteem nor socioeconomic status had any significant impact on aggression. Aggression is not a condition that depends on how much the person likes himself. Baumeister [22] considers that self-esteem relevance has been exaggerated as this construct is not the cause, but rather the consequence of many conditions with which it has traditionally been related. That would explain the lack of congruence between multiple studies in which both low and high self-esteem predicts aggression [20,22,99]. Other studies also affirm that there is no relationship between self-esteem and aggression [100].

Finally, regarding the socioeconomic level, there is no significant influence on aggression. In this case, the most important predictors of aggression have to do with the personal characteristics of adolescents and their interaction with parents, regardless of the socioeconomic level where this interaction occurs.

5. Conclusions

This study explored the precursors of aggression in a sample of Latino adolescents, considering environmental and personal variables resulting from the theoretical review. The results allowed us to point out that the most important predictors of aggression were openness, DM, and leadership value. Other significant predictors, with lesser effects, were the relationship with the mother. This parental figure plays an essential role in predicting aggression and becomes a risk factor when described as hostile, permissive, and with little involvement in the child's life. Concerning the father's practices, we found that punishments also increased aggression with a lesser effect.

The most significant factors inhibiting aggression were the biological sex, corroborating what has already been exposed by numerous studies, where women have lower levels of aggression than men. Moreover, values of conformity and transcendence were also found as aggression inhibitors. Other factors with lesser effects were personality traits like kindness and conscience, positive or inductive discipline from the father, and the induction of guilt and monitoring from both parents.

In this study, the personal adolescent's factors such as biological sex, personality, values, and moral disengagement had a more significant impact on aggression than family variables. This phenomenon may be related to a large part of the influence of family passes first towards personal factors and then towards aggression. In this sense, the development of values, for example, depends greatly on socialization in the family environment during early childhood. Later, the values will be introjected and appropriate by the subject.

On the other hand, and contrary to expectations, neither self-esteem nor socioeconomic level significantly influence aggression.

Finally, and through the proposed model, it was possible to explain aggression as a combination of attributes that allow adequate control over impulses and endow empathy and concern for the well-being of others.

Suggestions for Future Research

In order to further the field of research, it is important to take into account that these findings represent just a modest advance in research on aggressive behaviors. Much remains to be further studied, such as: What are the parents' differentiated influences in developing aggressive behaviors in adolescents? What other personal or contextual variables can moderate or mediate their development? How culture or other scenarios can affect its development?

The model presented in this study did not explain the total variance of aggression. Therefore, some recommendations could improve the predictive capacity of future alternative models.

First, it is recommended to continue working with variables associated with self-regulation and self-containment, as established in the present study. Therefore, future research should delve into these types of variables and how they can be potentiated. Including variables such as emotional intelligence, the capacity for introspection and experimentation with guilt, and even mirror neuron activity could be clarifying.

Additionally, it is proposed to incorporate dark personality traits, such as narcissism and Machiavellianism, or those that account for cynicism and the ability to manipulate and even question authority.

Research in parenting should continue delving into affection and discipline and the influence of each parent separately. In this regard, it is recommended to work with younger populations and longitudinal studies that reveal how the influence of socializing entities on this variable is developing. Another important aspect is to evaluate the influence of other contexts as the work was only done from within the family, and it could be interesting to explore the influence of the cultural and scholarly context. Finally, sociodemographic factors should continue to be included, albeit as a control measure.

6. Limitations

Some of the study's limitations were non-probabilistic sampling owing to difficulties in entering the schools and subsequent access to the population and the use of questionnaires or self-report measures that could affect the data owing to the social desirability of the participants.

Author Contributions: Conceptualization, C.A.R.-H., M.B.M.-G., L.M.I.-N., Y.A.F.-N. and J.J.A.-A.; methodology, C.A.R.-H. and J.J.A.-A.; formal analysis, C.A.R.-H.; investigation, C.A.R.-H., M.B.M.-G., L.M.I.-N., Y.A.F.-N. and J.J.A.-A.; resources, C.A.R.-H., M.B.M.-G., L.M.I.-N., Y.A.F.-N. and J.J.A.-A.; data curation, C.A.R.-H.; writing—original draft preparation, C.A.R.-H., M.B.M.-G., L.M.I.-N., Y.A.F.-N. and J.J.A.-A.; writing—review and editing, C.A.R.-H., M.B.M.-G., L.M.I.-N., Y.A.F.-N. and J.J.A.-A.; funding acquisition, C.A.R.-H. and J.J.A.-A. All authors have read and agreed to the published version of the manuscript.

Funding: This research was funded by Departamento Administrativo de Ciencia y Tecnología de Colombia, COLCIENCIAS, Ph.D. scholarship program.

Institutional Review Board Statement: The study was conducted according to the guidelines of the Declaration of Helsinki and approved by Universidad del Norte Ethics Committee (approval code 146 from 26 August 2016).

Informed Consent Statement: Informed consent was obtained from all subjects involved in the study.

Data Availability Statement: The data that support our results can be found through directly asking the first author.

Conflicts of Interest: The authors declare no conflict of interest.

References

1. Carrasco, M.A.; González, M.J. Aspectos conceptuales de la agresión: Definición y modelos explicativos [Theoretical issues on aggression: Concept and models]. *Acción Psicológica* **2006**, *4*, 7–38. [CrossRef]
2. Caprara, G.V.; Pastorelli, C. Toward a reorientation of research on aggression. *Eur. J. Personal.* **1989**, *3*, 121–138. [CrossRef]
3. Gallegos, W.L.A.; Pablo, U.C.S. Agresión y violencia en la adolescencia: La importancia de la familia. *Av. Psicol.* **2013**, *21*, 23–34. [CrossRef]
4. Martínez-González, M.; Turizo-Palencia, Y.; Arenas-Rivera, C.; Acuña-Rodríguez, M.; Gómez-López, Y.; Clemente-Suárez, V. Gender, Anxiety, and Legitimation of Violence in Adolescents Facing Simulated Physical Aggression at School. *Brain Sci.* **2021**, *11*, 458. [CrossRef] [PubMed]
5. Obermann, M.-L. Moral disengagement in self-reported and peer-nominated school bullying. *Aggress. Behav.* **2010**, *37*, 133–144. [CrossRef]
6. Ruiz, R.O.; Sánchez, V.; Menesini, E. Violencia Entre Iguales y Desconexión Moral: Un Análisis Transcultural. *Psicothema* **2002**, *14*, 37–49. Available online: http://dialnet.unirioja.es/servlet/articulo?codigo=4687146 (accessed on 12 September 2014).
7. Sánchez, M.A.F.M. La Agresividad Humana y sus Interpretaciones. *Albolafia Rev. Humanid. Cult.* **2020**, *20*, 427–441. Available online: https://dialnet.unirioja.es/servlet/articulo?codigo=7720611 (accessed on 7 April 2021).
8. Martínez-González, M.B.; Robles-Haydar, C.A.R.; Amar-Amar, J.J.; Crespo-Romero, F.A. Crianza y desconexión moral en infantes: Su relación en una comunidad vulnerable de Barranquilla. *Rev. Latinoam. Cienc. Soc. Niñez Juv.* **2016**, *14*, 315–330. [CrossRef]
9. Cardozo-Rusinque, A.A.; Martínez-González, M.B.; De La Peña-Leiva, A.A.; Avedaño-Villa, I.; Crissien-Borrero, T.J. Factores psicosociales asociados al conflicto entre menores en el contexto escolar. *Educ. Soc.* **2019**, *40*, e0189140. [CrossRef]
10. Elsaesser, C.; Kennedy, T.M.; Tredinnick, L. The role of relationship proximity to witnessed community violence and youth outcomes. *J. Commun. Psychol.* **2019**, *48*, 562–575. [CrossRef]
11. Schwartz, S.H.; Melech, G.; Lehmann, A.; Burgess, S.; Harris, M.; Owens, V. Extending the Cross-Cultural Validity of the Theory of Basic Human Values with a Different Method of Measurement. *J. Cross Cult. Psychol.* **2001**, *32*, 519–542. [CrossRef]
12. Shalom, H.S. The Hebrew University of Jerusalem an Overview of the Schwartz Theory of Basic Values. *Online Read. Psychol. Cult.* **2012**, *2*, 11. [CrossRef]

13. Paciello, M.; Fida, R.; Tramontano, C.; Cole, E.; Cerniglia, L. Moral dilemma in adolescence: The role of values, prosocial moral reasoning and moral disengagement in helping decision making. *Eur. J. Dev. Psychol.* **2013**, *10*, 190–205. [CrossRef]
14. Beramendi, M.; Espinosa, A.; Ara, S. Perfiles Axiológicos de Estudiantes de Tres Carreras Universitarias: Funciones Discriminantes de Tres Lecturas de la Teoría de Schwartz. *Liberabit* **2013**, *19*, 45–54. Available online: http://www.scielo.org.pe/scielo.php?script=sci_arttext&pid=S1729-48272013000100005&nrm=iso (accessed on 26 April 2021).
15. Benish-Weisman, M. The interplay between values and aggression in adolescence: A longitudinal study. *Dev. Psychol.* **2015**, *51*, 677–687. [CrossRef] [PubMed]
16. Hanel, P.H.; Wolfradt, U. The 'dark side' of personal values: Relations to clinical constructs and their implications. *Pers. Individ. Differ.* **2016**, *97*, 140–145. [CrossRef]
17. Seddig, D.; Davidov, E. Values, Attitudes Toward Interpersonal Violence, and Interpersonal Violent Behavior. *Front. Psychol.* **2018**, *9*, 604. [CrossRef]
18. Caprara, G.V.; Barbaranelli, C.; Borgogni, L.; Perugini, M. The "big five questionnaire": A new questionnaire to assess the five factor model. *Pers. Individ. Differ.* **1993**, *15*, 281–288. [CrossRef]
19. Sánchez-Teruel, D.; Robles-Bello, M.A. Model "Big Five" personality and criminal behavior. *Int. J. Psychol. Res.* **2013**, *6*, 102–109. [CrossRef]
20. Cava, M.J.; Musitu, G.; Murgui, S. Familia y Violencia Escolar: El rol Mediador de la Autoestima y la Actitud Hacia la Autoridad Institucional. *Psicothema* **2006**, *18*, 367–373. Available online: http://www.psicothema.com/pdf/3224.pdf (accessed on 11 March 2021).
21. Donnellan, M.B.; Trzesniewski, K.H.; Robins, R.W.; Moffitt, T.; Caspi, A. Low Self-Esteem Is Related to Aggression, Antisocial Behavior, and Delinquency. *Psychol. Sci.* **2005**, *16*, 328–335. [CrossRef] [PubMed]
22. Baumeister, R.; Bushman, B.J.; Campbell, W.K. Self-Esteem, Narcissism, and Aggression. *Curr. Dir. Psychol. Sci.* **2000**, *9*, 26–29. [CrossRef]
23. Baumeister, R.F.; Smart, L.; Boden, J. Relation of threatened egotism to violence and aggression: The dark side of high self-esteem. *Psychol. Rev.* **1996**, *103*, 5–33. [CrossRef]
24. Diamantopoulou, S.; Rydell, A.-M.; Henricsson, L. Can Both Low and High Self-esteem Be Related to Aggression in Children? *Soc. Dev.* **2008**, *17*, 682–698. [CrossRef]
25. Gámez-Guadix, M.; Almendros, C. Exposición a la Violencia entre los Padres, Prácticas de Crianza y Malestar Psicológico a Largo Plazo de los Hijos. *Psychosoc. Interv.* **2011**, *20*, 121–130. [CrossRef]
26. Rohner, R.P. The Parental "Acceptance-Rejection Syndrome": Universal Correlates of Perceived Rejection. *Am. Psychol.* **2004**, *59*, 830–840. [CrossRef] [PubMed]
27. Lila, M.; Garcia, F.; Gracia, E. Perceived paternal and maternal acceptance and children's outcomes in Colombia. *Soc. Behav. Pers. Int. J.* **2007**, *35*, 115–124. [CrossRef]
28. Huang, L.; Malone, P.S.; Lansford, J.E.; Deater-Deckard, K.; Di Giunta, L.; Bombi, A.S.; Bornstein, M.H.; Chang, L.; Dodge, K.A.; Oburu, P.; et al. Measurement invariance of discipline in different cultural contexts. *Fam. Sci.* **2011**, *2*, 212–219. [CrossRef]
29. Lansford, J.E.; Deater-Deckard, K. Childrearing Discipline and Violence in Developing Countries. *Child Dev.* **2012**, *83*, 62–75. [CrossRef]
30. Gershoff, E.T.; Grogan-Kaylor, A.; Lansford, J.E.; Chang, L.; Zelli, A.; Deater-Deckard, K.; Dodge, K.A. Parent Discipline Practices in an International Sample: Associations with Child Behaviors and Moderation by Perceived Normativeness. *Child Dev.* **2010**, *81*, 487–502. [CrossRef]
31. Hoffman, M.L. Erratum: "Moral Internalization, Parental Power, and the Nature of Parent-Child Interaction". *Dev. Psychol.* **1975**, *11*, 526. [CrossRef]
32. Bandura, A. Moral Disengagement in the Perpetration of Inhumanities. *Pers. Soc. Psychol. Rev.* **1999**, *3*, 193–209. [CrossRef] [PubMed]
33. Martín, E.G.; Alonso, C.H.; Palleja, J.M. Autoeficacia y delincuencia. *Psicothema* **2002**, *14*, 63–71.
34. Pozzoli, T.; Gini, G.; Vieno, A. Individual and Class Moral Disengagement in Bullying Among Elementary School Children. *Aggress. Behav.* **2012**, *38*, 378–388. [CrossRef]
35. Yang, J.; Wang, X.; Lei, L. Perceived school climate and adolescents' bullying perpetration: A moderated mediation model of moral disengagement and peers' defending. *Child. Youth Serv. Rev.* **2020**, *109*, 104716. [CrossRef]
36. Menesini, E.; Palladino, B.E.; Nocentini, A. Emotions of Moral Disengagement, Class Norms, and Bullying in Adolescence: A Multilevel Approach. *Merrill-Palmer Q.* **2015**, *61*, 124. [CrossRef]
37. Bussey, K.; Luo, A.; Fitzpatrick, S.; Allison, K. Defending victims of cyberbullying: The role of self-efficacy and moral disengagement. *J. Sch. Psychol.* **2020**, *78*, 1–12. [CrossRef]
38. Caprara, G.V.; Tisak, M.S.; Alessandri, G.; Fontaine, R.G.; Fida, R.; Paciello, M. The contribution of moral disengagement in mediating individual tendencies toward aggression and violence. *Dev. Psychol.* **2014**, *50*, 71–85. [CrossRef]
39. Kokkinos, C.M.; Voulgaridou, I.; Markos, A. Personality and relational aggression: Moral disengagement and friendship quality as mediators. *Pers. Individ. Differ.* **2016**, *95*, 74–79. [CrossRef]
40. White-Ajmani, M.L.; Bursik, K. Situational context moderates the relationship between moral disengagement and aggression. *Psychol. Violence* **2014**, *4*, 90–100. [CrossRef]

1. Rollero, C.; De Piccoli, N. Myths about Intimate Partner Violence and Moral Disengagement: An Analysis of Sociocultural Dimensions Sustaining Violence against Women. *Int. J. Environ. Res. Public Health* **2020**, *17*, 8139. [CrossRef]
2. D'Urso, G.; Petruccelli, I.; Grilli, S.; Pace, U. Risk Factors Related to Cognitive Distortions Toward Women and Moral Disengagement: A Study on Sex Offenders. *Sex. Cult.* **2018**, *23*, 544–557. [CrossRef]
3. Bandura, A. The role of selective moral disengagement in terrorism and counterterrorism. In *Understanding Terrorism: Psychosocial Roots, Consequences, and Interventions*; Moghaddam, F.M., Marsella, A.J., Eds.; American Psychological Association: Washington, DC, USA, 2004; pp. 121–150.
4. Buttlar, B.; Rothe, A.; Kleinert, S.; Hahn, L.; Walther, E. Food for Thought: Investigating Communication Strategies to Counteract Moral Disengagement Regarding Meat Consumption. *Environ. Commun.* **2021**, *15*, 55–68. [CrossRef]
5. Walters, G.D. Procedural justice, legitimacy beliefs, and moral disengagement in emerging adulthood: Explaining continuity and desistance in the moral model of criminal lifestyle development. *Law Hum. Behav.* **2018**, *42*, 37–49. [CrossRef]
6. Bandura, A. Social cognitive theory of self-regulation. *Organ. Behav. Hum. Decis. Process.* **1991**, *50*, 248–287. [CrossRef]
7. Moore, C.; Detert, J.R.; Treviño, L.K.; Baker, V.L.; Mayer, D.M. Why employees do bad things: Moral disengagement and unethical organizational behavior. *Pers. Psychol.* **2012**, *65*, 1–48. [CrossRef]
8. Bandura, A. Selective Moral Disengagement in the Exercise of Moral Agency. *J. Moral Educ.* **2002**, *31*, 101–119. [CrossRef]
9. Martínez-González, M.B.; Robles-Haydar, C.A.; Alfaro-Álvarez, J. Concepto de desconexion moral y sus manifestaciones contemporaneas/Moral disengagement concept and its contemporary manifestations. *Utop. Prax. Latinoam.* **2021**, *25*, 349. [CrossRef]
10. Bandura, A.; Barbaranelli, C.; Caprara, G.V.; Pastorelli, C. Mechanisms of moral disengagement in the exercise of moral agency. *J. Pers. Soc. Psychol.* **1996**, *71*, 364–374. [CrossRef]
11. Bao, Z.; Zhang, W.; Lai, X.; Sun, W.; Wang, Y. Parental attachment and Chinese adolescents' delinquency: The mediating role of moral disengagement. *J. Adolesc.* **2015**, *44*, 37–47. [CrossRef]
12. Bustamante, A.; Chaux, E. Reducing Moral Disengagement Mechanisms: A Comparison of Two Interventions. *J. Lat. Am. Stud.* **2014**, *6*, 52–54. [CrossRef]
13. De Caroli, M.E.; Sagone, E. Belief in a Just World, Prosocial Behavior, and Moral Disengagement in Adolescence. *Procedia Soc. Behav. Sci.* **2014**, *116*, 596–600. [CrossRef]
14. Pelton, J.; Gound, M.; Forehand, R.; Brody, G. The Moral Disengagement Scale: Extension with an American Minority Sample. *J. Psychopathol. Behav. Assess.* **2004**, *26*, 31–39. [CrossRef]
15. Mamazza, L. Lo Studio Della Personalità in Una Prospettiva Longitudinale: Misura e Relazioni con Intelligenza, Profitto Scolastico e Indicatori di Buono/Cattivo Adattamento. Ph.D. Thesis, Università degli Studi di Padova, Padova, Italy, 2012.
16. Barbaranelli, C.; Caprara, G.V.; Rabasca, A.; Pastorelli, C. A questionnaire for measuring the Big Five in late childhood. *Pers. Individ. Differ.* **2003**, *34*, 645–664. [CrossRef]
17. Ospino, G.A.C.; Barbosa, C.P.; Suescún, J.; Oviedo, H.C.; Herazo, E.; Arias, A.C. Validez y dimensionalidad de la escala de autoestima de Rosenberg en estudiantes universitarios. *Pensam. Psicológico* **2017**, *15*, 29–39. [CrossRef]
18. Supple, A.J.; Plunkett, S.W. Dimensionality and Validity of the Rosenberg Self-Esteem Scale for Use with Latino Adolescents. *Hisp. J. Behav. Sci.* **2010**, *33*, 39–53. [CrossRef]
19. Rohner, R.P.; Ali, S. Parental Acceptance-Rejection Questionnaire (PARQ). In *Encyclopedia of Personality and Individual Differences*; Zeigler-Hill, V., Shackelford, T.K., Eds.; Springer: Cham, Switzerland, 2016; pp. 1–4.
20. Barrio, V.D.; Ramírez-Uclés, I.; Romero, C.; Carrasco, M.Á. Adaptación del Child-PARQ/Control: Versiones Para el Padre y la Madre en Población Infantil y Adolescente Española. *Acción Psicológica* **2014**, *11*, 27–46. Available online: http://scielo.isciii.es/scielo.php?script=sci_arttext&pid=S1578-908X2014000200002&nrm=iso (accessed on 28 April 2021). [CrossRef]
21. Lansford, J.E.; Chang, L.; Dodge, K.A.; Malone, P.S.; Oburu, P.; Palmérus, K.; Bacchini, D.; Pastorelli, C.; Bombi, A.S.; Zelli, A.; et al. Physical Discipline and Children's Adjustment: Cultural Normativeness as a Moderator. *Child Dev.* **2005**, *76*, 1234–1246. [CrossRef]
22. Pastorelli, C.; Lansford, J.E.; Kanacri, B.P.L.; Malone, P.S.; Di Giunta, L.; Bacchini, D.; Bombi, A.S.; Zelli, A.; Miranda, M.C.; Bornstein, M.H.; et al. Positive parenting and children's prosocial behavior in eight countries. *J. Child Psychol. Psychiatry* **2016**, *57*, 824–834. [CrossRef]
23. Caprara, G.V.; Pastorelli, C. Early emotional instability, prosocial behaviour, and aggression: Some methodological aspects. *Eur. J. Pers.* **1993**, *7*, 19–36. [CrossRef]
24. del Barrio, V.; Rosset, C.M.; Martínez, R.L. Evaluación de la Agresión y la Inestabilidad Emocional en Niños Españoles: Su Relación con la Depression. *Clínica Salud* **2001**, *12*, 33–50. Available online: https://www.redalyc.org/articulo.oa?id=180618320002 (accessed on 22 January 2021).
25. Medrano, L.A.; Muñoz-Navarro, R. Aproximación conceptual y práctica a los modelos de ecuaciones estructurales. *Rev. Digit. Investig. Docencia Univ.* **2017**, *11*, 219–239. [CrossRef]
26. Hair, J.F.; Gómez Suárez, M. *Análisis Multivariante*; Prentice-Hall: Madrid, Spain, 2010.
27. Bernardes, T.; de Moraes, T.P. ¿Por qué los hombres presentan un comportamiento más agresivo que las mujeres? Por una antropología evelutiva del comportamiento agresivo. *Nómadas Crit. J. Soc. Jurid. Sci.* **2013**, *37*, 93–111. [CrossRef]
28. Eisenegger, C.; Naef, M.; Snozzi, R.; Heinrichs, M.; Fehr, E. Prejudice and truth about the effect of testosterone on human bargaining behaviour. *Nat. Cell Biol.* **2009**, *463*, 356–359. [CrossRef] [PubMed]

69. Vecchio, G.M.; Gerbino, M.; Di Giunta, L.; Castellani, V.; Pastorelli, C. Funzionamento morale e prosocialità: Valori, ragionamento e "agentività" morale. *Psicol. Dell'Educ.* **2008**, *2*, 21.
70. Schwartz, S.H. Universals in the Content and Structure of Values: Theoretical Advances and Empirical Tests in 20 Countries. *Adv. Exp. Soc. Psychol.* **1992**, *25*, 1–65. [CrossRef]
71. Schwartz, S.H.; Rubel, T. Sex differences in value priorities: Cross-cultural and multimethod studies. *J. Pers. Soc. Psychol.* **2005**, *89*, 1010–1028. [CrossRef]
72. Simkin, H.; Etchezahar, E.; Ungaretti, J. Personalidad y Autoestima Desde el Modelo y la Teoría de los Cinco Factores. *Hologramática* **2012**, *2*, 171–193. Available online: http://psicologiasocial.sociales.uba.ar/wp-content/uploads/sites/162/2013/06/Simkin__Etchezahar__Ungaretti_-_2012_-_Personalidad_y_Autoestima_desde_el_modelo_y_la_teoria_de_los_Cinco_Factores_1-libre.pdf (accessed on 14 April 2021).
73. Caprara, G.V.; Pastorelli, C.; Weiner, B. At-risk children's causal inferences given emotional feedback and their understanding of the excuse-giving process. *Eur. J. Pers.* **1994**, *8*, 31–43. [CrossRef]
74. Pinquart, M. Associations of Parenting Dimensions and Styles with Internalizing Symptoms in Children and Adolescents: A Meta-Analysis. *Marriage Fam. Rev.* **2016**, *53*, 613–640. [CrossRef]
75. Smetana, J.G. Current research on parenting styles, dimensions, and beliefs. *Curr. Opin. Psychol.* **2017**, *15*, 19–25. [CrossRef]
76. Álvarez Ramírez, E.; García Méndez, M. Estilos de Amor y Culpa Como Predictores de la Satisfacción Marital en Hombres y Mujeres. *Enseñ. Investig. Psicol.* **2017**, *22*, 76–85. Available online: https://www.redalyc.org/articulo.oa?id=29251161007 (accessed on 16 May 2021).
77. Rote, W.M.; Smetana, J.G. Situational and structural variation in youth perceptions of maternal guilt induction. *Dev. Psychol.* **2017**, *53*, 1940–1953. [CrossRef] [PubMed]
78. Abella, V.; Bárcena, C. PEN, Modelo de los Cinco Factores y Problemas de Conducta en la Adolescencia. *Acción Psicológica* **2014**, *11*, 55–67. Available online: http://scielo.isciii.es/scielo.php?script=sci_arttext&pid=S1578-908X2014000100006&nrm=iso (accessed on 7 May 2021). [CrossRef]
79. Landazabal, M.G.; Lazcano, J.A.; Martínez-Valderrey, V.; Mateo, C.M.; Iturrioz, E.B.; Alboniga-Mayor, J.J. Conducta antisocial: Conexión con emociones positivas y variables predictoras. *Apunt. Psicol.* **2013**, *31*, 123–133.
80. Gini, G.; Pozzoli, T.; Bussey, K. Collective moral disengagement: Initial validation of a scale for adolescents. *Eur. J. Dev. Psychol.* **2013**, *11*, 386–395. [CrossRef]
81. Barchia, K.; Bussey, K. Individual and collective social cognitive influences on peer aggression: Exploring the contribution of aggression efficacy, moral disengagement, and collective efficacy. *Aggress. Behav.* **2011**, *37*, 107–120. [CrossRef]
82. Bandura, A. Failures in Self-Regulation: Energy Depletion or Selective Disengagement? *Psychol. Inq.* **1996**, *7*, 20–24. [CrossRef]
83. Malik, N.M.; Lindahl, K.M. Aggression and dominance: The roles of power and culture in domestic violence. *Clin. Psychol. Sci. Pract.* **1998**, *5*, 409–423. [CrossRef]
84. Orellana, B.S.; Portalanza, C.A. Influencia del liderazgo sobre el clima organizacional. *Suma Neg.* **2014**, *5*, 117–125. [CrossRef]
85. Lozano, E.A.; Conesa, M.D.G.; Hernández, E.H. Relaciones Entre Estilos Educativos, Temperamento y Ajuste Social en la Infancia: Una Revision. *An. Psicol.* **2007**, *23*, 33–40. Available online: https://www.redalyc.org/articulo.oa?id=16723105 (accessed on 15 May 2021).
86. Scarpati, M.P.; Pertuz, M.S.; Silva, A.S. Límites, Reglas, Comunicación en Familia Monoparental con Hijos Adolescents. *Diversitas* **2014**, *10*, 225–246. Available online: http://www.scielo.org.co/scielo.php?script=sci_arttext&pid=S1794-99982014000200004&nrm=iso (accessed on 15 May 2021). [CrossRef]
87. Tur-Porcar, A.; Mestre, V. Crianza y agresividad de los menores: ¿es diferente la influencia del padre y de la madre? *Psicothema* **2012**, *24*, 284–288. [PubMed]
88. Kauth, A.R.; de Magallanes, L.M.; de Quintana, M.E.L. El Machismo en el Imaginario Social. *Rev. Latinoam. Psicol.* **1993**, *25*, 275–284. Available online: https://www.redalyc.org/articulo.oa?id=80525209 (accessed on 15 May 2021).
89. Wang, M.-T.; Kenny, S. Longitudinal Links Between Fathers' and Mothers' Harsh Verbal Discipline and Adolescents' Conduct Problems and Depressive Symptoms. *Child Dev.* **2013**, *85*, 908–923. [CrossRef] [PubMed]
90. Vissing, Y.M.; Straus, M.A.; Gelles, R.J.; Harrop, J.W. Verbal aggression by parents and psychosocial problems of children. *Child Abus. Negl.* **1991**, *15*, 223–238. [CrossRef]
91. Mulvaney, M.K.; Mebert, C.J. Parental corporal punishment predicts behavior problems in early childhood. *J. Fam. Psychol.* **2007**, *21*, 389–397. [CrossRef]
92. Wright, J.P.; Cullen, F.T.; Agnew, R.S.; Brezina, T. "The root of all evil"? An exploratory study of money and delinquent involvement. *Justice Q.* **2001**, *18*, 239–268. [CrossRef]
93. Kasser, T.; Ahuvia, A. Materialistic values and well-being in business students. *Eur. J. Soc. Psychol.* **2002**, *32*, 137–146. [CrossRef]
94. Kasser, T.; Ryan, R.M. A dark side of the American dream: Correlates of financial success as a central life aspiration. *J. Pers. Soc. Psychol.* **1993**, *65*, 410–422. [CrossRef]
95. Egan, V.; Hughes, N.; Palmer, E.J. Moral disengagement, the dark triad, and unethical consumer attitudes. *Pers. Individ. Differ.* **2015**, *76*, 123–128. [CrossRef]
96. Cassaretto, M. Relación entre la personalidad y el afrontamiento en estudiantes preuniversitarios. *Rev. Vanguard. Psicológica* **2011**, *1*, 202–225.

97. Bandura, A.; Barbaranelli, C.; Caprara, G.V.; Pastorelli, C. Self-Efficacy Beliefs as Shapers of Children's Aspirations and Career Trajectories. *Child Dev.* **2001**, *72*, 187–206. [CrossRef] [PubMed]
98. Del Barrio, V.; Carrasco, M.Á.; Holgado, F.P. Factor Structure Invariance in the Children's Big Five Questionnaire. *Eur. J. Psychol. Assess.* **2006**, *22*, 158–167. [CrossRef]
99. Martínez-Martínez, A.; Castro-Sánchez, M.; Rodríguez-Fernández, S.; Zurita-Ortega, F.; Chacón-Cuberos, R.; Espejo-Garcés, T. Violent behaviour, victimization, self-esteem and physical activity of Spanish adolescents according to place of residence: A structural equation model/Conducta violenta, victimización, autoestima y actividad física de adolescentes españoles en función del lugar de residencia: Un modelo de ecuaciones estructurales. *Rev. Psicol. Soc.* **2018**, *33*, 111–141. [CrossRef]
100. del Pino, C.L.; Burón, A.S.; Nieto, M.Á.P.; Fernández-Martín, M.P. Impulsiveness, self-esteem and cognitive control of the aggressiveness of adolescent. *Edupsykhé Rev. Psicol. Educ.* **2008**, *7*, 81–99.

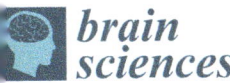

Article

Gender, Anxiety, and Legitimation of Violence in Adolescents Facing Simulated Physical Aggression at School

Marina B. Martínez-González [1,*], Yamile Turizo-Palencia [1], Claudia Arenas-Rivera [1], Mónica Acuña-Rodríguez [1], Yeferson Gómez-López [1] and Vicente J. Clemente-Suárez [2,3]

[1] Department of Social Science, Universidad de la Costa, Barranquilla 080001, Colombia; yturizo1@cuc.edu.co (Y.T.-P.); carenas@cuc.edu.co (C.A.-R.); macuna6@cuc.edu.co (M.A.-R.); ygomez22@cuc.edu.co (Y.G.-L.)
[2] Faculty of Sport Sciences, Universidad Europea de Madrid, 28670 Villaviciosa de Odón, Spain; vctxente@yahoo.es
[3] Grupo de Investigación Cultura, Educación y Sociedad, Universidad de la Costa, Barranquilla 080001, Colombia
* Correspondence: mmartine21@cuc.edu.co

Abstract: We analyzed gender and anxiety differences in middle school students facing a physical peer aggression situation. The participants were 1147 adolescents aged between 12 and 18 years (male: $n = 479$; female: $n = 668$) who watched a 12 s animation representing the situation and filled out a questionnaire to analyze the legitimation of violent behaviors and anxiety levels. We registered their decisions to solve the situation using a categorical scale that included assertive, avoidant, aggressive, submissive, and supportive behaviors. Gender was not associated with the adolescent's behaviors in facing a simulated peer aggression situation. However, male teenagers tended to perceive adults as sanctioners and neutrals; those who used the diffusion of responsibility and dehumanization to justify their behavior also showed a higher state of anxiety. Female teenagers who expected legitimation from their peers, presented higher anxiety as well. Educational interventions may use these results, helping adolescents to understand that their acts have substantial implications in the lives of others. It is essential to develop group interventions that modify how adolescents manage their conflicts and change gender stereotypes that significantly impact health. We highlight the need for linking families in educational programs facing the challenges of transforming the legitimization of violence in parental practices.

Keywords: bullying; moral disengagement; violence; disruptive behavior; peer aggression; social rules; socialization; externalizing symptoms

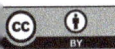

1. Introduction

Legitimation is a psychological construct used to analyze authority, power, blind obedience, sociopolitical violence, individual/state relationship, and social protest [1]. In the context of violence, this concept explains the justifying discourse that keeps people willing to commit punishable actions against others [2]. Internalization and institutionalization processes consolidate these beliefs in daily interpersonal relationships, assuming violence as inevitable and even admissible in a group or society [3].

Previous studies about violence legitimization in childhood highlighted the perception of legitimacy to use violence against provocation, based on the authority, and as a persuasive action when the situation is threatening [4–7]. These studies also analyzed the role of moral disengagement mechanisms and the expectations of legitimation perceived from peers and adults as behavioral determinants [7–9].

Regarding the use of moral disengagement mechanisms, Bandura [4,5] postulated eight cognitive mechanisms to maintain a positive self-concept, reducing guilt in immoral actions: (a) moral justification links a violent act to a heroic purpose; (b) euphemistic language reduces the harmful connotation of the act; (c) advantageous comparison minimizes the immoral act, contrasting it with another crueler act; (d) displacement of responsibility identifies an authority as responsible for the acts; (e) diffusion of responsibility is when the action of the group mitigates the perception of one's own responsibility; (f) distortion of consequences minimizes the harmful effects of a behavior; (g) attribution of blaming refers the victim as provocative; and (h) dehumanization removes people from their human qualities to facilitate mistreatment against them.

Growing up perceiving situations of violence both in the family and in the community has been associated with children's legitimation of violence [7,8,10,11]. A context that legitimizes violence reduces prosocial behaviors [12] and reduces the negative affect of the anxiety associated with witnessing these events and recognizing its manifestations [13]. For this reason, the social acceptance of violence exposes children to the risk of reproducing violence in their daily relationships [10,11,14], but also in the society that they will constitute in adulthood [15,16].

However, children and adolescents who live in violent situations are exposed to chronic stress that compromises their health [17,18]. Anxiety response refers to different physical and mental manifestations that are not attributable to real dangers and appears as crises or diffuse states [19]. Some authors distinguish between state anxiety and trait anxiety. The first consists of a transitory state facing current events with a higher probability of change over time. The second is considered more stable and durable [20]. These anxiety states could vary in intensity and durability according to the different situations or evolutionary stages that everyone goes through. However, adolescence is the time in life where there is a greater willingness to generate anxiety, with social, emotional, and behavioral effects [21,22]. These difficulties appear in building conflictive interpersonal relationships, less emotional control, rejection of criticism, little acceptance among peers, and victimization [23,24].

Previous researchers found higher levels of anxiety in women, especially in adolescence and childhood [25]. Likewise, a higher incidence of state anxiety has been reported in women than men, associated with maturational and reproductive processes (premenstrual cycle, pregnancy, menstrual delays, and the social pressure of adolescence, among others), and a higher rate of related negative affect with stress, anxiety, and depression [26–28]. Many of these situations involve school conflicts as the main interaction scenario in adolescence, a stage in which gender differences associated with aggression have been reported [29,30]. In this line, male teenagers are more aggressive than female teenagers when facing problems, tending to engage in antisocial behaviors as physical and verbal abuse and rule violations. On the other hand, female teenagers seem to have a prosocial orientation and inclination to solve problems assertively, empathize, and be concerned with others. However, new evidence has found no gender differences related to aggression manifestations [31], which could be associated with a generational and cultural change in parenting and relationship patterns [32].

The present research aimed to analyze gender and anxiety differences in middle school students' behavior facing a simulated physical peer aggression situation. The study hypotheses were (i) the gender of the participants, offenders, and the authorities would modulate the adolescent's behaviors in a simulated peer aggression situation; and (ii) the legitimization of violence would be present in males and participants with higher anxiety levels.

2. Materials and Methods

A total of 1147 volunteer adolescents participated in the present research, aged between 12 and 18 years (male: $n = 479$; M = 16.32; SD = 1.10; female: $n = 668$; M = 16.27; SD = 0.85), with a stratified random sampling of simple affixation, in which the sample was collected from schools at different socioeconomic levels from the city of Barranquilla

(Colombia). The procedure was conducted following the Helsinki Declaration (revised in Brazil, 2013) and approved by the university ethical committee (approval code 094).

The data were collected anonymously. Before participating, all participants, parental or guardian, and their professors were informed about the experimental procedures, indicating the right to withdraw from the study at any time and providing written informed consent.

2.1. Procedure

As a laboratory investigation, this study used animations that simulated physical peer aggression at school to assess different reactions from participants. Previous researchers have effectively used simulated scenarios of violence to assess participants' responses [33–37].

The adolescents were contacted in different schools. The final sample was conformed for those whose parents consented to participate. They completed the evaluation task in a computer room, in groups of 30 people, sitting randomly to face the different situations presented. First, they read the purpose of the study and gave consent to participate. Next, the instructions appeared, and the participants answered demographic questions. Then, instructions to watch the video and answer related questions were given.

The research was carried out with a cross-sectional evaluation using a multifactorial randomized block design. The adolescents were placed according to their gender in four possible stimulus combinations, as detailed below.

After observing the stimulus video, they answered how they would react to that situation and questions related to moral disengagement mechanisms to justify their action. In the end, all of the adolescents answered the anxiety questionnaires.

2.2. Instruments

An animation with a simulated physical peer aggression situation was shown. Participants watched a 12 s online animation representing a physical violence situation from peers at school. There were four different stimuli, with the gender of the offender and the teacher varying (see Figure 1). The stimulus consisted of an animation with a voiceover describing the situation to generate the participant's identification with the main character. The scene showed a group of students and the teacher in the classroom; then, the teacher went out to answer a call. In his/her absence, one of the students, described as a bully, pushed the character identified with the participant. Some images from the animation are presented in Figure 2.

Female Teenagers	Male teenagers
• Female offender - Female teacher • Female offender - Male teacher • Male offender - Female teacher • Male offender - Male teacher	• Female offender - Female teacher • Female offender - Male teacher • Male offender - Female teacher • Male offender - Male teacher

Figure 1. We used a randomized block design in the study, considering the gender of the participants and the animated version of the offenders and teachers.

After this, questions about the reaction in facing the situation and its justifications were presented. These questions were inspired by moral disengagement mechanism theory [4,5,38], and include questions about the legitimation of violence expected from their peers and adults as mediators in the conflict. The answers were registered using a categorical scale that included assertive, avoidant, aggressive, submissive, and supportive behaviors; then, the answers were integrated to analyze if participants tended to attack or not (assertive, avoidant, submissive, and supportive categories were integrated as "no attack" and the aggressive responses as "attack").

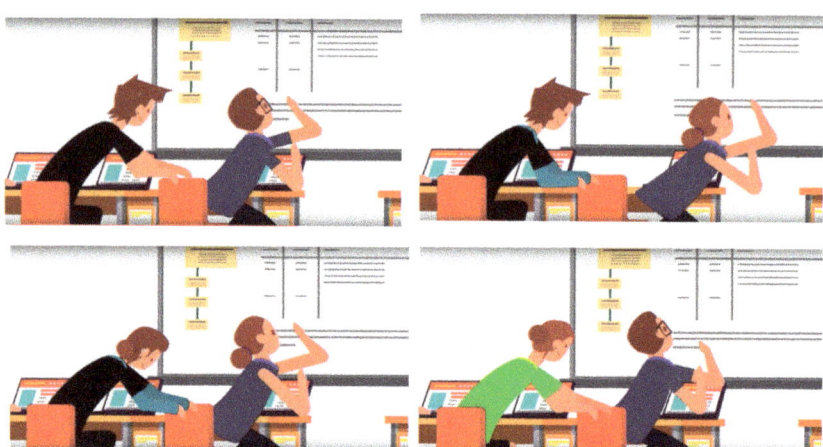

Figure 2. Images of stimulus simulating a peer's physical aggression at school. In each box, the offender's character is on the left, and the participant's character on the right.

The State-Trait Anxiety Inventory for children and adolescents was used to measure anxiety [39]. It is composed of two scales, the first to measure state anxiety, containing 20 items, and the second one to measure trait anxiety, with 20 more items. An example of a question is: "I am worried about things at school."

2.3. Statistical Analysis

JASP statistical software was used to analyze the data. The chi-square test was used to analyze the reactions according to gender, and ANOVA was used to analyze differences in anxiety levels according to the participant's gender and their reactions facing the proposed situation. The level of significance was set at $p \leq 0.05$.

3. Results

3.1. Adolescents' Behaviors in Facing the Simulated Physical Peer Aggression Situation by Gender

We found that 11.5% of males and 12.3% of females decided to attack as a reaction to the stimulus (Table 1). No significant differences were found in the tendency to attack by the participant's gender ($p = 0.683$), aggressor's gender ($p = 0.06$), teacher's gender ($p = 0.185$), or the combination of the aggressor's and teacher's gender ($p = 0.137$). There were also no significant differences in state anxiety ($p = 0.579$) and trait anxiety ($p = 0.72$) by gender.

3.2. Moral Disengagement Mechanisms Used by Gender

Regarding the mechanisms of moral disengagement used by the participants, no differences by gender were found for moral justification ($p = 0.336$), advantageous comparison ($p = 0.352$), displacement of responsibility ($p = 0.364$), distortion of consequences ($p = 0.458$), attribution of blaming ($p = 0.88$), or dehumanization ($p = 0.077$). Significant differences by gender were found for the mechanisms of euphemistic language and diffusion of responsibility, with males presenting both mechanisms in a higher proportion than females (Table 2).

Table 1. Comparison by gender for reactions facing the simulated physical peer aggression situation.

			Reaction to Stimulus		Total
			Attack	Does not Attack	
Participant gender					
	Male	Count	55.00	424.0	479.0
		% within column	40.1%	42.0%	41.8%
	Female	Count	82.00	586.0	668.0
		% within column	59.9%	58.0%	58.2%
	Total	Count	137.00	1010.0	1147.0
		% within column	100.0%	100.0%	100.0%
		Chi-Squared Tests	$X^2 = 0.167$	$p = 0.683$	
Offender gender					
	Male	Count	81.00	511.0	592.0
		% within column	59.1%	50.6%	51.6%
	Female	Count	56.00	499.0	555.0
		% within column	40.9%	49.4%	48.4%
	Total	Count	137.00	1010.0	1147.0
		% within column	100.0%	100.0%	100.0%
		Chi-Squared Tests	$X^2 = 3.515$	$p = 0.061$	
Teacher gender					
	Men	Count	80.00	529.0	609.0
		% within column	58.4%	52.4%	53.1%
	Women	Count	57.00	481.0	538.0
		% within column	41.6%	47.6%	46.9%
	Total	Count	137.00	1010.0	1147.0
		% within column	100.0%	100.0%	100.0%
		Chi-Squared Tests	$X^2 = 1.754$	$p = 0.185$	
Offender and Teacher gender combined					
	Men-Men	Count	46.00	280.0	326.0
		% within column	33.6%	27.7%	28.4%
	Men-Women	Count	46.00	325.0	371.0
		% within column	33.6%	32.2%	32.3%
	Women-Men	Count	23.00	155.0	178.0
		% within column	16.8%	15.3%	15.5%
	Women-Women	Count	22.00	250.0	272.0
		% within column	16.1%	24.8%	23.7%
	Total	Count	137.00	1010.0	1147.0
		% within column	100.0%	100.0%	100.0%
		Chi-Squared Tests	$X^2 = 5.534$	$p = 0.137$	

Designed by the authors.

Table 2. Comparison by gender for moral disengagement mechanisms (euphemistic language, diffusion of responsibility).

Moral Disengagement Mechanisms		Euphemistic Language			Diffusion of Responsibility		
Gender		Undecided	Absence	Presence	Undecided	Absence	Presence
Male	Count	325.0	66.00	88.00	136.0	304.0	39.00
	% within row	67.8%	13.8%	18.4%	28.4%	63.5%	8.1%
	% within column	40.3%	39.3%	50.9%	39.0%	41.8%	54.9%
Female	Count	481.0	102.00	85.00	213.0	423.0	32.00
	% within row	72.0%	15.3%	12.7%	31.9%	63.3%	4.8%
	% within column	59.7%	60.7%	49.1%	61.0%	58.2%	45.1%
Total	Count	806.0	168.00	173.00	349.0	727.0	71.00
	% within row	70.3%	14.6%	15.1%	30.4%	63.4%	6.2%
	% within column	100.0%	100.0%	100.0%	100.0%	100.0%	100.0%
Chi-Squared Tests	X^2	7.007		$p = 0.030$	X^2	6.182	$p = 0.045$

Designed by the authors.

Anxiety Related to Diffusion of Responsibility and Dehumanization by Gender of the Participants

Male participants showed higher state anxiety than female participants when the used diffusion of responsibility and dehumanization mechanisms (Table 3). No significant differences in state anxiety or trait anxiety by gender were found when the participants used euphemistic language ($p = 0.304$), as well as in trait anxiety for the mechanisms of diffusion of responsibility ($p = 0.718$) and dehumanization ($p = 0.834$).

Table 3. ANOVA for STAI-E related to diffusion of responsibility and dehumanization by the gender of the participants.

Moral Disengagement Mechanism	Gender	Mean	SD	n	F	p
Diffusion of responsibility						
Undecided	Male	28.71	2.740	136		
	Female	28.87	2.770	213		
Absence	Male	28.79	2.743	304	5.151	0.006
	Female	28.44	2.598	423		
Presence	Male	30.38	2.889	39		
	Female	28.28	2.517	32		
Dehumanization						
Undecided	Male	29.28	3.351	46		
	Female	28.12	2.590	41		
Absence	Male	28.77	2.625	405	4.003	0.019
	Female	28.62	2.687	592		
Presence	Male	30.11	3.665	28		
	Female	28.26	2.105	35		

Designed by the authors.

3.3. Legitimation of Violence Expected from Peers and Adults by Gender

Significant differences by gender in the legitimization of violence expected from peers and adults were found (Table 4). There was a lack of legitimization of violence expected from peers. However, females perceived them as legitimizers of their violent reaction. The perception of peers as sanctioners was minimal for both males and females. There was a lack of legitimation of violence perceived in adults, especially in females. Males were slightly more likely to perceive adults as sanctioners and neutral than females.

Table 4. Comparison by gender for the legitimation of violence perceived in peers and legitimation of violence perceived in adults.

Gender		Legitimation from Peers				Legitimation from Adults			
		Neutral	Absence	Presence	Sanction	Neutral	Absence	Presence	Sanction
Male	Count	191.0	241.0	45.00	2.00	29.00	357.0	5.00	88.00
	% within row	39.9%	50.3%	9.4%	0.4%	6.1%	74.5%	1.0%	18.4%
	% within column	48.6%	38.4%	36.6%	50.0%	55.8%	39.1%	41.7%	52.1%
Female	Count	202.0	386.0	78.00	2.00	23.00	557.0	7.00	81.00
	% within row	30.2%	57.8%	11.7%	0.3%	3.4%	83.4%	1.0%	12.1%
	% within column	51.4%	61.6%	63.4%	50.0%	44.2%	60.9%	58.3%	47.9%
Total	Count	393.0	627.0	123.00	4.00	52.00	914.0	12.00	169.00
	% within row	34.3%	54.7%	10.7%	0.3%	4.5%	79.7%	1.0%	14.7%
	% within column	100.0%	100.0%	100.0%	100.0%	100.0%	100.0%	100.0%	100.0%
Chi-Squared Tests		X^2	11.87	$p =$	0.008	X^2	14.33	$p =$	0.002

Designed by the authors.

Anxiety Related to Legitimation of Violence Expected from Peers and Gender of the Participants

Finally, trait anxiety was significantly higher in females, especially those who identified peers as legitimizers of their reaction (Table 5). No significant differences by gender were found in trait anxiety (0.663) and state anxiety (0.578) when adults were perceived as legitimizers of violence. No significant differences were found in state anxiety ($p = 0.257$) for the legitimation expected from peers associated with the gender of the participants.

Table 5. ANOVA for STAI-R related to the legitimation of violence perceived in peers and gender of the participants.

Peer Legitimation	Gender of the Participants	Mean	SD	n	F	p
Neutral	Male	24.69	4.344	191		
	Female	26.27	4.585	202		
Absence	Male	25.15	4.431	243	2.962	0.031
	Female	25.03	4.251	388		
Presence	Male	26.38	4.868	45		
	Female	26.67	4.755	78		

Designed by the authors.

4. Discussion

This study aimed to analyze gender and anxiety differences in middle school students' behavior facing a simulated physical peer aggression situation. The hypothesis (i) was not confirmed, since gender was not associated with the adolescent's behaviors in a simulated peer aggression situation; hypothesis (ii) was confirmed, since males presented higher moral disengagement mechanisms to justified violent reactions and a higher state anxiety when they used diffusion of responsibility and dehumanization mechanisms to justify their behavior.

The absence of gender differences in the use of violence in the present research was in line with previous research in this area [31]. Early studies about the prevalence of antisocial behavior in boys versus girls reported stronger genetic influences in girls and stronger environmental influences in boys. However, later meta-analyses found that antisocial behavior was equally heritable, but its etiology could differ across sex [40].

Generational and cultural changes in parenting and relationship patterns could impact new relationship forms that normalize violence without gender differences [29,32].

In this study, females evidenced a slightly higher expectation of legitimization from peers than males. This result coincides with previous studies, where females tend to be more concerned with social approval, afraid of abandonment [41,42], and worried about evaluation from their peers [28,43]. Our results also evidence that females with higher trait anxiety expected more legitimation from their peers. The higher trait anxiety levels could make them understand the violence as a catharsis, legitimizing it [44]. In this line, previous researchers found that girls were more at risk for internalizing adjustment problems as negative affect with stress, anxiety, and depression [26,27], and find adverse interpersonal events more stressful than males [45]. Relative to adults, girls did not perceive them as legitimizers or sanctioners. These results could be explained by adults' expectations about girls, who tend to evaluate them as less violent than boys [46].

We found that boys evidenced a higher expectation of neutrality and sanction from adults. These results could contradict previous studies that evidenced that many cultural parenting patterns promote male children's violence to solve conflicts [14]. However, neutrality expectations coincide with those studies, since many parents leave their children to decide when to use violence [7]. In consonant, it was reported that boys experience more advised violence from family, but even from non-family members, including neighbors and peers [10]. This fact could represent a stressful factor regarding the socially expected behavior of men facing conflicts. The social acceptance of violence exposes children to the risk of reproducing it in their daily relationships [10,11,47], and exposes them to chronic stress [17] and posttraumatic stress disorders in young adulthood [18]. In this study, male teenagers showed higher state anxiety associated with using moral disengagement mechanisms, such as diffusion of responsibility and dehumanization.

The diffusion of responsibility considers the group's role in the perception of individual responsibility for an act [4,5]. In this case, the increase of anxiety shows the possible social pressure experienced by boys facing interpersonal conflicts. Dehumanization is considered the worst violence justification [48], and its use has implications for the development of empathy by perceiving certain human beings as having fewer human qualities [49]. Usually, perceiving the other's suffering generates aversive sensations, but dehumanization reduces this empathy. Nevertheless, today, there is some doubt about the concept explaining this moral failure related to care about the other's suffering as not presupposing a cognitive failure to recognize their humanity. Contrarily, this remains an intensely human undertaking [50]. Thus, the link between dehumanization and state anxiety could be evidence of this cognitive contradiction.

Other moral disengagement mechanisms, such as euphemistic language and diffusion of responsibility, showed variations between males and females. Those mechanisms have been found with a strong presence in adolescents, increasing bullying perpetration. The adolescents who recur in these thoughts to justify their actions describe them as not severe and without significant consequences [49], which maintains these behaviors, preventing them from disappearing. Therefore, modification in the adolescent's perception in this sense appears to be essential to reduce bullying cases.

4.1. Limitations

The participants of this study were from Colombia. This country and its population have experienced more than 60 years of internal armed conflict, with consequently high exposure to violent content through the media and in many aspects of daily life. The generalizability of the results to other populations and contexts will need replication through cross-cultural investigations that favor a greater understanding of the phenomenon of the legitimization of violence in adolescence, and its relationships with anxiety.

4.2. Prevention and Policy Implications

The results obtained in this research can be used by educational interventions to improve coexistence and programs to change the justification of violent behaviors, helping adolescents to understand that their acts have substantial implications in the lives of others. Likewise, it is essential to develop group interventions that modify how adolescents' conflicts are managed, as the same as gender stereotypes that have a significant impact on health. Finally, we highlight the need for linking families in educational programs facing the challenges of transforming the legitimization of violence in parental practices.

5. Conclusions

The gender of the participants, offenders, and authorities was not associated with the adolescents' behaviors in a simulated peer aggression situation. Nevertheless, moral disengagement mechanisms, such as euphemistic language and diffusion of responsibility, were higher in males. Male teenagers showed a greater tendency to perceive adults as sanctioners and neutrals; males had higher state anxiety when they used diffusion of responsibility and dehumanization mechanisms to justify their behavior. Female teenagers presented higher trait anxiety when they expected legitimation from peers.

Author Contributions: Conceptualization, M.B.M.-G., C.A.-R., and Y.T.-P.; methodology, M.B.M.-G., V.J.C.-S., and C.A.-R.; formal analysis, M.B.M.-G. and V.J.C.-S.; resources, M.B.M.-G.; data curation, M.A.-R. and Y.G.-L.; writing—original draft preparation, M.B.M.-G., Y.T.-P., C.A.-R., M.A.-R., Y.G.-L., and V.J.C.-S.; writing—review and editing, M.B.M.-G. and V.J.C.-S.; supervision, M.B.M.-G.; project administration, M.B.M.-G. All authors have read and agreed to the published version of the manuscript.

Funding: This research received no external funding.

Institutional Review Board Statement: The study was conducted according to the Declaration of Helsinki guidelines and approved by the Ethics Committee of Universidad de la Costa; approval code 094 related to the project INV.140-01-001-13.

Informed Consent Statement: Informed consent was obtained from all subjects involved in the study.

Data Availability Statement: Data supporting reported results can be found asking directly of the first author.

Conflicts of Interest: The authors declare no conflict of interest.

References

1. Kelman, H.C. Reflections on the social and psychological processes of legitimization and delegitimization. In *The Psychology of Legitimacy: Emerging Perspectives on Ideology, Justice, and Intergroup Relations*; Jost, J.T., Major, B., Eds.; Cambridge University Press: Cambridge, UK, 2001; pp. 54–73.
2. Barreto, I.; Borja, H.; Serrano, Y.; López-López, W. La legitimación como proceso en la violencia política, medios de comunicación y construcción de culturas de paz. *Univ. Psychol.* **2009**, *8*, 737–748. Available online: http://www.scielo.org.co/scielo.php?script=sci_arttext&pid=S1657-92672009000300010&nrm=iso (accessed on 12 December 2020).
3. Galtung, J. Cultural Violence. *J. Peace Res.* **1990**, *27*, 291–305. [CrossRef]
4. Bandura, A. Moral Disengagement in the Perpetration of Inhumanities. *Personal. Soc. Psychol. Rev.* **1999**, *3*, 193–209. [CrossRef] [PubMed]
5. Bandura, A. Selective Moral Disengagement in the Exercise of Moral Agency. *J. Moral Educ.* **2002**, *31*, 101–119. [CrossRef]
6. Fernández Villanueva, I. Justificación y Legitimación de la Violencia en la Infancia: Un Estudio Sobre la Legitimación Social de las Agresiones en los Conflictos Cotidianos Entre Menores. Ph.D. Thesis, Universidad Complutense de Madrid, Servicio de Publicaciones, Madrid, Spain, 2009.
7. Martínez-González, M.B.; Amar, J.J. *Quién es el malo del Paseo?* 1st ed.; Editorial Universidad del Norte: Barranquilla, Colombia, 2016.
8. Cardozo-Rusinque, A.A.; Martínez-González, M.B.; Peña-Leiva, A.A.D.L.; Avedaño-Villa, I.; Crissien-Borrero, T.J. Factores psicosociales asociados al conflicto entre menores en el contexto escolar. *Educ. Soc.* **2019**, *40*, e0189140. [CrossRef]
9. Martínez-González, M.B.; Robles-Haydar, C.A.; Alfaro-Alvarez, J. Concepto de desconexion moral y sus manifestaciones contemporaneas/Moral disengagement concept and its contemporary manifestations. *Utopía Prax. Latinoam.* **2020**, *25*, 349–362.
10. Kim, J.; Lee, B.; Farber, N.B. Where do they learn violence? The roles of three forms of violent socialization in childhood. *Child. Youth Serv. Rev.* **2019**, *107*, 104494. [CrossRef]
11. Kim, J.; Kim, Y.K.; Farber, N.B. Multiple Forms of Early Violent Socialization and the Acceptance of Interpersonal Violence Among Chinese College Students. *Violence Vict.* **2019**, *34*, 474–491. [CrossRef]
12. Jiménez, J.S.F.G. Exposición a la violencia en adolescentes: Desensibilización, legitimación y naturalización. *Diversitas* **2018**, *14*, 55–67. [CrossRef]
13. Pino, M.; Montaño, S.; Agudelo, K.; Idárraga-Cabrera, C.; Fernández-Lucas, J.; Herrera-Mendoza, K. Emotion recognition in young male offenders and non-offenders. *Physiol. Behav.* **2019**, *207*, 73–75. [CrossRef] [PubMed]
14. Duman, S.; Margolin, G. Parents' Aggressive Influences and Children's Aggressive Problem Solutions With Peers. *J. Clin. Child Adolesc. Psychol.* **2007**, *36*, 42–55. [CrossRef]
15. Goodman, M.L.; Hindman, A.; Keiser, P.H.; Gitari, S.; Porter, K.A.; Raimer, B.G. Neglect, Sexual Abuse, and Witnessing Intimate Partner Violence During Childhood Predicts Later Life Violent Attitudes Against Children Among Kenyan Women: Evidence of Intergenerational Risk Transmission From Cross-Sectional Data. *J. Interpers. Violence* **2020**, *35*, 623–645. [CrossRef]
16. Mebarak, M.R.; Annicchiarico, G.C.; Castillo, L.F.; Molinares, N.Q. Análisis de las pautas de crianza y los tipos de autoridad, y su relación con el surgimiento de conductas criminales: Una revisión teórica. *Rev. Crim.* **2016**, *58*, 61–70. Available online: http://www.scielo.org.co/scielo.php?script=sci_arttext&pid=S1794-31082016000300006&nrm=iso (accessed on 15 July 2020).
17. Finegood, E.D.; Chen, E.; Kish, J.; Vause, K.; Leigh, A.K.K.; Hoffer, L.; Mille, G.E. Community violence and cellular and cytokine indicators of inflammation in adolescents. *Psychoneuroendocrinology* **2020**, *115*, 104628. [CrossRef]
18. Lee, H.; Kim, Y.; Terry, J. Adverse childhood experiences (ACEs) on mental disorders in young adulthood: Latent classes and community violence exposure. *Prev. Med.* **2020**, *134*, 106039. [CrossRef]
19. Sierra, J.C.; Ortega, V.; Zubeidat, I. Ansiedad, angustia y estrés: Tres conceptos a diferenciar. *Rev. Mal-Estar E Subj.* **2021**, *3*, 10–59. Available online: https://www.redalyc.org/articulo.oa?id=27130102 (accessed on 27 February 2021).
20. Spielberger, C.D.; Gorsuch, R.L.; Lushene, R.E. *STAI: Cuestionario de Ansiedad Estado-Rasgo*; TEA Ediciones: Madrid, Spain, 1999.
21. Corr, R.; Pelletier-Baldelli, A.; Glier, S.; Bizzell, J.; Campbell, A.; Belger, A. Neural mechanisms of acute stress and trait anxiety in adolescents. *NeuroImage Clin.* **2021**, *29*, 102543. [CrossRef]
22. Núñez, A.; Álvarez-García, D.; Pérez-Fuentes, M.-C. Anxiety and self-esteem in cyber-victimization profiles of adolescents. *Comunicar* **2021**, *29*, 47–59. [CrossRef]
23. Vega, A.; Cabello, R.; Megías-Robles, A.; Gómez-Leal, R.; Fernández-Berrocal, P. Emotional Intelligence and Aggressive Behaviors in Adolescents: A Systematic Review and Meta-Analysis. *Trauma Violence Abuse* **2021**, 152483802199129. [CrossRef] [PubMed]

24. Liu, Y.; Yue, S.; Hu, X.; Zhu, J.; Wu, Z.; Wang, J.; Wu, Y. Associations between feelings/behaviors during COVID-19 pandemic lockdown and depression/anxiety after lockdown in a sample of Chinese children and adolescents. *J. Affect. Disord.* **2021**, *284*, 98–103. [CrossRef] [PubMed]
25. Rodriguez, J.H.; Gregus, S.J.; Craig, J.T.; Pastrana, F.A.; Cavell, T.A. Anxiety Sensitivity and Children's Risk for Both Internalizing Problems and Peer Victimization Experiences. *Child Psychiatry Hum. Dev.* **2020**, *51*, 174–186. [CrossRef] [PubMed]
26. Mercader-Yus, E.; Neipp-López, M.C.; Gómez-Méndez, P.; Vargas-Torcal, F.; Gelves-Ospina, M.; Puerta-Morales, L.; León-Jacobus, A.; Cantillo-Pacheco, K.; Mancera-Sarmiento, M. Ansiedad, autoestima e imagen corporal en niñas con diagnóstico de pubertad precoz. *Rev. Colomb. Psiquiatr.* **2018**, *47*, 229–236. [CrossRef]
27. McLean, C.P.; Anderson, E.R. Brave men and timid women? A review of the gender differences in fear and anxiety. *Clin. Psychol. Rev.* **2009**, *29*, 496–505. [CrossRef] [PubMed]
28. Storch, E.A.; Brassard, M.R.; Masia-Warner, C.L. The relationship of peer victimization to social anxiety and loneliness in adolescence. *Child Study J.* **2003**, *33*, 1–18.
29. Reyes, H.L.M.; Foshee, V.A.; Chen, M.S.; Ennett, S.T. Patterns of Adolescent Aggression and Victimization: Sex Differences and Correlates. *J. Aggress. Maltreatment Trauma* **2019**, *28*, 1130–1150. [CrossRef] [PubMed]
30. Archer, J. Sex Differences in Aggression in Real-World Settings: A Meta-Analytic Review. *Rev. Gen. Psychol.* **2004**, *8*, 291–322. [CrossRef]
31. Slawinski, B.L.; Klump, K.L.; Burt, S.A. No sex differences in the origins of covariation between social and physical aggression. *Psychol. Med.* **2019**, *49*, 2515–2523. [CrossRef] [PubMed]
32. Lei, H.; Chiu, M.M.; Cui, Y.; Li, S.; Lu, M. Changes in aggression among mainland Chinese elementary, junior high, and senior high school students across years: A cross-temporal meta-analysis. *Aggress. Violent Behav.* **2019**, *48*, 190–196. [CrossRef]
33. Allen, A.B.; Cazeau, S.; Grace, J.; Banos, A.S. Self-Compassionate Responses to an Imagined Sexual Assault. *Violence Women* **2020**, 107780122090563. [CrossRef]
34. Martínez-González, R.; Robles-Haydar, M.B.; Amar-Amar, C.A.; Jabba-Molinares, J.J.; Ariza, D.P.; Abello-Llanos, J.G. Role-playing game as a computer-based test to assess the resolution of conflicts in childhood. *Interciencia* **2019**. Available online: https://www.redalyc.org/articulo.oa?id=33960068012 (accessed on 23 September 2020).
35. Anderson, R.E.; Brouwer, A.M.; Wendorf, A.R.; Cahill, S.P. Women's Behavioral Responses to the Threat of a Hypothetical Date Rape Stimulus: A Qualitative Analysis. *Arch. Sex. Behav.* **2016**, *45*, 793–805. [CrossRef]
36. Rovira, A. The use of virtual reality in the study of people's responses to violent incidents. *Front. Behav. Neurosci.* **2009**. [CrossRef]
37. Rayburn, N.R.; Jaycox, L.H.; McCaffrey, D.F.; Ulloa, E.C.; Zander-Cotugno, M.; Marshall, G.N.; Shelley, G.A. Reactions to dating violence among Latino teenagers: An experiment utilizing the Articulated Thoughts in Simulated Situations paradigm. *J. Adolesc.* **2007**, *30*, 893–915. [CrossRef] [PubMed]
38. Bandura, A. Failures in Self-Regulation: Energy Depletion or Selective Disengagement? *Psychol. Inq.* **1996**, *7*, 20–24. [CrossRef]
39. Moreno, D.A.C.; Copete, P.E.B. Validación del inventario de ansiedad estado-rasgo (STAIC) en niños escolarizados entre los 8 y los 15 años. *Acta Colomb. Psicol.* **2005**, *8*, 79–90. Available online: http://www.scielo.org.co/scielo.php?script=sci_arttext&pid=S0123-91552005000100005&nrm=iso (accessed on 7 July 2020).
40. Burt, S.A.; Slawinski, B.L.; Klump, K.L. Are there sex differences in the etiology of youth antisocial behavior? *J. Abnorm. Psychol.* **2018**, *127*, 66–78. [CrossRef] [PubMed]
41. Rose, A.J.; Rudolph, K.D. A review of sex differences in peer relationship processes: Potential trade-offs for the emotional and behavioral development of girls and boys. *Psychol. Bull.* **2006**, *132*, 98–131. [CrossRef] [PubMed]
42. Henrich, C.C.; Blatt, S.J.; Kuperminc, G.P.; Zohar, A.; Leadbeater, B.J. Levels of Interpersonal Concerns and Social Functioning in Early Adolescent Boys and Girls. *J. Pers. Assess.* **2001**, *76*, 48–67. [CrossRef]
43. Rudolph, K.D.; Conley, C.S. The Socioemotional Costs and Benefits of Social-Evaluative Concerns: Do Girls Care Too Much? *J. Pers.* **2005**, *73*, 115–138. [CrossRef]
44. Nanay, B. Catharsis and vicarious fear. *Eur. J. Philos.* **2018**, *26*, 1371–1380. [CrossRef]
45. Kawabata, Y.; Nakamura, M.S.; de Luna, M.J.F. A mediation model for relational aggression, victimization, attachment, and depressive symptoms in Guam: A gender-informed approach. *J. Pac. Rim Psychol.* **2020**, *14*, e8. [CrossRef]
46. Card, N.A.; Stucky, B.D.; Sawalani, G.M.; Little, T.D. Direct and Indirect Aggression During Childhood and Adolescence: A Meta-Analytic Review of Gender Differences, Intercorrelations, and Relations to Maladjustment. *Child Dev.* **2008**, *79*, 1185–1229. [CrossRef] [PubMed]
47. Elsaesser, C.; Kennedy, T.M.; Tredinnick, L. The role of relationship proximity to witnessed community violence and youth outcomes. *J. Community Psychol.* **2020**, *48*, 562–575. [CrossRef] [PubMed]
48. Blanco, A.; Caballero, A.; De la Corte, L. *Psicología de los Grupos*; Pearson Educación: Madrid, Spain, 2005.
49. Zych, I.; Llorent, V.J. Affective Empathy and Moral Disengagement Related to Late Adolescent Bullying Perpetration. *Ethics Behav.* **2019**, *29*, 547–556. [CrossRef]
50. Lang, J. The limited importance of dehumanization in collective violence. *Curr. Opin. Psychol.* **2020**, *35*, 17–20. [CrossRef] [PubMed]

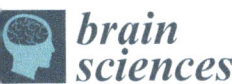

Article

The Relation of Callous–Unemotional Traits and Bullying in Early Adolescence Is Independent from Sex and Age and Moderated by Conduct Problems

Gennaro Catone [1], Luisa Almerico [2], Anna Pezzella [2], Maria Pia Riccio [3], Carmela Bravaccio [3], Pia Bernardo [4], Pietro Muratori [5], Antonio Pascotto [6], Simone Pisano [3,*,†] and Vincenzo Paolo Senese [2,†]

1. Department of Educational, Psychological and Communication Sciences, Suor Orsola Benincasa University, 80120 Naples, Italy; gennaro.catone@unisob.na.it
2. Department of Psychology, University of Campania "Luigi Vanvitelli", 80120 Naples, Italy; almericoluisa@hotmail.com (L.A.); anna.pezzella333@gmail.com (A.P.); vincenzopaolo.senese@unicampania.it (V.P.S.)
3. Department of Translational Medical Sciences, Federico II University, 80120 Naples, Italy; piariccio@gmail.com (M.P.R.); carmela.bravaccio@unina.it (C.B.)
4. Department of Neuroscience and Rehabilitation, Santobono-Pausilipon Children Hospital, 80120 Naples, Italy; pia.bernardo84@gmail.com
5. IRCCS Stella Maris, Calambrone, 56128 Pisa, Italy; pietro.muratori@fsm.unipi.it
6. Department of Mental and Physical Health and Preventive Medicine, University of Campania "Luigi Vanvitelli", 80120 Naples, Italy; prof.antoniopascotto@gmail.com
* Correspondence: pisano.simone@gmail.com; Tel.: +39-817463398-801
† These authors are joint last authors.

Abstract: In youths, callous–unemotional (CU) traits and conduct problems (CP) are independently associated with bullying perpetration and these effects are also observed when controlling for sex. Moreover, research indicates that the co-existence of high levels of both CU and CP further increase the risk. Although several studies have examined the relationship between CU traits and traditional bullying, few have also included a measure of cyberbullying and very few of them have focused the early adolescence. The aim of this study was to replicate and extend these findings in a large sample of Italian early adolescents considering both traditional and cyberbullying behaviors. Data were extracted from the Bullying and Youth Mental Health Naples study (BYMHNS) which included 2959 students of 10–15 years of age. CP, CU traits, traditional bullying behaviors, and cyberbullying behaviors were assessed by multi-item self-report scales. As expected, we replicated the significant and specific association between CU traits and traditional bullying, extending the findings to cyberbullying. In addition, in the latter case the effect was moderated by CP. The theoretical and clinical implications of these results were discussed.

Keywords: callous–unemotional traits; conduct problems; bullying; cyberbullying; gender

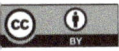

1. Introduction

1.1. CU Traits

Callous–unemotional (CU) traits identify a psychological construct characterized by the absence of concern for the feelings of others, lack of guilt or remorse feelings, lack of empathy, superficial or inadequate affectivity, and lack of concern for the consequence of one's actions [1–6]. In the literature, it has been shown that CU traits constitute the affective dimension of psychopathy in adults [7] and that in children and adolescents the presence of high levels of these traits is associated with a higher risk of deficits in affective processing and future development of antisocial behaviors and other negative outcomes [8–13]. Moreover, the latest version of the Diagnostic and Statistical Manual of Mental Disorders (DSM-V) includes CU traits as a specifier for the diagnosis of conduct disorder, designating a group characterized by "limited pro-social emotions" (LPE) [14].

Although CU traits have been mainly studied in populations of children and adolescents with conduct disorders, there is growing evidence that CU traits should be also considered in non-clinical samples given that high scores on this dimension can be observed in individuals not showing evident conduct problems [12,15–19]. For example, Pardini and Byrd [20] highlighted that children (mean age = 10.31; SD = 0.72; male = 47.9%) with higher CU traits have a unique and particular deviant social pattern that is not common to all aggressive children. Indeed, compared to children with aggressive behaviors but without high CU traits, those with high levels of CU traits use more aggression to dominate others, have more difficulty in anticipating discomfort and suffering in others, and show less concern for the others or for the consequences of their behavior. Moreover, data showed that independently of general conduct problems, CU traits are positively associated with aggression in both children and adolescents [15,21–26], including bullying behaviors [24,26–32]. Thus, high CU traits could be considered a general risk factor for the development of particularly severe, persistent, and treatment-resistant forms of conduct disorder [33].

1.2. Bullying

Among the various aggressive behaviors, bullying is one of the most studied. According to Olweus [34], bullying is defined as an intentional, reiterative, and aggressive behavior that an individual or group may make toward a person and that denotes an asymmetrical relationship, characterized by an imbalance of physical, intellectual, or strength power [34–38]. Prevalence of bullying varies depending on the study selected and worldwide. In this sample, we found a prevalence of traditional bullying victimization and perpetration ranging from 11.4% to 40.7% and 5.1% to 22%, respectively, depending on the assessment method [39] and a prevalence of cyberbullying victimization perpetration of 13.5/5.2% [40]. Recently, an Australian systematic review and meta-analysis detected a 12-month prevalence of traditional bullying victimization of 15.17% and perpetration of 5.275%, and a cyberbullying victimization and perpetration of lifetime prevalence of 7.02% and 3.45% [41].

Bullying is a widespread phenomenon that occurs in different social contexts and, more recently, in the online context. Aggressive bullying behaviors represent a serious risk factor for the psychological well-being of children who are victims [42], and for this reason bullying is considered a serious social problem in many countries [43], including in Italy [44–46].

In recent years, many studies have focused on intervention program for bullying behaviors. Zych et al. conducted a systematic review on community, school, family, peer, and individual protective factors that could be enhanced in bullying and cyberbullying preventive programs. They found that self-oriented personal competencies were protective against victimization, whereas good academic performance and other-oriented social competencies were protective against perpetration. Good peer interaction was a protective factor against the behavior of bully/victim and a low use of technology in terms of frequency was protective against cyberbullying [47]. In the same direction, Hinduja and Patchin found the construct of resilience a strong protective factor against bullying and cyberbullying behaviors [48]. Several intervention programs have been recognized as effective in reducing bullying behavior in school and other contexts [49–51].

Although several factors responsible for bullying behavior perpetration have been highlighted in the literature, it has recently been shown that CU traits seem to have a specific relationship with this behavior that would be independent of the sex, age, and manifestation of general conduct problems. Several international studies have shown that the CU trait is positively correlated with the perpetration of direct bullying [11,32,52] and that antisocial youth with high CU traits were more likely to perpetrate bullying than antisocial youth with low CU traits [15]. Furthermore, evidence has indicated that youths with high CU traits are less likely to respond positively to typical bullying interventions and show less concern for punishment, suggesting that anti-bullying intervention programs should take into account these traits [53].

1.3. Previous Studies on the Relationship between CU and Bullying

Even though the link between CU traits and bullying has been confirmed by some studies, the literature on the strength of their association and the role of factors influencing it (e.g., sex, age, conduct problems) is still scarce; moreover, it is very important to further study the relationship between CU traits and bullying in a valid way, by taking into account some important methodological aspects such as the assessment methodology and the context considered. Regarding the former, as stressed by several authors, for the detection of different bullying behaviors it is preferable to adopt a multi-item approach [54]. Indeed, a recent study [39] that compared single-item and multi-item measurements confirmed that the latter methodology offers a more valid detection and better captures the different degrees of bullying. As regards the context, it is worth noticing that most of the studies in the literature have investigated the process influencing bullying in traditional face-to-face contexts (e.g., school), whereas it is important to emphasize that with the wide spread of electronic communication and the use of computers and/or mobile phones by young people, bullying is no longer restricted to the face-to-face interactions but it is also observed in the virtual contexts [55]. Smith and colleagues introduced the term cyberbullying [56] to define bullying carried out through the use of digital technologies and the Internet (e.g., mobile phones, messaging platforms, social media, gaming platforms). Though some studies have provided evidence of an overlap between traditional bullying and cyberbullying [57,58], it has also been shown that cyberbullying differs from traditional bullying because it is characterized by the absence of spatio-temporal boundaries and the possibility of the anonymity of the perpetrator [59]. This latter aspect is particularly relevant given that the anonymity offered by the Internet leads adolescents to express themselves more recklessly and aggressively online than they would in face-to-face interactions [60].

As regards the negative effects of bullying and cyberbullying, if from one side data indicated that both are associated with the same consequences in the victims, such as anxiety, depression, substance abuse, suicidal ideation, and psychosis [61–64], on the other side, a study directly comparing the impact of traditional face-to-face bullying and cyberbullying on victims reported that the latter is associated with more frequent and intense anxiety and depressive symptoms than the former, particularly in terms of social anxiety [65]. Therefore, it is particularly important to also explore factors that may increase or decrease the risk of cyberbullying perpetration in adolescence.

Studies describing the association between CU traits and cyberbullying in adolescents showed that the two dimensions are significantly and positively associated [29,66–68], and that adolescents with high CU scores who manifest cyberbullying behavior tend to ignore the fear and the distress of the victims [69,70], thus increasing the risk in victims of developing symptoms of psychological distress [65,71–74]. For this reason, it is particularly important to study and prevent cyberbullying as it is easier to carry out than traditional bullying and leads to greater personal and social consequences [65]. This latter consideration is clearer if it is considered in the perspective of the interpersonal acceptance-rejection theory (IPARTheory) [75–77]. Indeed, according to the IPARTheory, the quality of individuals' interpersonal relationships, i.e., perceived acceptance–rejection, influences the general psychological adjustment and the expression of internalizing and externalizing problems. Therefore, because victims of traditional bullying and cyberbullying experience rejection from peers, they could manifest a psychological maladjustment and this, in turn, could lead them to engage inappropriate, aggressive, and problematic behaviors. In other terms, the expression of these negative behaviors increases the risk of its spreading since those who undergo bullying experiences could be led in turn to perpetrate them on others [78], for example using the virtual dimension for revenge for victimization [79,80]. Therefore, it is critically important to understand how much individual characteristics such as CU traits are specifically related to bullying behaviors and to what extent they may represent a general risk factor, to design targeted intervention programs aimed at reducing these phenomena, thus preventing their consequences.

In summary, the analysis of the literature on the relationship between bullying and CU traits indicates a need to replicate these studies by considering very large samples, to attain more replicable estimate of the effect sizes, and by considering bullying in both its traditional (face-to-face) and online (cyberbullying) forms, to better understand the extent to which the relationship is specific and whether it is moderated by other factors such as sex, age, the presence of conduct problems, and the context. Most research, indeed, focused exclusively on a single context of bullying behaviors (see for example [29,52]). Only very few studies have explored the relationship between CU traits and bullying in adolescence considering both the traditional and the cyber forms. Among these, Orue and Calvete [67] showed a significant predictive value of CU traits for both traditional and cyberbullying in a sample of 765 Spanish adolescents aged 14–18 years, and an Italian study, conducted on a sample of 540 subjects aged 10–16 years [27], showed that the presence of CU traits increased bullying behavior in both traditional and cyberbullying contexts.

Hypothesis for the present study: Starting from the abovementioned considerations, the aim of the present study was to replicate and extend the data present in the literature [27,52,67] responding to the need to verify the relationship between the presence of CU traits and bullying behavior on a very large sample, by using multi-item standardized measures and considering different bullying contexts. In particular, we wanted to investigate the predictive and specific role of CU traits independently of the sex, age, and presence of general conduct problems on bullying behaviors. To verify to what extent similar processes regulate both face-to-face and cyberbullying behaviors, both contexts of bullying were considered. In line with the previous literature, we expected to find a specific and significant relationship between CU traits and both forms of bullying and that this effect would be moderated by the conduct problems. In addition, a further objective of the study was to test the moderating effect of the sex and the age factors.

2. Methods

2.1. Participants

The data considered in this study were extracted from the Bullying and Youth Mental Health Naples study (BYMHNS), a larger cross-sectional study based on a sample of students gathered in the metropolitan city of Naples and in the surrounding areas. The data were collected during the 2015/2016 school years. Twelve schools comprising a total of 4444 students were contacted and agreed to participate. The final total sample of participants consisted of 2959 students of which 1426 (48.2%) were females and 1533 (51.8%) were males; with 44% of the participants belonging to schools in the city of Naples and 56.1% to those in the surrounding areas. As regards the class, 1048 (35.4%) students attended the first grade, 995 (33.6%) the second grade, and 916 (31%) the third grade. The mean age was 11.84 years ($SD = 0.97$, range: 10–15 years).

2.2. Procedure

Data were collected through the administration of self-assessment scales to obtain measures of traditional bullying, cyberbullying, and other demographics and psychopathological information. For each school, meetings were held with the headmaster and teachers to provide information about the study. In addition, the parents of the pupils received informed consent in which they express their agreement to the participation of their children in the research. During the administration of the protocol, which happened in the usual classroom and lasted about 1 h, the presence of at least one researcher was guaranteed to provide explanations and to answer any questions from the students. We had very few missing data (<1%) that were handled with means replacing. The Ethics Committee of the University of Campania "Luigi Vanvitelli" approved the study protocol (No. 500 of 29/04/2016). For more information about the whole project please refer to Catone et al. [39].

2.3. Measures

2.3.1. Conduct Problems

To attain a measure of general behavioral problems, responses to the conduct problems subscale of the Italian self-report version of the Strength and Difficulties Questionnaire for age 4–17 (SDQ) [81] were considered. The SDQ is a short self-report questionnaire useful for assessing the level of general psychopathology related to the last six months both in clinical and research settings [82]. It consists of 25 items divided into 5 subscales of 5 items each: emotional problems (no reversed); conduct problems (1 reversed); hyperactivity problems (2 reversed); peers problems (2 reversed); pro-social behavior (no reversed). In this study, only responses to the conduct problems subscale (e.g., "I get very angry and often lose my temper") were considered. Responses were collected on a 3-point Likert type scale: "not true" = 0, "somewhat true" = 1, "certainly true" = 2. A total score was computed for each participant (ranges: 0 to 10), with higher scores indicating higher conduct problems (CP). Cronbach's Alpha = 0.639; ω_t = 0.707.

2.3.2. Callous–Unemotional Traits

To measure callous and unemotional (CU) traits, the Italian 22-item version of the Inventory of Callous–Unemotional Traits (22-item ICU) [27,83] was administered. The 22-item ICU [23] evaluates a general callous–unemotional dimension and three sub-dimensions: callousness (9 items; 1 reversed), which refers to lack of empathy, remorse and guilt (e.g., "I do not care who I hurt to get what I want"); unemotionality (5 items; 3 reversed), indicating absence of emotional activation and expressiveness (e.g., "I do not show my emotions to others"); and uncaringness (8 items; all reversed), which is disinterest in the feelings of others and in the performance of daily activities (e.g., "I work hard on everything I do"). The score for each item is calculated on a 4-point Likert scale and ranges from 0 ("not at all true") to 3 ("definitely true"). A confirmatory factorial analysis carried out on the total sample confirmed that the best fitting factor structure identifies a general callous–unemotional factor and three specific factors, χ^2 (206) = 1424.13, $p < 0.001$, RMSEA = 0.045, 95% CI [0.043; 0.047], CFI = 0.794, SRMR = 0.046, N = 2959. Therefore, a total score was computed for each participant (ranges: 0 to 72), with higher scores indicating higher CU traits. Cronbach's Alpha = 0.697; ω_t = 0.692.

2.3.3. Traditional Bullying

To measure the traditional bullying perpetration, the Italian version of the bully subscale of the Illinois Bully Scale (IBS-B) [39] was administered. The Illinois Bully Scale [84] is a self-reported scale that includes 18 items divided into 3 subscales: bully (9-item; e.g., "I annoyed other students"), victim (4-item; e.g., "Other students beat and pushed me"), and fighting (5-item; e.g., "If someone beats me firstly, I will beat him/her"). In this study, for each item of the IBS-B, participants were asked to indicate the frequencies with which they carried out the described behavior. Responses were collected on a 5-point scale, which considered the following alternatives: "never" = 0, "1 or 2 times" = 1, "3 or 4 times" = 2, "5 or 6 times" = 3, "7 or more times" = 4. The good psychometric properties of the Italian IBS-B have been described in Catone et al. [39]. As indicated by Espelage and Holt [84] a total score of traditional bullying perpetration was computed for each participant (ranges: 0 to 36), with higher scores indicating higher self-reported bullying behaviors. Cronbach's Alpha = 0.824; ω_t = 0.859.

2.3.4. Cyberbullying

To measure the cyberbullying perpetration [40], the Italian version of the Smith's cyberbullying scale (SCBS) was administered. The SCBS [56] is a self-report scale assessing cyberbullying behaviors by considering seven different media (7-item): text messaging; pictures/photos or video clips; phone calls; email; chat rooms; instant messaging; and websites. Participants were preliminarily presented a definition of cyberbullying behaviors then were asked to indicate for each media if they bullied others through it during the last year. Responses were collected on a 5-points scale that considered the following alternatives: "never" = 0; "only once or twice" = 1; "two or three times a month" = 2; "about once a week" = 3; "several times a week" = 4). Although the Italian adaptation of the scale has been already used, its psychometric characteristics have not been described. For this reason, the dimensionality and reliability of the SCBS were preliminarily verified before running the main analyses of this study. A confirmatory factorial analysis carried out on the total sample confirmed the unidimensional structure of the scale, $\chi^2(14) = 205.31$, $p < 0.001$, RMSEA = 0.068, 90% CI [0.060; 0.076], CFI = 0.976, SRMR = 0.026, N = 2959; whereas the reliability analysis showed an adequate value, Cronbach's Alpha = 0.795; $\omega_t = 0.889$. Therefore, as indicated by Smith and colleagues [56], a total score of cyberbullying perpetration was computed for each participant (ranges: 0 to 28), with higher scores indicating higher self-reported cyberbullying behaviors.

2.4. Statistical Analyses

Prior to carrying out the main analysis, the descriptive statistics were computed to describe considered variables: demographics (sex, age, class, school), conduct problems (CP), CU traits, traditional bullying (IBS-B), and cyberbullying (SBCS) behaviors. Descriptive statistics are reported into Table 1. Data indicated that traditional bullying (IBS-B) and cyberbullying (SBCS) perpetration scores presented a severe deviation from non-normal distribution as indicated by skewness and kurtosis, and were therefore normalized by adding a constant of 1 and applying a logarithmic transformation [85]. All the analyses were performed on the transformed variables, but for descriptive purposes, untransformed data were used to report descriptive statistics. Then, correlation coefficients between the variables age, sex, conduct problems, CU traits, traditional bullying, and cyberbullying measures were computed to investigate the bivariate associations. According to Cohen (1988), for Pearson's r we considered indicative of small, medium, and large effects the values 0.10, 0.30, and 0.50, respectively. Finally, to investigate if the association between CU traits and bullying and cyberbullying perpetration is observed also when controlling for sex, age, and conduct problems, and if it was moderated by the context of bullying or the control variables, two hierarchical multiple regressions were carried out. In each regression, bullying (traditional or cyberbullying) was regressed on the control variables (sex, age, and conduct problems) and the ICU. In both regression models, all variables were included as z-scores, but sex was dummy-coded (males = 1; females = 0). In the first step, the sex and the age were included. In the second step, the conduct problem variable was added. In the third step, the ICU score was added, whereas, in the fourth and last step, the two-way interaction effects were added. When significant, the interaction effects were investigated by applying simple slope analysis and the Johnson and Neyman's (JN) approach [86] to define the lower and upper values of the moderator for which the effect of the predictor on the dependent variable was significant. All the analyses were performed with R 4.0.4 software and an Alpha level of 0.05 was used for all statistical tests.

Table 1. Summary of means, standard deviations, minimum, maximum, skewness, and kurtosis of the considered variables.

Variable	M	SD	Min	Max	Skewness	Kurtosis
Sex	-	-	0	1	-	-
Age	11.84	0.97	10	15	0.04	−0.66
Conduct	2.29	1.67	0	10	0.99	1.14
ICU	21.83	8.08	1	63	0.32	0.07
Traditional-B	3.05	4.14	0	36	3.09	13.91
Cyber-B	0.95	2.17	0	28	6.87	65.40

Note: $n = 2959$. Sex = participants' sex dummy coding (males = 1; females = 0); Age = age of participants in years; Conduct = conduct problems subscale of the SDQ; ICU = total score of the ICU; Traditional-B = total score of the bully subscale of the Illinois Bully Scale; Cyber-B = total score of the Smith's cyberbullying scale.

3. Results

The main descriptive statistics are reported into Table 1.

The results of the correlation analysis showed a strong association between the two measures of bullying ($r = 0.615$, $p < 0.001$) and that both measures were significantly associated with all the considered variables (see Table 2).

Table 2. Summary of intercorrelations (and 95% confidence intervals) for the considered variables.

Variable	1	2	3	4	5
1. Sex					
2. Age	0.018 [−0.02; 0.05]				
3. Conduct	−0.008 [−0.04; 0.03]	0.073 * [0.04; 0.11]			
4. ICU	0.127 * [0.09; 0.16]	0.128 * [0.09; 0.16]	0.360 * [0.33; 0.39]		
5. Traditional-B	0.176 * [0.14; 0.21]	0.101 * [0.07; 0.14]	0.485 * [0.46; 0.51]	0.338 * [0.31; 0.37]	
6. Cyber-B	0.079 * [0.04; 0.12]	0.086 * [0.05; 0.12]	0.376 * [0.35; 0.41]	0.292 * [0.26; 0.32]	0.615 * [0.59; 0.64]

Note: $n = 2959$; Sex = participants' sex dummy coding (males = 1; females = 0); Age = age of participants in years (z-score); Conduct = conduct problems subscale of the SDQ; ICU = total score of the ICU; Traditional-B = total score of the bully subscale of the Illinois Bully Scale; Cyber-B = total score of the Smith's cyberbullying scale; * $p < 0.001$. Note that for the correlation between sex and quantitative variables, a point biserial correlation coefficient was computed.

In particular, the analysis of the effect sizes showed that the two bullying measures were weakly associated with the control variables sex and age ($rs < 0.176$, $ps < 0.001$), while the association with conduct problems and CU traits was medium ($0.292 < r < 0.485$, $ps < 0.001$). Finally, data showed a medium association between conduct problems and CU traits ($r = 0.360$, $p < 0.001$). Therefore, male adolescents than females, older adolescents than younger, adolescents with higher conduct problems in the last six months and adolescents with higher scores on the CU trait had higher scores in both bullying and cyberbullying perpetration.

Results of hierarchical regressions are reported in Table 3. Results showed a similar pattern of effects for the two considered dependent variables.

3.1. Traditional Bullying

The results of the hierarchical regression analysis on the traditional bullying scores confirmed the positive association between the considered variables and the bullying behaviors, indicating that, over and above sex, age, and conduct problems, the CU trait had specific and additive effects on perpetration ($\beta = 0.167$, $p < 0.001$), although the effect size was small ($R^2_{diff} = 0.024$, $p < 0.001$) (see Step 3). Moreover, results of the last step (see Step 4) indicated that the effect of CU traits was not moderated by sex, age, or conduct problems.

3.2. Cyberbullying

The results of the hierarchical regression analysis carried out on the cyberbullying scores showed similar results to those observed for the traditional bullying scores. In particular, data confirmed the positive association between the considered variables and the bullying behaviors, indicating that, over and above sex, age, and conduct problems, the CU trait had a specific and additive effects on perpetration ($\beta = 0.174$, $p < 0.001$). Also in this domain, the observed effect size indicated a small effect ($R^2_{diff} = 0.026$, $p < 0.001$) (see Step 3). In contrast to previous findings, however, the data showed that the moderate model significantly increased the prediction of differences in the perpetration of cyberbullying ($R^2_{diff} = 0.016$, $p < 0.001$) (see Step 4). In particular, data showed a significant interaction between conduct problems and CU traits, indicating that the relationship between CU traits and cyberbullying became progressively stronger as conduct problems increased (see Figure 1). Therefore, the co-occurrence of conduct problems and CU traits increased the risk of issuing cyberbullying behaviors. The JN analysis indicated that the effect of CU traits was positive and significant when the conduct problems were higher than $-1.08\ SD$ from the mean, whereas it was negative and significant when the conduct problems were lower than $-2.34\ SD$ from the mean. As regards this latter case, it is worth noticing that in this study the range of observed standardized values of conduct problems was from -1.37 to 4.61.

Table 3. Hierarchical multiple regression analyses predicting traditional and cyberbullying from sex, age, conduct problems, ICU, and their interaction.

	Bullying					
	Traditional			Cyber		
Predictor	R^2_{diff}	b [95% CI]	β	R^2_{diff}	b [95% CI]	β
Step 1	0.045 **			0.021 **		
Sex		0.31 [0.25; 0.37]	0.188 **		0.10 [0.06; 0.14]	0.089 **
Age		0.08 [0.05; 0.11]	0.098 **		0.06 [0.04; 0.08]	0.112 **
Step 2	0.227 **			0.148 **		
Sex		0.32 [0.27; 0.37]	0.192 **		0.11 [0.07; 0.14]	0.093 **
Age		0.05 [0.03; 0.08]	0.063 **		0.05 [0.03; 0.07]	0.084 **
Conduct		0.39 [0.37; 0.42]	0.477 **		0.22 [0.20; 0.24]	0.386 **
Step 3	0.024 **			0.026 **		
Sex		0.28 [0.23; 0.33]	0.171 **		0.08 [0.04; 0.12]	0.071 **
Age		0.04 [0.01; 0.06]	0.046 *		0.04 [0.02; 0.06]	0.066 **
Conduct		0.34 [0.32; 0.37]	0.418 **		0.19 [0.17; 0.21]	0.324 **
ICU		0.14 [0.11; 0.17]	0.167 **		0.10 [0.08; 0.12]	0.174 **
Step 4	0.001			0.016 **		
Sex		0.28 [0.23; 0.33]	0.171 **		0.09 [0.05; 0.13]	0.077 **
Age		0.04 [0.01; 0.06]	0.047 *		0.04 [0.02; 0.06]	0.065 **
Conduct		0.34 [0.32; 0.37]	0.416 **		0.17 [0.15; 0.19]	0.304 **
ICU		0.12 [0.08; 0.16]	0.143 *		0.07 [0.04; 0.10]	0.125 **
Sex × ICU		0.03 [−0.02; 0.08]	0.029		0.03 [−0.01; 0.07]	0.042
Age × ICU		−0.01 [−0.03; 0.02]	−0.010		0.01 [−0.01; 0.03]	0.016
Conduct × ICU		0.01 [−0.01; 0.04]	0.021		0.06 [0.04; 0.07]	0.124 **
Total R2	0.297 **			0.211 **		

Note: n = 2959; Age = age of participants in years (z-score); Sex = participants' sex dummy coding (males = 1; females = 0); Conduct = conduct problem subscale of the SDQ; ICU = total score of the ICU; Traditional = total score of the bully subscale of the Illinois Bully Scale; Cyber = total score of the Smith's cyberbullying scale * $p < 0.01$; ** $p < 0.001$.

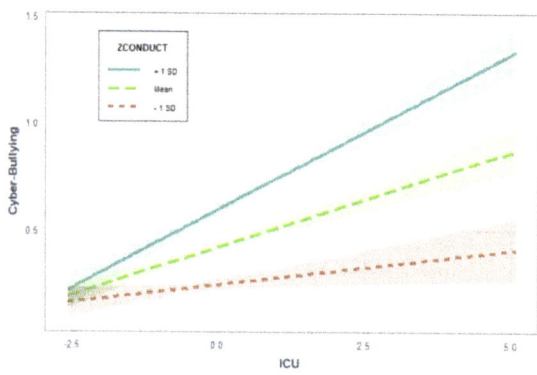

Figure 1. Interaction between CU traits and conduct problems on cyberbullying perpetration.

4. Discussion

In this study we sought to replicate and extend previous findings on the associations between CU traits and bullying perpetration in a large sample of adolescents, using standardized multi-item measures and by considering both traditional and cyberbullying. Results showed that the two bullying dimensions are remarkably similar and are influenced in a similar way by the variables considered, as indicated by the strong correlation between the traditional and cyberbullying perpetration and the presence of broadly alike correlations between both forms of bullying and conduct problems or CU traits. These results are in line with studies that reported a strong overlap between bullying and cyberbullying [87,88]; e.g., Modecki et al. affirmed that probably the two manifestations are different ways of implementing the same aggressive behavior [89]; whereas Przybylski and Bowes stated that probably cyberbullying almost always occurs together with traditional bullying [90]. However, it is important to emphasize that the data from this study also showed some differences between these two forms of bullying, in line with those authors who have found that the cyber context somehow facilitates such behaviors [59,60,65].

Related to the central point of this study, our results indicated that male, older adolescents, and adolescent with high scores on conduct problems or CU traits had higher scores on measures of traditional and cyberbullying perpetration. Furthermore, the results of the regression analysis indicated that CU traits were specifically associated with bullying perpetration in both traditional and cyber contexts. CU traits significantly increased the traditional bullying perpetration behaviors, and this association was independent of sex, age, or CP. At the same time, data indicated that, over and above sex, age, and conduct problems, CU traits also increased cyberbullying behavior perpetration and that in this latter case the association between conduct problems and cyberbullying perpetration was moderated by CU traits. In other terms, the simultaneous presence of CU traits and conduct problems can be considered a stronger risk factor for the involvement in cyberbullying perpetration.

These results confirm findings from other studies on the positive and significant association between CU traits and bullying aggressive behaviors [11,15,24,26–32,52]. In particular, Crapanzano et al. [28], in a sample of 284 students (age range 9–14 years), found a correlation between roles of perpetrators and conduct problems, positive CU traits, positive expectancies for aggression, and low levels of pro-social behavior. Fanti and Kimonis [30], considering a large sample ($N = 1214$), showed that adolescents with high CP and CU traits had a more severe pattern of bullying behaviors than adolescents with lower scores, arguing that the compresence of high CP and CU caused adolescents to pay less attention to the victim's distress and fear and this, in turn, reduced the possibility of spontaneously inhibiting the behavior. Moreover, these youths were also more likely to foresee that their aggression would result in more positive advantages for them. Golmaryami et al. [31] indicated that both perpetration and victimization were associated with CP, but when CU traits entered in the analysis, the association remained significant only for the group with low levels of victimization. Interestingly, Thornton et al. [26], by considering a sample of 284 ethnically diverse students (age range 9–14 years), showed that CU traits and CP interact in determining bullying proactive aggression; that students with high CP but low CU traits were more likely to express bullying reactive aggression and anger dysregulation, but that low CU traits were found in students who defended bullying victims.

At the same time, our findings slightly differed from those of Viding et al. [52]: While they found, in addition to the main effects that we also observed, that CU and CP interacted in predicting direct and indirect forms of bullying, we found the same pattern but only for cyberbullying. This may be explained in light of the fact that physical or verbal bullying, due to its characteristics of direct confrontation with the victim, was carried out more easily if the perpetrator had a lack of empathy and sensitivity. Cyberbullying can be assimilated more to indirect forms. In these behaviors, there is no direct confrontation with the victim's fear and distress. This has been called "lack of the emotional reactivity" and several authors have suggested that in cyberbullying, the reward resulting from one's perpetrated action is not immediate but delayed, and this implies that in an electronic context the perpetration has an intrapersonal purpose (essentially performing the action), rather than an interpersonal one (observing reactions, obtaining a positive outcome [62]). Munoz et al. [32] confirmed these results, showing that those with high CU traits and with low affective empathy were more involved in direct forms of bullying.

These results have some theoretical and practical implications. First, it is particularly important to better understand the factors that underlie aggressive behaviors such as bullying and to distinguish between traditional and digital forms. This can allow us to build psychological and social models capable of having a greater impact on prevention and intervention programs, which in turn can help to prevent some of the negative consequences that in the perspective of IPARTheory [75–77] are associated with the experiences of interpersonal rejection: hostility, aggression, passive aggression, or psychological problems with the management of hostility and aggression; emotional unresponsiveness; impaired self-esteem; impaired self-adequacy; emotional instability; and negative world-view. Namely, those personality dispositions which could become stable and that may increase the risk of showing internalizing or externalizing disturbances, respectively facilitating further risk of victimization or the tendency to bullying others as revenge [78–80]. Second, children and adolescents with CP and CU traits might request different forms of bullying intervention and prevention programs such as they tend to respond worse to standard treatments [91]. As already suggested by other authors [52], rather than only "educative" or "punitive" programs, a mixed methodology that includes rewards for adequate behaviors, adult or peer mentoring and education with empathy, and social training programs may be more suitable for youth high on CU and CP.

In addition to its merits, several limitations of this study must be also considered. First, our data were correlational and self-reported and this could threaten the internal validity; future studies need to consider different methodologies (e.g., longitudinal) and approaches (e.g., multi-informant) to improve the validity of the data. Our measure of traditional bullying did not differentiate between direct and indirect forms, and this could threaten the construct validity; future studies need to also consider these facets. Third, we did not gather data on socioeconomic status of participants, and thus we could not include this variable in the analysis; future studies need to consider this dimension.

5. Conclusions

In conclusion, in this study, we replicated in a large sample of Italian adolescent previous findings indicating that CU traits are significantly and positively associated with bullying behaviors, over and above age, sex, and general conduct problems. Our data confirmed that the specific association between CU traits and bullying behaviors is observed for both traditional and cyberbullying contexts and that in the cyber contexts, in particular, the compresence of CU traits and general conduct problems represents a further risk factor of bullying. Consequently, these results further draw attention to the need to assess the presence of CU traits in order to prevent the bullying phenomenon and, if needed, to design valid and efficacy targeted intervention programs.

Author Contributions: Conceptualization, G.C., S.P. and V.P.S.; data curation, G.C., A.P. (Antonio Pascotto), S.P. and V.P.S.; formal analysis, L.A., A.P. (Anna Pezzella) and V.P.S.; supervision, G.C., A.P. (Antonio Pascotto), C.B., S.P. and V.P.S.; writing—original draft, G.C., L.A., A.P. (Anna Pezzella), M.P.R., P.B., P.M., S.P. and V.P.S.; writing—review and editing, G.C., L.A., A.P. (Anna Pezzella), M.P.R., C.B., P.B., P.M., S.P. and V.P.S. All authors have read and agreed to the published version of the manuscript.

Funding: The research project was partially funded by "Fondazione Banco di Napoli".

Institutional Review Board Statement: The study was conducted in accordance with the guidelines of the Declaration of Helsinki, and approved by the Ethics Committee of the University of Campania "Luigi Vanvitelli" (protocol n. 500 of 29/04/2016).

Informed Consent Statement: Informed consent was obtained from the parents of the participants.

Data Availability Statement: The dataset that support the findings of this study is available from the corresponding author upon reasonable request.

Conflicts of Interest: The authors declare no conflict of interest.

References

1. Ciucci, E.; Baroncelli, A. The emotional core of bullying: Further evidences of the role of callous-unemotional traits and empathy. *Personal. Individ. Differ.* **2014**, *67*, 69–74. [CrossRef]
2. Fontaine, N.M.G.; McCrory, E.J.P.; Boivin, M.; Moffitt, T.E.; Viding, E. Predictors and outcomes of joint trajectories of callous-unemotional traits and conduct problems in childhood. *J. Abnorm. Psychol.* **2011**, *120*, 730–742. [CrossRef] [PubMed]
3. Fontaine, N.M.G.; Hanscombe, K.B.; Berg, M.T.; McCrory, E.J.; Viding, E. Trajectories of callous-unemotional traits in childhood predict different forms of peer victimization in adolescence. *J. Clin. Child Adolesc. Psychol.* **2018**, *47*, 458–466. [CrossRef]
4. Frick, P.J. Extending the construct of psychopathy to youths: Implications for understanding, diagnosing, and treating antisocial children and adolescents. *Can. J. Psychiatry* **2009**, *54*, 803–812. [CrossRef]
5. Van Geel, M.; Toprak, F.; Goemans, A.; Zwaanswijk, W.; Vedder, P. Are youth psychopathic traits related to bullying? Meta-analyses on callous-unemotional traits, narcissism, and impulsivity. *Child Psychiatry Hum. Dev.* **2017**, *48*, 768–777. [CrossRef]
6. Pisano, S.; Muratori, P.; Gorga, C.; Levantini, V.; Iuliano, R.; Catone, G.; Coppola, G.; Milone, A.; Masi, G. Conduct disorders and psychopathy in children and adolescents: Aetiology, clinical presentation and treatment strategies of callous-unemotional traits. *Ital. J. Pediatr.* **2017**, *43*. [CrossRef]
7. Frick, P.J.; Hare, R.D. *The Antisocial Process Screening Device*; Multi-Health Systems: Toronto, ON, Canada, 2001.
8. Blair, R.J.R.; Peschardt, K.S.; Budhani, S.; Mitchell, D.G.V.; Pine, D.S. The development of psychopathy. *J. Child Psychol. Psychiatry* **2006**, *47*, 262–276. [CrossRef]
9. Lynam, D.R.; Gudonis, L. The development of psychopathy. *Annu. Rev. Clin. Psychol.* **2005**, *1*, 381–407. [CrossRef] [PubMed]
10. Bezdjian, S.; Raine, A.; Baker, L.A.; Lynam, D.R. Psychopathic personality in children: Genetic and environmental contributions. *Psychol. Med.* **2011**, *41*, 589–600. [CrossRef] [PubMed]
11. Essau, C.A.; Sasagawa, S.; Frick, P.J. Callous-unemotional traits in a community sample of adolescents. *Assessment* **2006**, *13*, 454–469. [CrossRef]
12. Frick, P.J.; Cornell, A.H.; Bodin, S.D.; Dane, H.E.; Barry, C.T.; Loney, B.R. Callous-unemotional traits and developmental pathways to severe conduct problems. *Dev. Psychol.* **2003**, *39*, 246–260. [CrossRef]
13. Rogers, J.C.; De Brito, S.A. Cortical and subcortical gray matter volume in youths with conduct problems: A meta-analysis. *JAMA Psychiatry* **2016**, *73*, 64–72. [CrossRef] [PubMed]
14. American Psychiatric Association. *Diagnostic and Statistical Manual of Mental Disorders*, 5th ed.; American Psychiatric Association: Washington, DC, USA, 2013.
15. Fanti, K.A.; Demetriou, C.A.; Kimonis, E.R. Variants of callous-unemotional conduct problems in a community sample of adolescents. *J. Youth Adolesc.* **2013**, *42*, 964–979. [CrossRef] [PubMed]
16. Herpers, P.C.M.; Rommelse, N.N.J.; Bons, D.M.A.; Buitelaar, J.K.; Scheepers, F.E. Callous-unemotional traits as a cross-disorders construct. *Soc. Psychiatry Psychiatr. Epidemiol.* **2012**, *47*, 2045–2064. [CrossRef]
17. Kumsta, R.; Sonuga-Barke, E.; Rutter, M. Adolescent callous-unemotional traits and conduct disorder in adoptees exposed to severe early deprivation. *Br. J. Psychiatry* **2012**, *200*, 197–201. [CrossRef]
18. Rowe, R.; Maughan, B.; Moran, P.; Ford, T.; Briskman, J.; Goodman, R. The role of callous and unemotional traits in the diagnosis of conduct disorder: Callousness and conduct disorder. *J. Child Psychol. Psychiatry* **2010**, *51*, 688–695. [CrossRef]
19. Viding, E.; McCrory, E.J. Why should we care about measuring callous–unemotional traits in children? *Br. J. Psychiatry* **2012**, *200*, 177–178. [CrossRef]
20. Pardini, D.A.; Byrd, A.L. Perceptions of aggressive conflicts and others' distress in children with callous-unemotional traits: "I'll show you who's boss, even if you suffer and I get in trouble": Perceptions of aggressive conflicts. *J. Child Psychol. Psychiatry* **2012**, *53*, 283–291. [CrossRef]
21. Ansel, L.L.; Barry, C.T.; Gillen, C.T.A.; Herrington, L.L. An analysis of four self-report measures of adolescent callous-unemotional traits: Exploring unique prediction of delinquency, aggression, and conduct problems. *J. Psychopathol. Behav. Assess.* **2015**, *37*, 207–216. [CrossRef]
22. Fanti, K.A.; Vanman, E.; Henrich, C.C.; Avraamides, M.N. Desensitization to media violence over a short period of time. *Aggress. Behav.* **2009**, *35*, 179–187. [CrossRef]
23. Kimonis, E.R.; Frick, P.J.; Skeem, J.L.; Marsee, M.A.; Cruise, K.; Munoz, L.C.; Aucoin, K.J.; Morris, A.S. Assessing callous-unemotional traits in adolescent offenders: Validation of the inventory of callous-unemotional traits. *Int. J. Law Psychiatry* **2008**, *31*, 241–252. [CrossRef]
24. Kimonis, E.R.; Fanti, K.A.; Frick, P.J.; Moffitt, T.E.; Essau, C.; Bijttebier, P.; Marsee, M.A. Using self-reported callous-unemotional traits to cross-nationally assess the DSM-5 "With Limited Prosocial Emotions" specifier. *J. Child Psychol. Psychiatry* **2015**, *56*, 1249–1261. [CrossRef] [PubMed]
25. Stickle, T.R.; Kirkpatrick, N.M.; Brush, L.N. Callous-unemotional traits and social information processing: Multiple risk-factor models for understanding aggressive behavior in antisocial youth. *Law Hum. Behav.* **2009**, *33*, 515–529. [CrossRef] [PubMed]

26. Thornton, L.C.; Frick, P.J.; Crapanzano, A.M.; Terranova, A.M. The incremental utility of callous-unemotional traits and conduct problems in predicting aggression and bullying in a community sample of boys and girls. *Psychol. Assess.* **2013**, *25*, 366–378. [CrossRef] [PubMed]
27. Ciucci, E.; Baroncelli, A.; Franchi, M.; Golmaryami, F.N.; Frick, P.J. The association between callous-unemotional traits and behavioral and academic adjustment in children: Further validation of the inventory of callous-unemotional traits. *J. Psychopathol. Behav. Assess.* **2014**, *36*, 189–200. [CrossRef]
28. Crapanzano, A.M.; Frick, P.J.; Childs, K.; Terranova, A.M. Gender differences in the assessment, stability, and correlates to bullying roles in middle school children: Gender and bullying. *Behav. Sci. Law* **2011**, *29*, 677–694. [CrossRef]
29. Fanti, K.A.; Demetriou, A.G.; Hawa, V.V. A longitudinal study of cyberbullying: Examining riskand protective factors. *Eur. J. Dev. Psychol.* **2012**, *9*, 168–181. [CrossRef]
30. Fanti, K.A.; Kimonis, E.R. Bullying and victimization: The role of conduct problems and psychopathic traits. *J. Res. Adolesc.* **2012**, *22*, 617–631. [CrossRef]
31. Golmaryami, F.N.; Frick, P.J.; Hemphill, S.A.; Kahn, R.E.; Crapanzano, A.M.; Terranova, A.M. The social, behavioral, and emotional correlates of bullying and victimization in a school-based sample. *J. Abnorm. Child. Psychol.* **2016**, *44*, 381–391. [CrossRef]
32. Muñoz, L.C.; Qualter, P.; Padgett, G. Empathy and bullying: Exploring the influence of callous-unemotional traits. *Child Psychiatry Hum. Dev.* **2011**, *42*, 183–196. [CrossRef]
33. Frick, P.J.; Ray, J.V.; Thornton, L.C.; Kahn, R.E. Can callous-unemotional traits enhance the understanding, diagnosis, and treatment of serious conduct problems in children and adolescents? A Comprehensive Review. *Psychol. Bull.* **2014**, *140*, 1–57. [CrossRef]
34. Olweus, D. *Bullying at School: What We Know and What We Can Do*; Blackwell: Oxford, UK, 1993.
35. Smith, P.K. *The Nature of School Bullying: A Cross-National Perspective*; Routledge: London, UK, 1999.
36. Salmivalli, C. Bullying and the peer group: A review. *Aggress. Violent Behav.* **2010**, *15*, 112–120. [CrossRef]
37. Hart, T.C.; Hart, J.L.; Miethe, T.D. Situational context of student bullying victimization and reporting behavior: A conjunctive analysis of case configurations. *Justice Res. Policy* **2013**, *15*, 43–73. [CrossRef]
38. Paez, G.R. Cyberbullying among adolescents: A general strain theory perspective. *J. Sch. Violence* **2018**, *17*, 74–85. [CrossRef]
39. Catone, G.; Signoriello, S.; Pisano, S.; Siciliano, M.; Russo, K.; Marotta, R.; Carotenuto, M.; Broome, M.R.; Gritti, A.; Senese, V.P.; et al. Epidemiological pattern of bullying using a multi-assessment approach: Results from the Bullying and Youth Mental Health Naples Study (BYMHNS). *Child Abus. Negl.* **2019**, *89*, 18–28. [CrossRef] [PubMed]
40. Catone, G.; Senese, V.P.; Pisano, S.; Siciliano, M.; Russo, K.; Muratori, P.; Marotta, R.; Pascotto, A.; Broome, M.R. The drawbacks of information and communication technologies: Interplay and psychopathological risk of nomophobia and cyber-bullying, results from the Bullying and Youth Mental Health Naples Study (BYMHNS). *Comput. Hum. Behav.* **2020**, *113*, 106496. [CrossRef]
41. Jadambaa, A.; Thomas, H.J.; Scott, J.G.; Graves, N.; Brain, D.; Pacella, R. Prevalence of traditional bullying and cyberbullying among children and adolescents in Australia: A systematic review and meta-analysis. *Aust. N. Z. J. Psychiatry* **2019**, *53*, 878–888. [CrossRef] [PubMed]
42. Singham, T.; Viding, E.; Schoeler, T.; Arseneault, L.; Ronald, A.; Cecil, C.M.; McCrory, E.; Rijsdijk, F.; Pingault, J.-B. Concurrent and longitudinal contribution of exposure to bullying in childhood to mental health: The role of vulnerability and resilience. *JAMA Psychiatry* **2017**, *74*, 1112–1119. [CrossRef]
43. Chan, H.C.O.; Wong, D.S.W. Traditional school bullying and cyberbullying in Chinese societies: Prevalence and a review of the whole-school intervention approach. *Aggress. Violent Behav.* **2015**, *23*, 98–108. [CrossRef]
44. Gini, G. Associations between bullying behaviour, psychosomatic complaints, emotional and behavioural problems. *J. Paediatr. Child Health* **2008**, *44*, 492–497. [CrossRef]
45. Menesini, E.; Calussi, P.; Nocentini, A. Cyberbullying and traditional bullying: Unique, additive, and synergistic effects on psychological health symptoms. In *Cyberbullying in the Global Playground*; Wiley-Blackwell: Oxford, UK, 2012; pp. 245–262.
46. Catone, G.; Gritti, A.; Russo, K.; Santangelo, P.; Iuliano, R.; Bravaccio, C.; Pisano, S. Details of the contents of paranoid thoughts in help-seeking adolescents with psychotic-like experiences and continuity with bullying and victimization: A pilot study. *Behav. Sci.* **2020**, *10*, 122. [CrossRef]
47. Zych, I.; Farrington, D.P.; Ttofi, M.M. Protective factors against bullying and cyberbullying: A systematic review of meta-analyses. *Aggress. Violent. Behav.* **2019**, *45*, 4–19. [CrossRef]
48. Hinduja, S.; Patchin, J.W. Cultivating youth resilience to prevent bullying and cyberbullying victimization. *Child Abuse Negl.* **2017**, *73*, 51–62. [CrossRef]
49. Cantone, E.; Piras, A.P.; Vellante, M.; Preti, A.; Daníelsdóttir, S.; D'Aloja, E.; Lesinskiene, S.; Angermeyer, M.C.; Carta, M.G.; Bhugra, D. Interventions on bullying and cyberbullying in schools: A systematic review. *Clin. Pract. Epidemiol. Ment. Health* **2015**, *11* (Suppl. 1 M4), 58–76. [CrossRef] [PubMed]
50. Ortega-Barón, J.; Buelga, S.; Ayllón, E.; Martínez-Ferrer, B.; Cava, M.J. Effects of intervention program Prev@Cib on traditional bullying and cyberbullying. *Int. J. Environ. Res. Public Health* **2019**, *16*, 527. [CrossRef] [PubMed]
51. Ferrer-Cascales, R.; Albaladejo-Blázquez, N.; Sánchez-SanSegundo, M.; Portilla-Tamarit, I.; Lordan, O.; Ruiz-Robledillo, N. Effectiveness of the TEI program for bullying and cyberbullying reduction and school climate improvement. *Int. J. Environ. Res. Public Health* **2019**, *16*, 580. [CrossRef] [PubMed]

52. Viding, E.; Simmonds, E.; Petrides, K.V.; Frederickson, N. The contribution of callous-unemotional traits and conduct problems to bullying in early adolescence. *J. Child Psychol. Psychiatry* **2009**, *50*, 471–481. [CrossRef] [PubMed]
53. Wang, C.-W.; Musumari, P.M.; Techasrivichien, T.; Suguimoto, S.P.; Tateyama, Y.; Chan, C.-C.; Ono-Kihara, M.; Kihara, M.; Nakayama, T. Overlap of traditional bullying and cyberbullying and correlates of bullying among Taiwanese adolescents: A cross-sectional study. *BMC Public Health* **2019**, *19*, 1756. [CrossRef]
54. Menesini, E.; Nocentini, A. Cyberbullying definition and measurement: Some critical considerations. *J. Psychol.* **2009**, *217*, 230–232. [CrossRef]
55. Juvonen, J.; Gross, E.F. Extending the school grounds? Bullying experiences in cyberspace. *J. Sch. Health* **2008**, *78*, 496–505. [CrossRef]
56. Smith, P.K.; Mahdavi, J.; Carvalho, M.; Fisher, S.; Russell, S.; Tippett, N. Cyberbullying: Its nature and impact in secondary school pupils. *J. Child Psychol. Psychiatry* **2008**, *49*, 376–385. [CrossRef]
57. Beran, T.; Li, Q. Cyber-harassment: A study of a new method for an old behavior. *J. Educ. Comput. Res.* **2005**, *32*, 265–277.
58. Li, Q. Bullying in the new playground: Research into cyberbullying and cyber victimisation. *Australas. J. Educ. Technol.* **2007**, *23*, 435–454. [CrossRef]
59. Patchin, J.W.; Hinduja, S. Bullies move beyond the schoolyard: A preliminary look at cyberbullying. *Youth Violence Juv. Justice* **2006**, *4*, 148–169. [CrossRef]
60. Ybarra, M.L.; Mitchell, K.J. Online aggressor/targets, aggressors, and targets: A comparison of associated youth characteristics. *J. Child Psychol. Psychiatry* **2004**, *45*, 1308–1316. [CrossRef] [PubMed]
61. Bauman, S. Cyberbullying in a rural intermediate school: An exploratory study. *J. Early Adolesc.* **2010**, *30*, 803–833. [CrossRef]
62. Kowalski, R.M.; Giumetti, G.W.; Schroeder, A.N.; Lattanner, M.R. Bullying in the digital age: A critical review and meta-analysis of cyberbullying research among youth. *Psychol. Bull.* **2014**, *140*, 1073–1137. [CrossRef] [PubMed]
63. Juvonen, J.; Graham, S.; Schuster, M.A. Bullying among young adolescents: The strong, the weak, and the troubled. *Pediatrics* **2003**, *112 Pt 1*, 1231–1237. [CrossRef]
64. Catone, G.; Marwaha, S.; Kuipers, E.; Lennox, B.; Freeman, D.; Bebbington, P.; Broome, M. Bullying victimisation and risk of psychotic phenomena: Analyses of British national survey data. *Lancet Psychiatry* **2015**, *2*, 618–624. [CrossRef]
65. Wang, J.; Nansel, T.R.; Iannotti, R.J. Cyber and traditional bullying: Differential association with depression. *J. Adolesc. Health* **2011**, *48*, 415–417. [CrossRef]
66. Orue, I.; Andershed, H. The youth psychopathic traits inventory-short version in spanish adolescents—Factor structure, reliability, and relation with aggression, bullying, and cyber bullying. *J. Psychopathol. Behav. Assess.* **2015**, *37*, 563–575. [CrossRef]
67. Orue, I.; Calvete, E. Psychopathic Traits and moral disengagement interact to predict bullying and cyberbullying among adolescents. *J. Interpers. Violence* **2019**, *34*, 2313–2332. [CrossRef]
68. Wright, M.F.; Harper, B.D.; Wachs, S. The associations between cyberbullying and callous-unemotional traits among adolescents: The moderating effect of online disinhibition. *Personal. Individ. Differ.* **2019**, *140*, 41–45. [CrossRef]
69. Kimonis, E.R.; Frick, P.J.; Fazekas, H.; Loney, B.R. Psychopathy, aggression, and the processing of emotional stimuli in non-referred girls and boys. *Behav. Sci. Law* **2006**, *24*, 21–37. [CrossRef]
70. Pardini, D.A.; Lochman, J.E.; Frick, P.J. Callous/unemotional traits and social-cognitive processes in adjudicated youths. *J. Am. Acad. Child Adolesc. Psychiatry* **2003**, *42*, 364–371. [CrossRef] [PubMed]
71. Ybarra, M.L. Linkages between depressive symptomatology and internet harassment among young regular internet users. *Cyberpsychol. Behav.* **2004**, *7*, 247–257. [CrossRef]
72. Vieno, A.; Lenzi, M.; Gini, G.; Pozzoli, T.; Cavallo, F.; Santinello, M. Time trends in bullying behavior in Italy. *J. Sch. Health* **2015**, *85*, 441–445. [CrossRef] [PubMed]
73. Holfeld, B.; Sukhawathanakul, P. Associations between Internet attachment, cyber victimization, and internalizing symptoms among adolescents. *Cyberpsychol. Behav. Soc. Netw.* **2017**, *20*, 91–96. [CrossRef]
74. Schneider, S.K.; O'Donnell, L.; Stueve, A.; Coulter, R.W.S. Cyberbullying, school bullying, and psychological distress: A regional census of high school students. *Am. J. Public Health* **2012**, *102*, 171–177. [CrossRef] [PubMed]
75. Rohner, R.P. *The Warmth Dimension: Foundations of Parental Acceptance-Rejection Theory*; Sage Publications: Newbury Park, CA, USA, 1986.
76. Rohner, R.P.; Lansford, J.E. Deep structure of the human affectional system: Introduction to interpersonal acceptance-rejection theory. *J. Fam. Theory Rev.* **2017**, *9*, 426–440. [CrossRef]
77. Rohner, R.P.; Khaleque, A. *Handbook for the Study of Parental Acceptance and Rejection*, 4th ed.; Rohner Research Publications: Storrs, CT, USA, 2005.
78. Lozano-Blasco, R.; Cortés-Pascual, A.; Latorre-Martínez, M.P. Being a cybervictim and a cyberbully—The duality of cyberbullying: A meta-analysis. *Comput. Hum. Behav.* **2020**, *111*, 106444. [CrossRef]
79. King, J.E.; Walpole, C.E.; Lamon, K. Surf and turf wars online—Growing implications of internet gang violence. *J. Adolesc. Health* **2007**, *41* (Suppl. 1), S66–S68. [CrossRef] [PubMed]
80. König, A.; Gollwitzer, M.; Steffgen, G. Cyberbullying as an act of revenge? *Aust. J. Guid. Couns.* **2010**, *20*, 210–224. [CrossRef]
81. Goodman, R. The strengths and difficulties questionnaire: A research note. *J. Child. Psychol. Psychiatry* **1997**, *38*, 581–586. [CrossRef] [PubMed]
82. Bonichini, S. *La Valutazione Psicologica dello Sviluppo*; Carocci Editore: Rome, Italy, 2017.

83. Pisano, S.; Senese, V.P.; Bravaccio, C.; Santangelo, P.; Milone, A.; Masi, G.; Catone, G. Cyclothymic-hypersensitive temperament in youths: Refining the structure, the way of assessment and the clinical significance in the youth population. *J. Affect. Disord.* **2020**, *271*, 272–278. [CrossRef]
84. Espelage, D.L.; Holt, M.K. Bullying and victimization during early adolescence: Peer influences and psychosocial correlates. *J. Emot. Abus.* **2001**, *2*, 123–142. [CrossRef]
85. Tabachnick, B.G.; Fidell, L.S. *Using Multivariate Statistics*; Allyn & Bacon: Boston, MA, USA, 2001.
86. Johnson, P.O.; Neyman, J. Tests of certain linear hypotheses and their applications to some educational problems. *Stat. Res. Mem.* **1936**, *1*, 39–57.
87. Zych, I.; Ortega-Ruiz, R.; Del Rey, R. Systematic review of theoretical studies on bullying and cyberbullying: Facts, knowledge, prevention, and intervention. *Aggress. Violent Behav.* **2015**, *23*, 1–21. [CrossRef]
88. Casas, J.A.; Del Rey, R.; Ortega-Ruiz, R. Bullying and cyberbullying: Convergent and divergent predictor variables. *Comput. Hum. Behav.* **2013**, *29*, 580–587. [CrossRef]
89. Modecki, K.L.; Minchin, J.; Harbaugh, A.G.; Guerra, N.G.; Runions, K.C. Bullying prevalence across contexts: A meta-analysis measuring cyber and traditional bullying. *J. Adolesc. Health* **2014**, *55*, 602–611. [CrossRef]
90. Przybylski, A.K.; Bowes, L. Cyberbullying and adolescent well-being in England: A population-based cross-sectional study. *Lancet Child. Adolesc. Health* **2017**, *1*, 19–26. [CrossRef]
91. Hawes, D.J.; Dadds, M.R. The treatment of conduct problems in children with callous-unemotional traits. *J. Consult. Clin. Psychol.* **2005**, *73*, 737–741. [CrossRef] [PubMed]

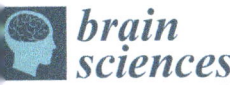

Article

Psychopathic Traits in Childhood: Insights from Parental Warmth and Fearless Temperament via Conscience Development

Laura López-Romero [1,*], Olalla Cutrín [1], Lorena Maneiro [1,2], Beatriz Domínguez-Álvarez [1] and Estrella Romero [1]

1 Department of Clinical Psychology and Psychobiology, Universidade de Santiago de Compostela, 15782 Santiago de Compostela, Spain; olalla.cutrin@usc.es (O.C.); lorena.maneiro@usc.es (L.M.); beatrizdominguez.alvarez@usc.es (B.D.-Á.); estrella.romero@usc.es (E.R.)
2 Institute of Education and Child Studies, Leiden University, 2333 AK Leiden, The Netherlands
* Correspondence: laura.lopez-romero@usc.es

Abstract: The role of psychopathic traits in predicting more serious and persistent patterns of child conduct problems has been well documented. The jointly presence of interpersonal (grandiose–deceitful), affective (e.g., callous–unemotional), and behavioral psychopathic traits (impulsive–need of stimulation) identifies a group of children at increased risk of psychosocial maladjustment. The present study aims to disentangle the underlying mechanisms by examining how early parenting (i.e., warmth) and child temperament (i.e., fearlessness) predict later psychopathic traits, via conscience development (CD). Data were collected in a large sample of children (n = 2.266; 48.5% girls), aged 3 to 6 at the onset of the study (M_{age} = 4.25; SD = 0.91), who were followed up one and two years later. The results showed direct effects from fearlessness to interpersonal and behavioral psychopathic traits. Parental warmth, fearless temperament, and their interaction, predicted CD, which, in turn, showed a negative effect on psychopathic traits. The indirect effects indicated significant negative mediation effects of warmth through CD on psychopathic traits, which seem to be stronger when children present lower levels of fearlessness. Overall, these results contribute to better understand the development of child psychopathic traits and provide additional insight on effective strategies that will help to restrain the potential development of a high-risk profile in early childhood.

Keywords: psychopathic traits; childhood; fearlessness; parental warmth; conscience development

Citation: López-Romero, L.; Cutrín, O.; Maneiro, L.; Domínguez-Álvarez, B.; Romero, E. Psychopathic Traits in Childhood: Insights from Parental Warmth and Fearless Temperament via Conscience Development. *Brain Sci.* 2021, 11, 923. https://doi.org/10.3390/brainsci11070923

Academic Editors: Annarita Milone and Gianluca Sesso

Received: 16 June 2021
Accepted: 9 July 2021
Published: 13 July 2021

Publisher's Note: MDPI stays neutral with regard to jurisdictional claims in published maps and institutional affiliations.

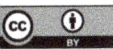

Copyright: © 2021 by the authors. Licensee MDPI, Basel, Switzerland. This article is an open access article distributed under the terms and conditions of the Creative Commons Attribution (CC BY) license (https://creativecommons.org/licenses/by/4.0/).

1. Introduction

Child conduct problems, involving a heterogeneous pattern of deviant behaviors such as aggression, rule-breaking, and oppositional or destructive behavior [1,2], have a negative impact on children's socio-emotional development, as well as on family, school, and peer interactions, with an important cost for society [3,4]. In an attempt to further identify specific factors that may place a child at increased risk for being involved in an early-onset, severe and stable pattern of conduct problems, some authors have proposed the study of psychopathic personality at early developmental stages [5–7]. Psychopathic traits have been traditionally defined as a constellation of co-occurring interpersonal (i.e., grandiose–deceitful (GD)), affective (i.e., callous–unemotional (CU)) and behavioral/lifestyle (i.e., impulsive–need of stimulation (INS)) traits [8–11]. Over the past two decades, psychopathic traits have been consistently linked to more serious and persistent patterns of conduct problems and aggression, later antisocial behavior and delinquency, lower levels of social competence and prosocial behavior, and even to adult psychopathy [11–13], with some of these results being also replicated in early childhood [14–16]. Given the lasting negative consequences of early psychopathic traits, additional understanding on how they develop, by identifying potential underlying etiological mechanisms, is needed. Considering that children with conduct problems who also show psychopathic traits tend to benefit less from traditional interventions (e.g., parenting programs) [17–19], advancing our knowledge on this topic will shed new light on the development of effective strategies, tailored to the unique characteristics of children with psychopathic traits, for both prevention and intervention purposes.

1.1. Developmental Models of Psychopathic Traits

Psychopathic personality has been defined as a developmental disorder with its roots in early childhood [12,20]. The full array of interpersonal, affective, and behavioral psychopathic traits has been reliably identified at early developmental stages [9,21]. As was consistently observed, high levels of psychopathic traits identify a group of children at increased risk for more serious and persistent problems, showing a closer association with long-lasting behavioral and psychosocial disturbances, as well as with distinctive etiological mechanisms (see the compendious reviews [11,12]).

Comprehensive developmental models on the etiology and later development of psychopathic traits have suggested that certain temperamental styles, such as behavioral disinhibition or fearlessness, are linked with problems in conscience development (CD), these associations being critical for understanding the emergence of psychopathic traits (see [22]). The construct of conscience, refers to the development, maintenance, and application of generalizable, internal regulators of one's behavior [23]. While the broader concept is multifaceted, comprising diverse affective (e.g., moral emotions), regulatory (e.g., self-control capacities), motivational (e.g., responsiveness to socialization) and cognitive (e.g., moral cognitions) components and processes [24,25], conscience has been often defined by guilt and empathy [26]. These moral emotions represent, as well, two of the hallmarks of the construct of psychopathy, and play an important role in a child's development by promoting prosocial development whilst restraining antisocial behavior. From this theoretical perspective, problems in CD would be largely due to problems in the development of guilt and empathy, which in turn would be influenced by certain temperamental styles, including fearlessness, insensitivity to punishment or low responsiveness to cues of distress [27,28]. More specifically, children characterized by a fearless and disinhibited temperament tend to seek out novel situations to test limits, and usually do not fear the consequences of misbehavior, which places them at greater risk to engage in dangerous activities [29]. This temperamental style, characterized by a poor autonomic arousal in the presence of punitive stimuli, contributes, across development, to failure in interiorizing parental and societal norms, rules and regulations, restraining the appearance of internal states and emotions that would ensure compliance and commitment to the norms and demands that come from the environment (i.e., the development of moral and emotional consciousness) [23,30]. This multiple chain of deficits could also be on the basis of the development of psychopathic traits [31,32]. In support of this assumption is the evidence revealing that children high on psychopathic traits also tend to show a fearless temperament [28,33,34], and a pronounced lack of remorse and empathy [35]. As suggested by Blair and Cipolotti [36], a general emotional impairment may affect the development of moral emotions, eventually leading to dishonest and careless behavior, which is also a core element in the psychopathy definition [37].

Notwithstanding the importance of temperamental factors in the development of psychopathic traits, it should be noted that they are supposed to be largely due to biological deficits and, therefore, might be difficult to avoid or prevent. When practical implications are prioritized, the identification, assessment, and management of those factors able to enhance, maintain, or restrain such developmental process gain more prominence. In this regard, the role of parenting practices in the development of psychopathic traits has been evidenced as particularly influential (see [38]), with parental warmth predicting a reduction, whilst parental harshness favoring an increase, in overall psychopathic [39] and more specific CU traits [40–43] across childhood and adolescence. Parenting practices have also shown a clinical value not only in reducing problematic behavior in children with high psychopathic traits [44], but also in favoring a significant reduction in all affective, interpersonal, and behavioral features of psychopathic personality [45].

In this context, after evidencing that not all children showing a fearless and uninhibited temperament will invariable manifest deficits in moral emotions, most theories of CD have also considered the role of parenting, which interacts with a child's temperament in a complex dynamic process [46]. In this regard, it has been suggested that parenting practices, particularly those relying on parental warmth, affection, and other positive qualities, may be especially influential for CD in fearless children [46,47]. Similar interactions have been replicated in current developmental models on the etiology of CU traits, suggesting that highly positive parenting buffered the risk that fearlessness posed to the development of CU behaviors [48,49].

1.2. The Present Study

Based on the foregoing, it can be suggested that child temperament interacts with parental practices to increase or buffer the risk for later psychopathic traits [50], with these effects being potentially driven by changes in CD. Nevertheless, it should be noted that most of the aforementioned literature has focused on the development of CU traits, which represents the affective dimension of the psychopathy construct. Even considering that research from the CU perspective has provided a great knowledge in the field, studying psychopathic personality from a multidimensional perspective (i.e., including all interpersonal, affective, and behavioral traits) has proven to be effective in identifying children at increased risk for later maladjustment, even when compared to children just high on CU traits [16,51,52]. Therefore, if we aim to better identify this high-risk profile early in development, psychopathic personality, with all its dimensions, should be taken into account [53,54]. Current research on the multidimensional construct in young children has basically examined its internal structure and predictive value, with studies aimed at identifying distinctive etiological mechanisms mainly conducted in older samples (see [11]). In this regard, it is important to test whether previous findings on CU traits can be extrapolated to other psychopathy dimensions or, in turn, whether a combination of high interpersonal, affective, and behavioral psychopathic traits may identify a distinctive etiological subgroup of children at increased risk for later maladjustment. It is also important to examine these questions in early childhood because this is a key period for developmental foundations of empathy and conscience [47], and when severe trajectories of child conduct problems emerge [55]. Answering these questions will help to clarify the mechanisms underlying the development of psychopathic traits, with potential practical implications relevant to assessment, diagnostic classification, and tailored interventions.

The main purpose of the current study was, therefore, to unravel the etiological mechanisms leading to psychopathic traits in childhood by testing a developmental model where parenting practices and fearless temperament interact to predict psychopathic traits, via CD. Since guilt and empathy can be identified early in life, and because they play an important role in the development of psychopathic traits [9,35], the current study only focused on the emotional components of CD. Furthermore, because parental warmth has proven to be relevant in the development of both CD and psychopathic traits [38,47,56], being also an important target for recent adaptations to intervene with children high on psychopathic traits [57], it was included as a measure of parenting. We expected that both parental warmth and fearlessness would drive effects on psychopathic traits via CD. Based on previous research, we hypothesized that parental warmth would have effects on both CD and psychopathic traits, particularly at lower levels of fearlessness [46].

2. Materials and Methods

2.1. Participants

The Estudio Longitudinal para una Infancia Saludable (Longitudinal Study for a Healthy Childhood; (ELISA)) is a prospective longitudinal study conducted in Galicia (NW Spain) with the aim of better understanding the behavioral, emotional, personality, and psychosocial development from early childhood to adolescence. For the purposes of the current study, parent-reported information collected in the first three waves of study were included in the analyses. Data collection started when children were in preschool (i.e., children aged 3 to 6 years old), encompassing children born in 2011–2013. Only children with available data in some of the main study variables, namely fearlessness, parental warmth, guilt and empathy, and psychopathic traits, were included in the present study, resulting in an initial sample of 2266 children (48.5% girls), who were on average 4 years old (M_{age} = 4.25; SD = 0.91). A total of 72 public (79.2%), charter (18.1%), and private (2.8%) schools participated in the study, which were located in predominantly working-class communities, with no diversity in terms of ethnicity (93.9% of children were Spanish). Regarding children's family background, 23.7% of mothers and 39.8% of fathers completed compulsory education, 47.4% and 31.2% completed higher education, and 28.9% and 29% completed vocational training studies.

Two follow-ups were conducted within one-year intervals. Thus, the first follow-up (T2) was conducted one year after the initial wave of data collection and the second follow-up (T3) was conducted two years after the first wave of the study. The level of attrition is considered adequate, since 88.6% of respondents who participated in T1 participated in T2, and 76.3% of respondents who participated in T1 also participated in T3. As commonly observed in longitudinal studies, attrition was derived from death or frailty, withdrawal, lack of success in additional contacts for a follow-up survey, or by non-returning a survey by some participants [58]. Comparisons between participating families and families who dropped out of one wave of the study revealed no significant differences in terms of age $F_{(2248)}$ = 2.51, p = 0.082, and initial (T1) levels of conduct problems $F_{(2227)}$ = 0.30, p = 0.741. However, differences in terms of gender and SES were found between groups. Specifically, there was a higher proportion of boys in families who dropped out of one wave of the study ($\chi^2_{(2)}$ = 11.88, p < 0.01); whereas higher levels of SES were found in families who participated in all three waves of the study ($F_{(2249)}$ = 16.27, p < 0.001), a result consistently found in previous longitudinal research [58]. Even though, in longitudinal studies spanning different developmental periods, one may expect other developmental variables being also affecting participation rates [59].

2.2. Measures

To assess the intended constructs, measures specifically developed for being used with preschool children were selected. Moreover, the use of validated measures with a Spanish version were prioritized. In case it was not available at the time of data collection, items were adapted and translated by the research group, according to the standard guidelines for translation and adaptation of instruments [60].

Covariates. In addition to the gender of the child (1 = boy; 2 = girl), we accounted for the socioeconomic status (SES) of the family in the first wave of study. The SES variable was created by combining the scores on a set of items related to the socioeconomic background of the family (i.e., academic level of the mother and academic level of the father, monthly income, and parent's concerns about the family economic situation).

2.2.1. Baseline Variables (T1)

Parental warmth. A parent-reported scale based on the Warmth subscale from the Child Rearing Scale (CRS) [61,62], included in previous studies with preschool children [63], was used to assess the levels of parental warmth. This scale is composed of 6 items (α = 0.82; e.g., "You express affection by hugging, kissing, and holding your child", "You have warm, close times together with your child"), scored in a 5-point scale (1 = *never* to 5 = *very often*).

Fearlessness. The level of child's fearlessness was reported by parents through a scale consisting of six items (α = 0.85; e.g., "He/she does not seem to be afraid of anything", "He/she does not seem to be afraid when someone is trying to frighten him/her"), developed for being used from age three, and used in previous studies, including the ELISA project [9,16]. Parents scored each item on a four-point scale, ranging from 1 (*Does not apply at all*) to 4 (*Applies very well*).

2.2.2. Mediating Variable (T2)

A latent variable of CD was defined by the composite score of two observed variables, namely guilt and empathy.

Guilt. A parent-reported scale composed of 5 items ($\alpha = 0.64$; e.g., "Doesn't act very upset when he/she has done something wrong", "He/she seems to feel guilty after breaking a rule") was used to measure the level of guilt displayed by the child. The items were scored in a 7-point scale from 1 (*Definitely false*) to 7 (*Definitely true*). This scale was adapted from the guilt/shame scale that was developed and included in the long form of the Children's Behavior Questionnaire (CBQ) [64,65] as an additional measure to assess specific social behavior patterns. The items were adapted from the Spanish (European) version of the standard CBQ retrieved, under request, from the author's official website. The guilt/shame scale was originally composed of 14 items [64], however, for the purposes of the current study, only the items corresponding to the facet of guilt were considered.

Empathy. A parent-reported scale adapted from the Griffith Empathy Measure (GEM) [66], a measure intended to assess empathy from preschool years onwards, was used to assess child's empathy. Parents rated six items, adapted and translated by the research team, referring to cognitive empathy (3 items; e.g., "Doesn't seem to understand why people get upset", "Rarely understands why other people cry") and affective empathy (3 items; e.g., "Feels sad when other children or people are upset", "Feels happy when someone else is happy"), in a four-point scale from 0 (*Totally disagree*) to 3 (*Totally agree*). The global empathy score was used in the present study ($\alpha = 0.67$).

2.2.3. Longitudinal Outcomes (T3)

Psychopathic traits. The parent-reported version of the Spanish Child Problematic Traits Inventory (CPTI) [9,67] was used for the assessment of child's psychopathic traits. The scale is composed of 28 items, specifically developed to be used in children from age 3, and grouped in three subscales: eight items to measure the interpersonal or grandiose–deceitful (GD) psychopathy component ($\alpha = 0.83$; e.g., "Thinks that he or she is better than everyone on almost everything"), 10 items to measure the affective or callous–unemotional (CU) psychopathy component ($\alpha = 0.88$; e.g., "Never seems to have bad conscience for things that he or she has done"), and 10 items to measure the behavioral or impulsive–need of stimulation (INS) psychopathy component ($\alpha = 0.86$; e.g., "Provides himself or herself with different things very fast and eagerly"). Parents rated the CPTI items in a response scale ranging from 1 (*Does not apply at all*) to 4 (*Applies very well*).

2.3. Procedure

This study was approved by the Bioethics Committee at the Universidade de Santiago de Compostela, and the Spanish Ministry of Economy and Competitiveness. A total of 126 public, charter and private schools were initially contacted in order to ask for potential collaboration. The contacts were initially conducted by phone, and information letters were subsequently sent by email. If a school accepted to take part in the study, families were contacted and invited to participate via information letters and group meetings in the schools. An active consent form was filled out by families (i.e., mother, father, or main caregiver) for each child who participate in the study. The informed consents were collected by preschool teachers, who handed out the information to the parents. In all the waves of study, participants were given a month to fill out the questionnaires. After that period, some reminders were sent to those who were late, firstly by the preschool teacher and then directly by the ELISA staff via email. Families did not receive any monetary compensation for their participation in the study. Nonetheless, as a reward for their participation, all the schools received a set of educational games for preschoolers in T1, whilst both families and schools participated in a draw of several sets of books and educational games, valued between EUR 50 and 100, at the end of the third wave data collection (T3).

2.4. Data Analyses

Firstly, descriptive statistics and zero-order correlations among all the study variables were analyzed. To test the conditional indirect effects of parental warmth, fearlessness, and CD on psychopathic traits, an SEM model was conducted in Mplus 7.4 [68]. The model included parental warmth as the predictor, fearlessness as the moderator (i.e., low, moderate, and high), the interaction between parental warmth and fearlessness, CD as the mediating variable, and the three psychopathic traits (i.e., GD, CU, and INS) as endogenous variables (see the conceptual model depicted in Figure 1). The predictor variables were mean-centered prior to the creation of the interaction term (i.e., warmth × fearlessness) in order to account for multicollinearity among variables [69]. The model was estimated using Full Information Maximum Likelihood (FIML), considered the least biased method of estimating missing information when indicators are missing at random [70]. Model fit was assessed using the root mean square error of approximation (RMSEA), standardized root mean squared residual (SRMR), comparative fit index (CFI), and the Tucker–Lewis index (TLI). According to Hu and Bentler's [71] suggestions, RMSEA and SRMR values lower or equal to 0.05, and TLI and CFI values of 0.95 or higher were considered indicators of a good model fit, whereas RMSEA and SRMR values smaller than 0.08, and TLI and CFI larger than 0.90 indicated an adequate model fit.

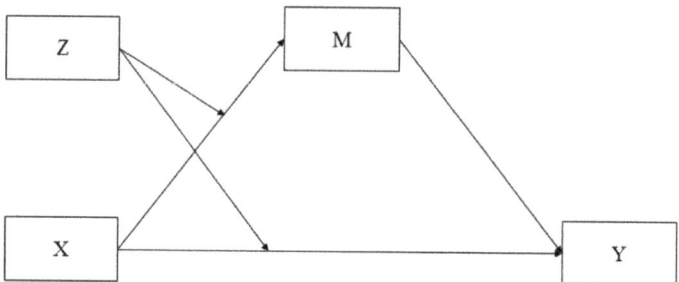

Figure 1. Conceptual model of conditional indirect effects. Model representing X as a predictor, Z as a moderator, M as a mediator, and Y as a dependent variable.

3. Results

3.1. Descriptive Statistics and Zero-Order Correlations

Descriptive statistics and bivariate correlations among all the study variables are displayed in Table 1. Parents reported very high levels of parental warmth and high levels of guilt and empathy in their children, as indicated by means very close or slightly close to the maximum rating. Parents reporting their children showed low to mid-levels of fearlessness and impulsive (INS) traits and very low levels of interpersonal (GD) and affective (CU) psychopathic traits. Parental warmth and children's empathy and guilt were significantly and positively related, whereas they were negatively related to fearlessness and all the psychopathic traits. Fearlessness and all the psychopathic traits showed a significant positive correlation.

Table 1. Descriptive statistics and bivariate correlations among the study variables.

	M (SD)	Range	1	2	3	4	5	6	7
1. Warmth T1	4.70 (0.38)	1–5	1						
2. Fearless T1	1.79 (0.66)	1–4	−0.05 *	1					
3. Guilt T2	5.08 (1.10)	1–7	0.17 ***	−0.23 ***	1				
4. Emp T2	2.19 (0.47)	0–3	0.10 ***	−0.19 ***	0.35 ***	1			
5. GD T3	1.37 (0.45)	1–4	−0.11 ***	0.22 ***	−0.33 ***	−0.16 ***	1		
6. CU T3	1.32 (0.43)	1–4	−0.14 ***	0.24 ***	−0.40 ***	−0.37 ***	0.59 ***	1	
7. INS T3	2.06 (0.60)	1–4	−0.10 ***	0.40 ***	−0.29 ***	−0.22 ***	0.53 ***	0.48 ***	1

Note: Fearless—fearlessness; Emp—empathy; GD—grandiose–deceitful; CU—callous–unemotional; INS—impulsive–need of stimulation; T1—wave 1; T2—wave 2; T3—wave 3. *** $p < 0.001$. * $p < 0.05$.

3.2. Conditional Indirect Effects

Figure 2 shows the structural equation model (SEM) computed to test the conceptual model of conditional indirect effects on psychopathic traits (i.e., GD, CU, INS) at T3. This model included parental warmth as the predictor and fearlessness as the moderator, both of them measured at T1; and CD as the mediator, which is a latent variable created from empathy ($\lambda = 0.55$, $p < 0.001$) and guilt ($\lambda = 0.63$, $p < 0.001$), both measured at T2. This model showed an adequate model fit, $\chi^2_{(6)} = 48.381$, $p < 0.001$; CFI = 0.98; TLI = 0.90; RMSEA = 0.06; SRMR = 0.01. All the psychopathic traits are significantly correlated in the SEM ($r_{GD\text{-}CU} = 0.45$, $p < 0.001$; $r_{GD\text{-}INS} = 0.42$, $p < 0.001$; $r_{CU\text{-}INS} = 0.30$, $p < 0.001$).

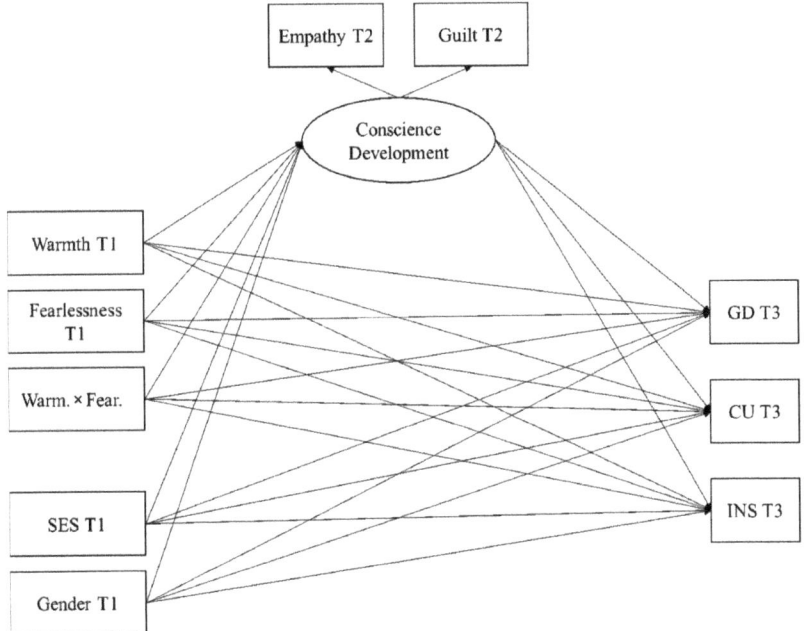

Figure 2. Structural equation model computed to test conditional indirect effects in the current study. The model considers parental warmth as the predictor, fearlessness as the moderator, conscience development as the mediator; Grandiose–Deceitful (GD), Callous–Unemotional (CU), Impulsive–Need of Stimulation (INS) traits as the dependent variables; and socioeconomic status (SES) and gender as the control variables.

The standardized results regarding the direct relationships modeled in Figure 2 are shown in Table 2. Control variables (SES and gender) significantly predicted CD, with higher levels of SES and being female predicting higher levels of CD in children. Parental warmth significantly and positively predicted CD; i.e., higher levels of warmth predicted higher levels of CD in children. Children's fearlessness significantly predicted CD negatively, and GD and INS traits positively; that is, higher levels of fearlessness predicted lower levels of CD and higher levels of interpersonal and behavioral traits in children. For its part, CD significantly and negatively predicted all three psychopathy dimensions in children. Finally, a negative interaction between parental warmth and fearlessness significantly predicted CD. The interaction term reflects that the positive relationship of warmth with CD tends to be stronger when children show low levels of fearlessness (see Figure 3). However, the very low magnitude of the interaction prevents us from clearly visualizing the differential tendency on the slopes.

Table 2. Standardized direct effects from the SEM testing the conceptual model of conditional indirect effects.

	CD T2	GD T3	CU T3	INS T3
	β	β	β	β
SES T1	0.08 **	−0.00	−0.02	−0.03
Gender (0-male, 1-female) T1	0.12 ***	0.01	−0.02	−0.03
Warmth T1	0.22 ***	−0.02	0.02	−0.01
Fearless T1	−0.33 ***	0.08 **	0.01	0.28 ***
Warmth × Fearless T1	−0.04 *	0.01	−0.03	0.02
CD T2	-	−0.39 ***	−0.64 ***	−0.32 ***

Note: SES—socio-economic status; Fearless—fearlessness; CD—conscience development; GD—grandiose-deceitful; CU—callous-unemotional; INS—impulsive-need of stimulation; T1—wave 1; T2—wave 2; T3—wave 3. Warmth and fearlessness at T1 are mean-centered variables. Conscience development is a latent variable created by the observed variables guilt and empathy at T2. *** $p < 0.001$. ** $p < 0.01$. * $p < 0.05$.

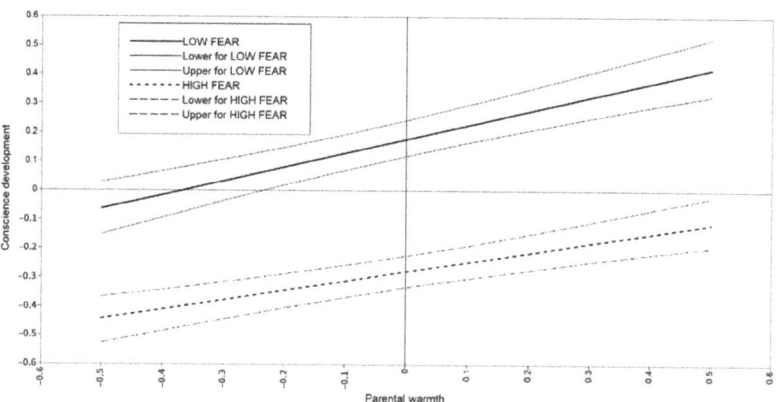

Figure 3. Estimated conscience development at T2 by the interaction of parental warmth and fearlessness at T1.

The conditional indirect effects computed in the model can help to interpret all these associations, which can be summarized in the following terms. Warmth directly predicted CD (mediator) which directly predicted all psychopathic traits (i.e., potential mediation effects), while the relationship between warmth and CD was moderated by fearlessness (i.e., potential moderated mediation effects). Because the direct effects of warmth on psychopathic traits were not moderated by the level of fearlessness, mediated moderation effects were discarded; i.e., regardless of the level of fearlessness, parental warmth is not directly related to GD, CU, and INS. As shown in Table 3, and in line with the interaction plot displayed in Figure 3, the unstandardized results of indirect effects indicated the significant presence of negative mediation effects of warmth through CD on psychopathic traits, which seem to be stronger when children present lower levels of fearlessness.

Table 3. Unstandardized indirect mediation effects of parental warmth (T1) on psychopathic traits (T3) through conscience development (T2) moderated by the level of fearlessness (T1).

Warmth through CD with	GD T3		CU T3		INS T3	
	Est.	95% CI	Est.	95% CI	Est.	95% CI
Low fearless.	−0.12 ***	−0.16, −0.09	−0.18 ***	−0.23, −0.14	−0.13 ***	−0.17, −0.09
Medium fearless.	−0.10 ***	−0.14, −0.08	−0.15 ***	−0.19, −0.13	−0.11 ***	−0.14, −0.09
High fearless.	−0.08 ***	−0.10, −0.06	−0.12 ***	−0.15, −0.10	−0.09 ***	−0.12, −0.07

Note: Fearless—fearlessness. CD—conscience development. GD—grandiose–deceitful. CU—callous–unemotional. INS—impulsive–need of stimulation. CI—confidence interval. *** $p < 0.001$.

Lastly, because fearlessness has been traditionally related with both CD and psychopathic traits [28,47], and taking into account the very low moderation effect previously observed, the potential mediation effects of fearlessness on children's psychopathic traits through CD was also tested. As reported in Table 2, fearlessness significantly negatively predicted CD ($\beta = -0.33$, $p < 0.001$; path a), which, in turn, significantly predicted GD ($\beta = -0.39$, $p < 0.001$; path b_1), CU ($\beta = -0.64$, $p < 0.001$; path b_2), and INS ($\beta = -0.32$, $p < 0.001$; path b_3). These relationships might be indicative of mediation effects (a * b_i) of fearlessness through CD on GD ($\beta = 0.13$), CU ($\beta = 0.21$), and INS ($\beta = 0.11$). The Sobel test indicated that all these mediation effects were statistically significant ($Z_{GD} = 7.43$, $p < 0.001$; $Z_{CU} = 7.99$, $p < 0.001$; $Z_{INS} = 7.32$, $p < 0.001$).

4. Discussion

Psychopathic personality has emerged as an important construct for better understanding child conduct problems [72]. Through a burgeoning line of research, psychopathic traits have been linked with a large set of problematic behaviors and negative outcomes from early childhood onwards [11,12]. Although most researchers usually define psychopathic personality as a constellation of co-occurring interpersonal, affective and behavioral traits [8,9], research conducted in childhood has mainly focused on the role of the affective dimension (i.e., CU traits), with the broader construct of psychopathy being still underrepresented [53,54,73]. This is particularly true as pertaining the etiological mechanisms leading to the development of psychopathic traits at early developmental stages. Advancing this knowledge might offer great utility to optimize our research and clinical practice [54], delving into more sophisticated developmental models of psychopathic personality and conduct problems. This would inspire the design of new intervention strategies that may lead to prevention and reduction of psychopathic traits and, therefore, to restrain the development of severe and persistent patterns of problematic behavior.

4.1. Fearlessness, Warmth, and Conscience Development: Unraveling the Paths to Psychopathic Traits

From a developmental model that posits the effect of temperamental variables (i.e., fearlessness) and parenting practices (i.e., parental warmth) in the development of psychopathic traits, the current study intended to account for person-by-context interactions that are supposed to interplay in a dynamic process that could influence the basis of both CD [46] and, subsequently, psychopathic traits [49]. Overall, results revealed that parental warmth did not have direct effects on psychopathic traits, although there would be indirect effects, totally mediated by CD, on all three psychopathy dimensions. More specifically, current results suggested that higher levels of parental warmth in preschool years (T1; ages 3 to 6) would predict higher levels of CD one year later (T2; ages 4 to 7), which, in turn, would potentially restrain the development of psychopathic traits at T3 (ages 5 to 8). Even considering that all indirect effects were significant irrespective of the level of fearlessness, a marginal interaction effect showed that higher levels of parental warmth predicted increases in CD particularly at lower levels of fearlessness. This result largely converges with previous studies on the developmental basis of CD, indicating that positive parenting practices (i.e., parental warmth), would be particularly influential for CD in fearless children [46,47]. Similar findings, yet revealing the inverse pattern, were shown in previous research examining the role of fearlessness and parenting practices (i.e., parental warmth, and parental harshness) in the development of CU traits. Thus, in a sample of low-income boys, child fearlessness only predicted early CU traits in the context of low positive parenting [49], a result also replicated in an adoption design that showed that early fearlessness, which was mainly inherited from biological mothers, was predictive of CU traits when adoptive parents showed lower levels of positive parenting [48].

Interestingly, our results evidenced the same conditional effects for all psychopathy dimensions, suggesting that previous findings linked to CU traits could be expanded, at least as pertaining to this model, to all three psychopathy dimensions. Although preliminary, this is an important result since most of previous research has examined the effects of both fearlessness and parental warmth on CU traits, without accounting for the potential shared effects with both GD and INS traits. It should be noted that current results showed direct effects of fearlessness on GD and INS traits, but not the expected direct effects on CU traits [28,34]. Although this result might be initially unexpected, it could largely converge with previous research, with the effects of fearlessness on CU traits being potentially mediated by CD. As was previously mentioned, empathy and guilt have been defined as components of conscience [26], as well as two of the hallmarks of CU traits [35]. Additionally, temperamental features related with CU traits, such as fearlessness, have been considered risk factors for impairments in empathy and, therefore, in the normal development of conscience and morality in children [27,28]. Based on the foregoing, a fearless temperament would be linked to CD by underpinning potential deficits in the development of empathy and guilt, which in turn, would be predictive of later CU traits.

4.2. Theoretical and Practical Implications

From a developmental psychopathology perspective, the development of a psychopathic personality is usually viewed as a dynamic, changing, and ongoing process [22]. Which factors are influencing its development, being capable to potentiate, maintain or alter its course, is still an ongoing challenge in this field. The basic developmental principle of *equifinality* is likely to be pertinent in the etiological mechanisms involved in psychopathic personality. Thus, it is not expected that a single factor—at the genetic, neurobiological, neurocognitive, developmental or environmental level—would act in an isolated way in the etiology and developmental pathway of psychopathic traits [74]. Dynamic interactive processes are probably behind the developmental underpinnings of the construct, being the associations between the temperament and environment complex and, probably, in a bidirectional way [40,63]. Moreover, it should be noted that the links between parenting practices and psychopathic traits could reflect gene–environment interactions [75], with psychopathic traits being potentially rooted via heritable patterns [76], whereas parenting would play a role as a potential environmental-mediated predictor of psychopathic traits [49]. Even considering the progress made in linking CD theories with the development of psychopathy traits, new advances are required to improve developmental models of psychopathic personality, integrating all the most relevant knowledge in a coherent paradigm that may help to further understand the early underpinnings and later developmental patterns of psychopathic traits. In this regard, Waller and Wagner [77] have proposed the Sensitivity to Threat and Affiliative Reward Model (STAR) as a comprehensive model to delve into the etiology of CU traits. It posits that both fearless temperament and low affiliative reward would be the two psychobiological and mechanistic precursors to CU traits, with their interaction being uniquely predictive of CU traits when compared to GD and INS [78]. Assuming the promising value of the STAR model for the development of CU traits, new efforts are needed to disentangle the mechanisms leading to both GD and INS and, even more interesting, to test whether these specific mechanisms are also central when all psychopathic traits are present.

Finally, current results would also derive some practical implications. Since psychopathic traits seem to be identifiers of youths within serious and long-standing pathways of problematic behavior, they should be primarily identified in clinical settings. To maximize results, these programs should be tailored to the unique characteristics that define this specific group (e.g., remorseless, lack of empathy, manipulation), and should include those factors that have been proven to be potential mechanisms of change in psychopathic personality (e.g., parental warmth). Some promising results from the applied context have shown that focusing on improving parental warmth, whilst declining inconsistent and coercive parenting, may have clinical value not only in reducing problematic behavior in children with high psychopathic traits, but also in favoring a significant reduction in all affective, interpersonal, and behavioral features of psychopathic personality [45,57]. Based on current findings, these effects could be also strengthened by stimulating the development of conscience through specific socioemotional training, favoring emotion recognition and affective responsivity [79].

4.3. Limitations and Future Lines of Research

To our knowledge, this is one of the first studies linking the developmental model of CD to psychopathic personality, accounting for all its dimensions. It involves a large sample of children from a prospective longitudinal study, conducted across two years, and starting at the preschool years, which is considered a key stage in the development of empathy and conscience [47]. Even though, there are some limitations that should be acknowledge in order to address future research. First, we only relied on parents' reports, which could have inflated some effects due to shared method variance. Second, we only focused on the affective component of conscience (i.e., moral emotions), making it necessary to further examine how other dimensions (e.g., moral reasoning), as well as the whole construct, are shaped from early socialization experiences in interaction with temperamental styles. From this chain of influences, it would be interesting to further examine how they finally contribute to the development of psychopathic traits and related disruptive behavior. Third, only fearlessness and parental warmth were included as predictors, making difficult to elaborate a comprehensive developmental model that would require some additional temperamental (e.g., affiliative reward), cognitive (e.g., emotion recognition) and environmental variables (e.g., parental harshness), including the quality of parent–child interactions, to delineate all the process and mechanisms leading to the construction of self and, in turn, to the development of psychopathic traits. Fourth, current results showed that gender may account for some of the effects, suggesting that additional research should take a gender perspective in order to examine whether there might be differences across groups in developmental mechanisms of psychopathic traits, which may also vary across development. Fifth, although a prospective longitudinal design was used, one might prevent to derive causal effects that should be examined in future research accounting for additional person-by-context interactions. Finally, additional studies addressing all psychopathy dimensions are particularly needed to further understand the etiological mechanisms underlying the development of specific psychopathic traits, and overall psychopathic personality, from early childhood onwards.

5. Conclusions

Current results allow strengthening developmental models of psychopathic traits, with parenting practices based on warmth and affection emerging as environmental mechanisms able to prompt changes in psychopathic traits across development [39], particularly at lower levels of fearlessness, and via CD. In this regard, it could be suggested that, whereas temperamental mechanisms (i.e., fearlessness) may underpin the most relevant features of psychopathic personality, environmental factors in general, and parenting practices in particular, would be able to either enhance or hinder their development across their lifespan [11], with CD as a potential mediator of these effects. It reinforces the possibility of designing new intervention strategies specifically tailored to the unique features of children with psychopathic traits, and the mechanisms able to drive some changes across development, leading to also prevent the development of serious patterns of problematic behaviors.

Author Contributions: Conceptualization, L.L.-R.; methodology, O.C. and L.M.; software, O.C., L.M. and B.D.-Á.; formal analysis, L.L.-R., O.C. and L.M.; investigation, L.L.-R., B.D.-Á. and E.R.; resources, E.R.; data curation, L.L.-R.; writing—original draft preparation, L.L.-R. and O.C.; writing—review and editing, L.M. and B.D.-Á.; supervision, L.L.-R. and E.R.; project administration, L.L.-R. and E.R.; funding acquisition, E.R. All authors have read and agreed to the published version of the manuscript.

Funding: This research was funded by FEDER/Ministerio de Ciencia, Innovación y Universidades—Agencia Estatal de Investigación/Grants (PSI2015-65766-R and 2019-PN103), and by Xunta de Galicia, under the Programa de Axudas á Etapa Posdoutoral da Xunta de Galicia 2017, 2019, and 2021, and Axudas para a Consolidación e Estruturación de Unidades de Investigación Competitivas e outras Accións de Fomento nas Univeridades; GRC, 2018 (Consellería de Cultura, Educación e Ordenación Universitaria).

Institutional Review Board Statement: The study was conducted according to the guidelines of the Declaration of Helsinki and approved by the Bioethics Committee at the Universidade de Santiago de Compostela (17/06/2016) and the Spanish Ministry of Economy and Competitiveness.

Informed Consent Statement: Informed consent was obtained from all subjects involved in the study.

Data Availability Statement: Data presented in this study are available upon request to the corresponding author.

Acknowledgments: The authors would like to thank all the members of the ELISA Project team for contributing to data collection and preparation. We would also like to extend our gratitude to the many families and schools who supported and participated in this study.

Conflicts of Interest: The authors declare no conflict of interest.

References

1. Blair, R.J.R.; Leibenluft, E.; Pine, D. Conduct disorder and callous-unemotional traits is youth. *N. Engl. J. Med.* **2014**, *371*, 2207–2216. [CrossRef] [PubMed]
2. Frick, P.J.; Matlasz, T. Disruptive, impulse-control, and conduct disorders. In *Developmental Pathways to Disruptive, Impulse-Control and Conduct Disorders*; Martel, M., Ed.; Academic Press: Cambridge, MA, USA, 2018; pp. 3–20.
3. Reef, J.; Diamantopoulou, S.; van Meurs, I.; Verhulst, F.C.; van der Ende, J. Developmental trajectories of child to adolescent externalizing behavior and adult DSM-IV disorder: Results of a 24-year longitudinal study. *Soc. Psychiatry Psychiatr. Epidemiol.* **2011**, *46*, 1233–1241. [CrossRef]
4. Rivenbark, J.G.; Odgers, C.L.; Caspi, A.; Harrington, H.; Hogan, S.; Houts, R.M.; Poulton, R.; Moffitt, T.E. The high societal costs of childhood conduct problems: Evidence from administrative records up to age 38 in a longitudinal birth cohort. *J. Child Psychol. Psychiatry* **2018**, *59*, 703–710. [CrossRef] [PubMed]
5. Frick, P.J. Developmental pathways to conduct disorder: Implications for future directions in research, assessment, and treatment. *J. Clin. Child Adolesc. Psychol.* **2012**, *41*, 378–389. [CrossRef]
6. Pardini, D.; Frick, P.J. Multiple developmental pathways to conduct disorder: Current conceptualizations and clinical implications. *J. Can. Acad. Child Adolesc. Psychiatry* **2013**, *22*, 20–25.
7. Waller, R.; Hyde, L.W.; Grabell, A.S.; Alves, M.L.; Olson, S.L. Differential associations of early callous-unemotional, oppositional, and ADHD behaviors: Multiple domains within early-starting conduct problems? *J. Child Psychol. Psychiatry* **2015**, *56*, 657–666. [CrossRef] [PubMed]
8. Cooke, D.J.; Michie, C. Refining the construct of psychopathy: Towards a hierarchical model. *Psychol. Assess.* **2001**, *13*, 171–188. [CrossRef] [PubMed]
9. Colins, O.F.; Andershed, H.; Frogner, L.; Lopez-Romero, L.; Veen, V.; Andershed, A.K. A New Measure to Assess Psychopathic Personality in Children: The Child Problematic Traits Inventory. *J. Psychopathol. Behav. Assess.* **2014**, *36*, 4–21. [CrossRef]
10. Hare, R.D.; Neumann, C.S. Psychopathy as a Clinical and Empirical Construct. *Annu. Rev. Clin. Psychol.* **2008**, *4*, 217–246. [CrossRef]
11. Salekin, R.T. Research Review: What do we know about psychopathic traits in children? *J. Child Psychol. Psychiatry* **2017**, *58*, 1180–1200. [CrossRef]

2. Frick, P.J.; Ray, J.V.; Thornton, L.C.; Kahn, R.E. Can callous-unemotional traits enhance the understanding, diagnosis, and treatment of serious conduct problems in children and adolescents? A comprehensive review. *Psychol. Bull.* **2014**, *40*, 1–57. [CrossRef]
3. Lynam, D.R.; Caspi, A.; Moffitt, T.E.; Loeber, R.; Stouthamer-Loeber, M. Longitudinal evidence that psychopathy scores in early adolescence predict adult psychopathy. *J. Abnorm. Psychol.* **2007**, *116*, 155–165. [CrossRef] [PubMed]
4. Colins, O.F.; Andershed, H.; Hellfeldt, K.; Fanti, K. The incremental usefulness of teacher-rated psychopathic traits in 5- to 7-year olds in predicting teacher-, parent-, and child self-report antisocial behavior at six-year follow-up. *J. Crim. Justice* **2021**, 101771. [CrossRef]
5. Ezpeleta, L.; de la Osa, N.; Granero, R.; Penelo, E.; Domènech, J.M. Inventory of callous-unemotional traits in a community sample of preschoolers. *J. Clin. Child Adolesc. Psychol.* **2013**, *42*, 91–105. [CrossRef]
6. López-Romero, L.; Colins, O.F.; Fanti, K.; Salekin, R.T.; Romero, E.; Andershed, H. Testing the predictive and incremental validity of callous-unemotional versus the multidimensional psychopathy construct in preschool children. *J. Crim. Justice* **2020**, 101744. [CrossRef]
7. Haas, S.M.; Waschbusch, D.A.; Pelham, W.E., Jr.; King, S.; Andrade, B.F.; Carrey, N.J. Treatment response in CP/ADHD children with callous/unemotional traits. *J. Abnorm. Child Psychol.* **2011**, *39*, 541–552. [CrossRef]
8. Hawes, D.J.; Dadds, M.R. The treatment of conduct problems in children with callous-unemotional traits. *J. Consult. Clin. Psychol.* **2005**, *73*, 737–741. [CrossRef]
9. Waschbusch, D.A.; Walsh, T.M.; Andrade, B.F.; King, S.; Carrey, N.J. Social problem solving, conduct problems, and callous-unemotional traits in children. *Child Psychiatry Hum. Dev.* **2007**, *37*, 293–305. [CrossRef]
10. Raine, A. *The Anatomy of Violence: The Biological Roots of Crime*; Penguin Books Limited: London, UK, 2013.
11. Blair, R. A cognitive neuroscience perspective on child and adolescent psychopathy. In *Handbook of Child and Adolescent Psychopathy*; Salekin, R.T., Lynam, D.R., Eds.; The Guildford Press: New York, NY, USA, 2010; pp. 156–178.
12. Frick, P.J.; Ray, J.V.; Thornton, L.C.; Kahn, R.E. A developmental psychopathology approach to understanding callous-unemotional traits in children and adolescents with serious conduct problems. *Child Psychol. Psychiatry* **2014**, *55*, 532–548. [CrossRef] [PubMed]
13. Kochanska, G.; Thompson, R.A. The emergence and development of conscience in toddlerhood and early childhood. In *Parenting and Children's Internalization of Values: A Handbook of Contemporary Theory*; Grusec, J.E., Kuczynski, L., Eds.; John Wiley & Sons Inc.: Hoboken, NJ, USA, 1997; pp. 53–77.
14. Aksan, N.; Kochanska, G. Conscience in Childhood: Old Questions, New Answers. *Dev. Psychol.* **2005**, *41*, 506–516. [CrossRef] [PubMed]
15. Kochanska, G.; Aksan, N. Conscience in childhood: Past, present, and future. In *Appraising the Human Developmental Sciences: Essays in Honor of Merrill-Palmer Quarterly*; Ladd, G.W., Ed.; Wayne State University Press: Detroit, MI, USA, 2007; pp. 238–249.
16. Thompson, R.A.; Newton, E.K. Emotion in early conscience. In *Emotions, Aggression, and Morality in Children: Bridging Development and Psychopathology*; Arsenio, W.F., Lemerise, E.A., Eds.; American Psychological Association: Washington, DC, USA, 2010; pp. 13–31.
17. Kochanska, G. Toward a synthesis of parental socialization and child temperament in early development of conscience. *Child Dev.* **1993**, *64*, 325–347. [CrossRef]
18. Lykken, D.T. Psychopathic personality: The scope of the problem. In *Handbook of Psychopathy*; Patrick, C., Ed.; Guilford Press: New York, NY, USA, 2006; pp. 3–13.
19. Calkins, S.D.; Blandon, A.Y.; Williford, A.P.; Keane, S.P. Biological, behavioral, and relational levels of resilience in the context of risk for early childhood problems. *Dev. Psychopathol.* **2007**, *19*, 675–700. [CrossRef]
20. Kochanska, G.; Koenig, J.L.; Barry, R.A.; Kim, S.; Yoon, J.E. Children's conscience during toddler and preschool years, moral self, and a competent, adaptive developmental trajectory. *Dev. Psychol.* **2010**, *46*, 1320–1332. [CrossRef] [PubMed]
21. Dadds, M.R.; Allen, J.L.; Oliver, B.R.; Faulkner, N.; Legge, K.; Moul, C.; Woolgar, M.; Scott, S. Love, eye contact, and the developmental origins of empathy v. psychopathy. *Br. J. Psychiatry* **2012**, *200*, 191–196. [CrossRef] [PubMed]
22. Rutter, M. Psychopathy in childhood: Is there a meaningful diagnosis? *Br. J. Psychiatry* **2012**, *200*, 175–176. [CrossRef] [PubMed]
23. Glenn, A.L.; Raine, A.; Venables, P.H.; Mednick, S.A. Early temperamental and psychophysiological precursors of adult psychopathic personality. *J. Abnorm. Psychol.* **2007**, *116*, 508–518. [CrossRef]
24. Goffin, K.C.; Boldt, L.J.; Kim, S.; Kochanska, G. A Unique Path to Callous-Unemotional Traits for Children who are Temperamentally Fearless and Unconcerned about Transgressions: A Longitudinal Study of Typically Developing Children from age 2 to 12. *J. Abnorm. Child Psychol.* **2018**, *46*, 769–780. [CrossRef] [PubMed]
25. Waller, R.; Wagner, N.J.; Barstead, M.G.; Subar, A.; Petersen, J.L.; Hyde, J.S.; Hyde, L.W. A meta-analysis of the associations between callous-unemotional traits and empathy, prosociality, and guilt. *Clin. Psychol. Rev.* **2020**, *75*, 101809. [CrossRef] [PubMed]
26. Blair, R.J.; Cipolotti, L. Impaired social response reversal. A case of 'acquired sociopathy'. *Brain* **2000**, *123*, 1122–1141. [CrossRef]
27. Paciello, M.; Ballarotto, G.; Cerniglia, L.; Muratori, P. Does the Interplay of Callous-Unemotional Traits and Moral Disengagement Underpin Disruptive Behavior? A Systematic Review. *Adolesc. Health Med. Ther.* **2020**, *11*, 9–20. [CrossRef]
28. Waller, R.; Gardner, F.; Hyde, L.W. What are the associations between parenting, callous-unemotional traits and antisocial behavior in youth? A systematic review of evidence. *Clin. Psychol. Rev.* **2013**, *33*, 593–608. [CrossRef] [PubMed]
29. Backman, H.; Laajasalo, T.; Jokela, M.; Aronen, E.T. Parental Warmth and Hostility and the Development of Psychopathic Behaviors: A Longitudinal Study of Young Offenders. *J. Child Fam. Stud.* **2021**, *30*, 955–965. [CrossRef]

40. Waller, R.; Gardner, F.; Viding, E.; Shaw, D.S.; Dishion, T.J.; Wilson, M.N.; Hyde, L.W. Bidirectional associations between parental warmth, callous unemotional behavior, and behavior problems in high-risk preschoolers. *J. Abnorm. Child Psychol.* **2014**, *42*, 1275–1285. [CrossRef] [PubMed]
41. Mills-Koonce, W.R.; Willoughby, M.T.; Garrett-Peters, P.; Wagner, N.; Vernon-Feagans, L. Family Life Project Key Investigators. The interplay among socioeconomic status, household chaos, and parenting in the prediction of child conduct problems and callous-unemotional behaviors. *Dev. Psychopathol.* **2016**, *28*, 757–771. [CrossRef]
42. Pasalich, D.; Dadds, M.; Hawes, D.; Brennan, J. Callous-unemotional traits moderate the relative importance of parental coercion versus warmth in child conduct problems: An observational study. *J. Child Psychol. Psychiatry* **2011**, *52*, 1308–1315. [CrossRef]
43. López-Romero, L.; Romero, E.; Gómez-Fraguela, J.A. Delving into callous-unemotional traits: Concurrent correlates and early parenting precursors. *J. Child Fam. Stud.* **2015**, *24*, 1451–1468. [CrossRef]
44. Kimonis, E.R.; Bagner, D.M.; Linares, D.; Blake, C.; Rodriguez, G. Parent training outcomes among young children with callous–unemotional conduct problems with or at risk for developmental delay. *J. Child Fam. Stud.* **2014**, *23*, 437–448. [CrossRef]
45. McDonald, R.; Dodson, M.C.; Rosenfield, D.; Jouriles, E.N. Effects of a parenting intervention on features of psychopathy in children. *J. Abnorm. Child Psychol.* **2011**, *39*, 1013–1023. [CrossRef]
46. Kochanska, G.; Aksan, N.; Joy, M.E. Children's fearfulness as a moderator of parenting in early socialization: Two longitudinal studies. *Dev. Psychol.* **2007**, *43*, 222–237. [CrossRef]
47. Kochanska, G. Multiple pathways to conscience for children with different temperaments: From toddlerhood to age 5. *Dev. Psychol.* **1997**, *33*, 228–240. [CrossRef]
48. Waller, R.; Trentacosta, C.J.; Shaw, D.S.; Neiderhiser, J.M.; Ganiban, J.M.; Reiss, D.; Leve, L.D.; Hyde, L.W. Heritable temperament pathways to early callous-unemotional behaviour. *Br. J. Psychiatry* **2016**, *209*, 475–482. [CrossRef]
49. Waller, R.; Shaw, D.S.; Hyde, L.W. Observed fearlessness and positive parenting interact to predict childhood callous-unemotional behaviors among low-income boys. *J. Child Psychol. Psychiatry* **2017**, *58*, 282–291. [CrossRef]
50. Waller, R.; Hyde, L.W. Callous-unemotional behaviors in early childhood: The development of empathy and prosociality gone awry. *Curr. Opin. Psychol.* **2018**, *20*, 11–16. [CrossRef] [PubMed]
51. Colins, O.F.; Andershed, H.; Salekin, R.T.; Fanti, K.A. Comparing different approaches for subtyping children with conduct problems: Callous-unemotional traits only versus the multidimensional psychopathy construct. *Psychopathol. Behav. Assess.* **2018**, *40*, 6–15. [CrossRef] [PubMed]
52. Frogner, L.; Gibson, C.L.; Andershed, A.K.; Andershed, H. Childhood psychopathic personality and callous–unemotional traits in the prediction of conduct problems. *J. Abnorm. Child Psychol.* **2003**, *88*, 211–225. [CrossRef]
53. Lilienfeld, S.O. The multidimensional nature of psychopathy: Five recommendations for research. *Psychopathol. Behav. Assess.* **2018**, *40*, 79–85. [CrossRef]
54. Salekin, R.T.; Andershed, H.; Batky, B.D.; Bontemps, A.P. Are callous unemotional (CU) traits enough? *Psychopathol. Behav. Assess.* **2018**, *40*, 1–5. [CrossRef]
55. Shaw, D.S.; Gilliom, M.; Ingoldsby, E.M.; Nagin, S. Trajectories leading to school-age conduct problems. *Dev. Psychol.* **2003**, *39*, 189–200. [CrossRef] [PubMed]
56. Muratori, P.; Lochman, J.E.; Lai, E.; Milone, A.; Nocentini, A.; Pisano, S.; Righini, E.; Masi, G. Which dimension of parenting predicts the change of callous unemotional traits in children with disruptive behavior disorder? *Compr. Psychiatry* **2016**, *69*, 202–210. [CrossRef]
57. Fleming, G.E.; Kimonis, E.R. PCIT for children with callous-unemotional traits. In *Handbook of Parent-Child Interaction Therapy*; Niec, L.N., Ed.; Springer: New York, NY, USA, 2018; pp. 19–34.
58. Young, A.F.; Powers, J.R.; Bell, S.L. Attrition in longitudinal studies: Who do you lose? *Aust. N. Z. J. Public Health* **2006**, *30*, 353–361. [CrossRef]
59. Launes, J.; Hokkanen, L.; Laasonen, M.; Tuulio-Henriksson, A.; Virta, M.; Lipsanen, J.; Tienari, P.J.; Michelsson, K. Attrition in a 30-year follow-up of a perinatal birth risk cohort: Factors change with age. *PeerJ* **2014**, *2*, e480. [CrossRef]
60. World Health Organization. *Process of Translation and Adaptation of Instruments*; World Health Organization: Geneva, Switzerland, 2016.
61. Paterson, G.; Sanson, A. The association of behavioural adjustment to temperament, parenting and family characteristics among 5-year-old children. *Soc. Dev.* **1999**, *8*, 293–309. [CrossRef]
62. Zubrick, S.R.; Lucas, N.; Westrupp, E.M.; Nicholson, J.M. *Parenting Measures in the Longitudinal Study of Australian Children: Construct Validity and Measurement Quality, Waves 1 to 4*; Department of Social Services: Greenway, Australia, 2014.
63. López-Romero, L.; Domínguez-Álvarez, B.; Isdahl-Troye, A.; Romero, E. Bidirectional Effects between Psychopathic Traits and Conduct Problems in Early Childhood: Examining Parenting as Potential Mediator. *Rev. Psicol. Clínica Niños Adolesc.* **2021**, *8*, 9–16. Available online: https://www.revistapcna.com/ (accessed on 8 June 2021).
64. Rothbart, M.K.; Ahadi, S.A.; Hershey, K.L. Temperament and social behavior in childhood. *Merrill-Palmer Q.* **1994**, *40*, 21–39.
65. Rothbart, M.K.; Ahadi, S.A.; Hershey, K.L.; Fisher, P. Investigations of temperament at 3–7 years: The Children's Behavior Questionnaire. *Child Dev.* **2001**, *72*, 1394–1408. [CrossRef] [PubMed]
66. Dadds, M.R.; Hunter, K.; Hawes, D.J.; Frost, A.D.J.; Vassallo, S.; Bunn, P.; Merz, S.; El Masry, Y. A measure of cognitive and affective empathy in children using parent ratings. *Child Psychiatry Hum. Dev.* **2008**, *39*, 111–122. [CrossRef]

67. López-Romero, L.; Maneiro, L.; Colins, O.F.; Andershed, H.; Romero, E. Psychopathic traits in early childhood: Further multi-informant validation of the Child Problematic Traits Inventory (CPTI). *J. Psychopathol. Behav. Assess.* **2019**, *41*, 366–374. [CrossRef]
68. Muthen, L.; Muthen, B. Mplus Version 7.4 Software. Available online: https://statmodel.com/ (accessed on 18 May 2021).
69. Marsh, H.W.; Wen, Z.; Hau, K.T.; Little, T.D.; Bovaird, J.A.; Widaman, K.F. Unconstrained structural equation models of latent interactions: Contrasting residual-and mean-centered approaches. *Struct. Equ. Modeling* **2007**, *14*, 570–580. [CrossRef]
70. Cham, H.; Reshetnyak, E.; Rosenfeld, B.; Breitbart, W. Full information maximum likelihood estimation for latent variable interactions with incomplete indicators. *Multivar. Behav. Res.* **2017**, *52*, 12–30. [CrossRef]
71. Hu, L.T.; Bentler, P.M. Cutoff criteria for fit indexes in covariance structure analysis: Conventional criteria versus new alternatives. *Struct. Equ. Modeling* **1999**, *6*, 1–55. [CrossRef]
72. Salekin, R.T.; Lynam, D.R. *Handbook of Child and Adolescent Psychopathy*; The Guilford Press: New York, NY, USA, 2010.
73. Colins, O.F.; Andershed, H. Childhood and adolescent psychopathy. In *Routledge International Handbook of Psychopathy and Crime*; DeLisi, M., Ed.; Routledge: New York, NY, USA, 2019; pp. 166–184.
74. Ribeiro da Silva, D.; Rijo, D.; Salekin, R.T. Child and adolescent psychopathy: A state-of-the-art reflection on the construct and etiological theories. *J. Crim. Justice* **2012**, *40*, 269–277. [CrossRef]
75. Hyde, L.W.; Waller, R.; Trentacosta, C.J.; Shaw, D.S.; Neiderhiser, J.M.; Ganiban, J.M.; Reiss, D.; Leve, L.D. Heritable and Nonheritable Pathways to Early Callous-Unemotional Behaviors. *Am. J. Psychiatry* **2016**, *173*, 903–910. [CrossRef] [PubMed]
76. Viding, E.; Blair, R.J.; Moffitt, T.E.; Plomin, R. Evidence for substantial genetic risk for psychopathy in 7-year-olds. *J. Child Psychol. Psychiatry* **2005**, *46*, 592–597. [CrossRef] [PubMed]
77. Waller, R.; Wagner, N. The Sensitivity to Threat and Affiliative Reward (STAR) model and the development of callous-unemotional traits. *Neurosci. Biobehav. Rev.* **2019**, *107*, 656–671. [CrossRef]
78. Domínguez-Álvarez, B.; Romero, E.; López-Romero, L.; Isdahl-Troye, A.; Wagner, N.J.; Waller, R. A Cross-Sectional and Longitudinal Test of the Low Sensitivity to Threat and Affiliative Reward (STAR) Model of Callous-Unemotional Traits among Spanish Preschoolers. *Res. Child Adolesc. Psychopathol.* **2021**, *49*, 877–889. [CrossRef] [PubMed]
79. Dadds, M.R.; English, T.; Wimalaweera, S.; Schollar-Root, O.; Hawes, D.J. Can reciprocated parent-child eye gaze and emotional engagement enhance treatment for children with conduct problems and callous-unemotional traits: A proof-of-concept trial. *Child Psychol. Psychiatry* **2019**, *60*, 676–685. [CrossRef] [PubMed]

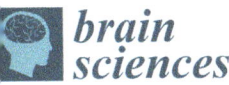

Article

Parenting and Sibling Relationships in Family with Disruptive Behavior Disorders. Are Non-Clinical Siblings More Vulnerable for Emotional and Behavioral Problems?

Martina Smorti [1,*], Emanuela Inguaggiato [2], Lara Vezzosi [1] and Annarita Milone [2]

1. Department of Surgical, Medical and Molecular Pathology and Critical Care Medicine, University of Pisa, 56126 Pisa, Italy; lara.vezzosi2@gmail.com
2. Department of Child Psychiatry and Psychopharmacology, IRCCS Stella Maris Foundation, 56018 Pisa, Italy; emanuela.inguaggiato@fsm.unipi.it (E.I.); annarita.milone@fsm.unipi.it (A.M.)
* Correspondence: martina.smorti@unipi.it; Tel.: +39-050-992-370

Abstract: Disruptive Behavior Disorders (DBD) are the most common mental health disorders in the school-aged child population. Although harsh parenting is a key risk factor in the shaping of DBD, studies neglect the presence of siblings and differential parenting. This study aims to compare: (1) parenting style and sibling relationship in sibling dyads of clinical families, composed of a DBD child and a non-clinical sibling, with control families composed of two non-clinical siblings; (2) parenting style, sibling relationship, and emotional and behavioral problems in DBD child, non-clinical sibling, and non-clinical child of control group. Sixty-one families (composed of mother and sibling dyads), divided into clinical ($n = 27$) and control ($n = 34$) groups, completed the APQ, SRI, and CBCL questionnaires. Results indicated differential parenting in clinical families, compared to control group families, with higher negative parenting toward the DBD child than the sibling; no difference emerged in sibling relationship within sibling dyads (clinical vs. control). Finally, externalizing and internalizing problems were higher in DBD children and their siblings, compared to control, indicating DBD sibling psychopathology vulnerability. Findings suggest inclusion of siblings in the clinical assessment and rehabilitative intervention of DBD children, given that the promotion of positive parenting could improve mental health in the offspring.

Keywords: disruptive behavior disorders; parenting style; sibling relationship; emotional and behavioral problems

Citation: Smorti, M.; Inguaggiato, E.; Vezzosi, L.; Milone, A. Parenting and Sibling Relationships in Family with Disruptive Behavior Disorders. Are Non-Clinical Siblings More Vulnerable for Emotional and Behavioral Problems? *Brain Sci.* **2021**, *11*, 1308. https://doi.org/10.3390/brainsci11101308

Academic Editor: Maria Pia Bucci

Received: 21 July 2021
Accepted: 27 September 2021
Published: 1 October 2021

Publisher's Note: MDPI stays neutral with regard to jurisdictional claims in published maps and institutional affiliations.

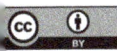

Copyright: © 2021 by the authors. Licensee MDPI, Basel, Switzerland. This article is an open access article distributed under the terms and conditions of the Creative Commons Attribution (CC BY) license (https://creativecommons.org/licenses/by/4.0/).

1. Introduction

Disruptive Behavior Disorders (DBDs) including Oppositional Defiant Disorder (ODD) and Conduct Disorder (CD), are a challenging mental health issue and represent the most common mental health reason for referral for school-aged youths [1–3]. DBDs, according to Diagnostic and Statistical Manual of Mental Disorders, Fifth Edition, are a cluster of disorders defined by the presence of a persistent pattern of negative, defiant, aggressive, rule-breaking or disruptive behaviors, such as a repetitive and persistent pattern of behavior that violates the basic rights of others or violates major age-appropriate societal rules or norms [4]. These characteristics often emerge early in development and persist into adolescence and adulthood, leading to widespread difficulties, causing clinically significant impairment in the youth's social, academic, familial, or personal functioning [4–7].

DBD children and adolescents are at risk of developing many severe psychopathological outcomes in adolescence and as adults (mood and bipolar disorders, psychopathy, and antisocial personality), with worsening prognosis and social costs [8–10]. The risk of later psychopathology (ADHD, mood disorders, substance use, suicidality), and poor overall functioning, is increased in DBDs in the presence of deficits of emotion regulation, characterized by lack of temper control, affective lability, mood instability, and emotional overreaction [11–16].

DBD is a multi-determined condition involving both biological and environmental factors; in fact, genetic, temperamental, environmental, social, and family factors, and the interaction between "nature" and "nurture", seem to influence developmental risk for DBD in children [17–21]. In the text the term child/children will be used to refer to offspring whether these are children or adolescents.

Regarding biological factors, several studies show moderate influence of these factors in the etiology of DBD, especially in the early-onset form, pervasive conduct disorder, and in relation to callous-unemotional traits. Molecular genetic studies, also conducted in twins, have shown associations between genetic variants of genes of the dopaminergic and serotonergic systems and DBD [22,23].

Previous studies have indicated that parenting styles are key factors in shaping DBD in children. Specifically, the use of harsh parenting, which includes coercive, controlling, and punitive methods, the use of verbal and physical aggression [24–27], combined with low warmth and poor positive parenting [28–30], are associated with DBDs as well as more general externalizing disorders in children and adolescents [31,32]. Despite the absolute level of negative parenting, children who report harsher and less supportive parenting tend to manifest more externalizing behaviors compared to their siblings [33–38]. Studies on family risk factors have mainly focused on the effect of specific parenting styles on DBD child adjustment [39,40], neglecting the presence of siblings. A perspective that takes into consideration parenting style on sibling dyads may allow the identification of risk and protective factors for the psychological adjustment of offspring in the same family, to better address preventive intervention [40].

Despite the large amount of literature on the effects of parental practices that are directed unequally among siblings (differential parenting [41]) and on externalizing behaviors in children from the same family, less is known about the effect of differential parenting on externalizing behaviors reported by children and adolescents in families with a DBD child. It must be noted that DBDs present specific features that increase the risk for several negative outcomes, such as acts of aggression, violence, and risk taking, in addition to the risk for psychopathology [42–44].

This study aimed to explore the impact of both parenting style and differential parenting on emotional and behavioral problems of DBD siblings and non-clinical siblings who shared the same environment. In Italy, where we conducted this study, mothers still maintain the central role of main caregivers of children below 18 years, despite the recent increased involvement of fathers in childcare activities [45]. In addition to the task of child-rearing, Italian mothers also have the role of providing guidance and the transmission of norms [46]. Moreover, the quality of the adolescent's relationship with the mother has a much stronger effect on adolescent risk behavior [47,48] compared to the paternal relationship. Therefore, in the current study we focus on maternal parenting.

This study also aimed to compare maternal parenting styles in families in which one sibling was diagnosed with DBD, while the other did not receive any psychiatric diagnoses, and control families with two non-clinical siblings. This comparison was aimed to identify if parenting styles in clinical families were characterized by more harsh and differential parenting towards clinical than non-clinical children/adolescents compared to control families. We expected higher differential parenting in families of the clinical sample compared to control families, with more negative parenting reported towards the DBD child compared to sibling.

Moreover, we aimed to compare maternal parenting style and emotional and behavioral problems reported in DBD siblings (DBDs), non-clinical siblings (S-DBDs), and non-clinical siblings of control families (CONTR), for early evaluation whether non-clinical siblings in families with DBD would present a higher risk for harsh and negative parenting, externalizing problems, and emotion dysregulation, compared to families without DBD. We expected that non-clinical siblings in families with DBD would report a lower level of negative parenting and externalizing problems compared to their DBD siblings, but higher compared to that reported in control group families.

Another aspect that has been largely neglected in the literature on DBDs until now is the role of sibling relationship quality. Previous studies, using a dyadic perspective, have shown that sibling relationship is linked to differential parenting, and that differential parenting has negative effects on sibling relationship. In fact, although a certain degree of differential parenting is normal and depends on a child's characteristics, such as age, gender, and temperament [49], differential treatment is linked with more negative sibling relationship as greater conflict and less affection between siblings [49,50], and as more externalizing behaviors, aggression, depressed mood, anxiety, and low self-esteem [40,50,51]. Moving from this consideration, we expected higher levels of conflict reported by siblings of the clinical group compared to the control group. Higher levels of conflict were expected based on parental differential treatment and on characteristics of the DBDs; in fact, typical patterns of externalizing disorders, such as negative, defiant, aggressive, rule-breaking, or disruptive behaviors, can also be implemented in families.

2. Materials and Methods

2.1. Sample

Our sample included two groups of families (clinical and control) composed of: (a) two biological siblings aged 6–16 years; and (b) their mother. In line with other studies, in which age spacing of four years between siblings is recognized as a strong correlate of differential parenting [52,53], only sibling dyads with age spacing of four years or less were considered for this study.

To be included in this study, participants (mother and offspring) had a good comprehension of the Italian language, gave consent to participate in the study, and completed the battery of questionnaires.

Additional inclusion criterion for the clinical-family sample were: (a) the presence of a child with a diagnosis of DBD according to DSM 5 criteria with Full IQ Scale greater than 85 and no comorbidity with Autism Specter Disorder diagnosis; (b) a sibling without any clinical diagnosis.

For the control group, an additional inclusion criterion was: pairs of siblings in which neither have been submitted to a clinical consultation.

The clinical group was enrolled in the Department of Child and Adolescent Psychiatry of a third level hospital (FSM Stella Maris Foundation in Pisa), which provides care to patients from all over Italy. Recruitment took place in the clinic for the diagnosis and treatment of behavioral disorders in developmental age called "Beyond the clouds". Families were consecutively recruited during the diagnosis process by the person responsible for this study. Following the diagnosis of DBD, an evidence-based multimodal treatment was offered to the clinical families.

Diagnoses of DBD, based on DSM-5 diagnostic criteria, were made by using historical information, a structured clinical interview, and the Italian version of the Schedule for Affective Disorders and Schizophrenia for School-Age Children—Present and Lifetime Version (K-SADS-PL) [54], administered by child psychiatry trainees under the supervision of the senior child psychiatrist. Diagnoses were definitively confirmed by consensus of a multidisciplinary board.

The Italian version of the Wechsler Intelligence Scale for Children—Fourth Edition (WISC-IV) [55], was administered to all patients to assess IQ.

The control group was recruited during leisure and sports activities in the metropolitan area of Central Italy. Participants (parents and children) were randomly selected among participants of leisure activities and approached when they finished. They were informed about the goals of the survey, and were told they had the option to drop out at any given moment if they wished to do so. Written informed consent from parents was obtained for all participants.

Of the 66 families who were contacted for this study that met inclusion criteria, three (two belonging to control group and one to clinical group) refused to participate due to lack of time. Two families (belonging to clinical group) could not be included in the final sample due to incomplete data (missing questionnaire about one sibling).

The final sample of the study was made up of 61 families: (a) 61 mothers, and (b) 61 couples of siblings, for a total of 122 children (87 males and 43 females), aged between 6 and 15.7 years (Mage = 9.8; SD = 2.1). The sample was divided into two groups, according to inclusion criteria.

The clinical group was composed of 27 families: (a) 27 mothers, and (b) 27 couples of siblings, for a total of 54 children (40 males, 14 females), aged between 6 and 14.8 (Mage = 9.9; SD = 2.0). For each pair of siblings, we labelled DBD the target child who reported the clinical diagnosis, and S-DBD the older sibling of the DBD, closest in age, with no clinical diagnosis.

For the control group, we considered a child comparable in age to DBD, labelled CONTR-1, and an older sibling, labelled CONTR-2. The control group was composed of 34 families: (a) 34 mothers, and (b) 34 pairs of siblings, for a total of 68 children (41 males, 27 females), aged between 6 and 15.7 (Mage = 9.8; SD 2.2). This sample has not been used in previous studies.

The investigator responsible for the study informed participants about the main study aims, specified that anonymity was guaranteed, participation was voluntary, they could withdraw from participation in any moment, and no monetary reward was given. A signed statement attesting to informed consent for study participation was obtained from all subjects. After the informed consent was signed, according to the study protocol, the mother filled in the questionnaire about parenting style and psychological problems for each child/adolescent, and each child/adolescent completed a specific questionnaire to evaluate the perception of the quality of the sibling relationship. Participants completed all questionnaires, and no missing data were reported.

The study conformed to the Declaration of Helsinki. The Regional Ethics Committee for Clinical Trials of Tuscany, Pediatric Ethics Committee section, approved the study (ethical approval code: GENCU/03/2019). Recruitment took place from April 2019 to October 2020 and lasted 18 months.

2.2. Measures

Mothers completed the Child Behavior Check List (CBCL) parent report form and Alabama Parenting Questionnaire (APQ) for each child. Each child/adolescent completed a questionnaire that evaluates the perception of the quality of sibling relationship: Sibling Relationship Inventory (SRI).

Socio-demographic, clinical, and socio-economic status were collected from the mother using an ad hoc questionnaire.

The CBCL [56–58] was used to explore and record emotional and behavioral problems and skills in children aged 6–18 years. It is a 118-item scale, asking parents how often his/her child engages in problematic behaviors (i.e., item 28 "Breaks rules at home, school, or elsewhere"). According to questionnaire norms [56–58], CBCL presents 8 different syndrome scales, 6 different DSM-Oriented scales, a total problem score, and two broad-band scores designated as internalizing problems and externalizing problems. The reliability coefficients (Cronbach's alpha) were 0.82, 0.81, and 0.82, respectively.

The CBCL calculates a specific profile correlated to poor self-regulation in children and adolescents by summing the T Score of CBCL scale Anxious/Depressed, Attention Problems, and Aggression Behaviors. Emotional Self-Regulation (DESR) profile is given to those who present a summed score > 180 but < 210 and Dysregulation Profile (DP) as those who present a summed score $\geq$ 210 [59,60]. The DESR profile has been related to maladaptive behaviors in response to frustration or negative emotions, impulsivity, elevated irritability and anger, and high rates of anxiety and disruptive behavior disorders [61]. The DP has demonstrated usefulness as a marker of dysregulation and psychopathology severity in children and adolescents, and has been associated with severe psychopathology, self-harm and suicidal behaviors [59,62], and substance use disorders [63].

The APQ [64,65], was used to assess parenting practices and quality of the parent-child relationship. The APQ includes 42 items requiring parents to indicate the frequency with which they implement the parenting practices using a 5-point Likert scale, ranging from 1 (never) to 5 (always). According to Italian validation of the APQ [65], the parenting domains measured by this instrument are: (1) positive parenting (PP), comprising parental involvement and positive parenting (i.e., item 2: "You let your child know when he/she is doing a good job with something"); (2) negative parenting (NP), comprising poor monitoring/supervision, inconsistent discipline (i.e., item 24: "You get so busy that you forget where your child is and what he/she is doing"); (3) corporal punishment (CP) (i.e., item 33: "You spank your child with your hand when he/she has done something wrong"). The subscale score is derived by a sum of the items. Higher scores indicate adequate parenting practices for the positive scale, inadequate parenting practices for the negative scale, and corporal punishment. In this study, the Cronbach α coefficients were 0.73 for Positive Parenting, 0.68 for Negative Parenting, and 0.74 for Corporal Punishment.

The SRI [66,67] was used to assess the quality of sibling relationship. This is a 17-item questionnaire developed to assess the child's perception of own behavior and own feelings towards sibling. The SRI assesses 3 qualitative dimensions of sibling relationship: (1) Affection, referring to behaviors of support, help, sharing and admiration between siblings (i.e., item 1: "Do you happen to take care of your brother or sister or deal with him/her if there are no adults?"), (2) Conflict, defined as disagreement and quarrels (i.e., item 3: "Do you happen to be very angry with your brother/sister?"); (3) Rivalry, which is the perception that children have of differential treatment from their parents (i.e., item 11: "Do you also think that your mother treats your brother/sister better than you?"). Individuals are required to indicate how often they experience content of item on a 5-point Likert scale ranging from 1 (never) to 5 (always). Total score is obtained summing the scores for the three dimensions. The questionnaire was proposed to each child as an interview, preceded by an opening statement with the aim of normalizing a certain behavior or feeling, which allows comparison of the representation that children have of the sibling relationship. The interviews were carried out by a graduate student. The Italian version of the SRI confirmed the three-factor structure of the original version and its reliability to assess qualitative aspects of the sibling relationship [67]. In this study, Cronbach's alpha values of Affection, Conflict, and Rivalry dimensions were 0.73, 0.71, and 0.71, respectively.

2.3. Data Analysis

Data were analyzed using the Statistical Package for Social Sciences (SPSS), version 24 (2017). A post hoc power analysis was conducted using the software package, GPower 3.1.9.4. This post hoc analyses revealed the statistical power for this study was 0.98.

Descriptive statistics of quantitative data was performed for all dimensions. The normality of the dimensions was tested, using the directions of Curran and colleagues as criterion, which identified an accepted range for skewness from -2 to $+2$ and for kurtosis from -7 to $+7$ [68].

In order to verify whether the child and his/her sibling scored significantly different from each other in parenting style dimensions and sibling relationship we conducted, a t-test for paired sample separately for clinical and control group inserting the mean value of APQ and SRI dimensions reported by child and his/her sibling as paired variable.

Moreover, in order to verify whether there was a difference between clinical child (DBD), non-clinical siblings of DBD (S-DBD) and children of control group (CONTR), in parenting style, sibling relationship and psychopathological disorders, a series of one-way Analysis of CoVariance (ANCOVA) have been conducted inserting groups of children (DBD, S-DBD and CONTR) as factor, study variables (parenting style dimensions of APQ, sibling relationship dimensions of SRI, psychopathological disorders subscales of CBCL) as dependent variables, and gender as covariate. We decided to insert gender as covariate because wide literature showed that DBD is highly prevalent in males than females. For multiple comparisons, Bonferroni corrections were applied. Finally, post hoc tests were performed to evaluate how three groups differ in parenting style, sibling relationship and psychopathological disorders. The alpha level was set to $p = 0.05$ for all tests with confidence interval at 95%.

Finally, in order to verify whether there was a difference between clinical child (DBD), non-clinical siblings of DBD (S-DBD) and children of control group (CONTR), in distribution of presence and absence of CBCL-Dysregulation Profile a Chi-square was performed.

3. Results

3.1. Difference between Clinical and Control Group Families

Socio-demographic features of two groups are reported in Table 1.

Table 1. Comparison between Clinical and control group families in socio-demographic features.

	Clinical Group $n = 27$	Control Group $n = 34$	Statistics
Parental marital status			$Chi^2(1) = 1.23$; n.s.
Married	20 (74%)	28 (82%)	
Divorced	7 (26%)	6 (18%)	
N children for family			$Chi^2(3) = 4.42$; n.s.
2	15 (56%)	25 (74%)	
3	8 (30%)	6 (17%)	
4	3 (5%)	2 (6%)	
5	1 (4%)	1 (3%)	
Maternal SES			$Chi^2(3) = 6.66$; n.s.
salariat	6 (22.2%)	9 (26.5%)	
intermediate	15 (55.6%)	22 (64.7%)	
working class	2 (7.4%)	0 (0%)	
unemployed	4 (14.8%)	3 (8.8%)	
Paternal SES			$Chi^2(3) = 6.18$; n.s.
salariat	9 (33.3%)	8 (23.5%)	
intermediate	10 (37%)	19 (55.9%)	
working class	7 (25.9%)	7 (10.6%)	
unemployed	1 (3.7%)	0 (0%)	

Note: SES: Socio Economic Status.

T test and Chi square test were performed in order to verify if differences existed between clinical and control group in demographic variables. Results showed no difference in families of clinical and control group respect to parental marital status, number of children for family, maternal socio-economic level and paternal socio-economic level. All participants came from traditional families (mother-father), irrespectively by parental marital status reported (married or divorced).

Difference between offspring of clinical and control group.

Concerning offspring characteristics, data analysis showed no difference for age (clinical group M = 9.9; DS = 2; control group M = 9.8; DS = 2.2; t(120) = 0.34; n.s.), gender composition (% of males in clinical group = 49.4% versus control group = 50.6% $Chi^2(1) = 2.56$; n.s.), and years of scholarship (clinical group M = 4.65; DS = 1.9 versus control group M = 4.62; DS = 2.1; t(120) = 0.08; n.s.).

All DBD children (27; 100%) received a clinical diagnosis of ODD with a prevalence of comorbidity with ADHD (19; 70.4%).

In line with the literature and characteristics of the disorder, the DBD group was mainly composed of males (25; 93%). A Chi-square test showed that there were differences in gender composition within clinical group sibling dyad ($Chi^2(1) = 9.63$; $p = 0.002$) because males were 93% of DBD versus 56% of S-DBDs. On the contrary no difference has been found for gender composition in control group (56% of males in CONTR-1 versus 65% in CONTR-2; $Chi^2(1) = 0.553$; n.s.).

3.2. Difference within Sibling Dyad

APQ and SRI mean scores reported by pair of siblings in clinical and control group are reported in Table 2.

Table 2. Mean (SD) reported by clinical sibling (DBD), non-clinical sibling of clinical family (S-DBD), control sibling 1 (CONTR-1) and control sibling 2 (CONTR-2) in APQ and SRI subscales. Results of t test are reported for both groups.

	Clinical Group		t(26)	p	Control Group		t(33)	p
	DBD	S-DBD			CONTR-1	CONTR-2		
APQ positive parenting	47.67 (4.60)	47.37 (4.65)	0.497	n.s.	46.65 (5.01)	47.23 (5.26)	−1.31	n.s.
APQ negative parenting	14.67 (4.22)	12.14 (4.14)	2.58	0.016	10.79 (3.59)	10.73 (3.54)	0.208	n.s.
APQ corporal punishment	4.41 (2.20)	4.33 (1.68)	0.311	n.s.	3.53 (0.896)	3.91 (1.28)	−1.97	n.s.
SRI affection	21.72 (6.96)	24.36 (5.74)	−1.51	n.s.	24.38 (3.29)	22.52 (4.86)	1.88	n.s.
SRI conflict	15.76 (4.09)	13.89 (3.55)	1.659	n.s.	13.41 (4.01)	14.08 (4.01)	−0.99	n.s.
SRI rivalry	8.04 (3.86)	7.88 (3.44)	0.148	n.s.	6.85 (3.40)	6.58 (2.54)	0.40	n.s.

A t-test for paired sample was performed separately for clinical and control group to verify whether sibling dyad differ in parenting style (APQ subscales), sibling relationship (SRI subscales). Results of t-test are reported in Table 2.

Concerning the APQ, no difference within the sibling dyad was found in the clinical group in positive parenting or corporal punishment. On the contrary, a difference emerged in negative parenting, with the parent reporting more negative parenting toward DBD child than S-DBD.

Moreover, no difference within the sibling dyad was found in the control group in positive parenting, negative parenting or corporal punishment.

Concerning to SRI no difference within sibling dyad was found in the clinical or control group in affection, conflict and rivalry.

3.3. Difference between Clinical, Non-Clinical Siblings and Control Group

APQ, SRI and CBCL subscale scores reported by DBD, S-DBD and CONTR are showed in Table 3.

Table 3. Mean (SD) reported by clinical sibling (DBD), non-clinical sibling of clinical family (S-DBD) and non-clinical sibling of control group (CONTR) in APQ, SRI and CBCL subscales. Results of one-way ANCOVA are reported.

	DBD M (SD)	S-DBD M (SD)	CONTR M (SD)	F (2117)	p	Adjusted η²	Post-Hoc
APQ							
Positive parenting	47.67 (4.60)	47.37 (4.65)	47.10 (5.12)	0.182	n.s.	0.003	
Negative parenting	14.67 (4.22)	12.14 (4.14)	10.76 (3.54)	9.00	0.000	0.132	DBD > CONTR
Corporal punishment	4.41 (2.20)	4.33 (1.68)	3.72 (1.12)	2.44	n.s.	0.040	
SRI							
Affection	21.72 (6.96)	24.36 (5.74)	23.46 (4.23)	2.16	n.s.	0.036	
Conflict	15.76 (4.09)	13.89 (3.55)	13.75 (4.0)	2.91	n.s.	0.026	
Rivalry	8.04 (3.86)	7.88 (3.44)	6.69 (2.98)	2.50	n.s.	0.041	
CBCL							
Internalizing	62.56 (8.75)	56.62 (9.41)	49.82 (10.54)	13.57	0.000	0.188	DBD > S-DBD > CONTR
Externalizing	66.93 (8.45)	54.0 (8.29)	46.48 (7.65)	55.67	0.000	0.488	DBD > S-DBD > CONTR
Anxious/depressed	64.78 (8.87)	57.81 (6.90)	54.30 (5.74)	18.22	0.000	0.238	DBD > S-DBD > CONTR
Withdrawn/Depressed	60.93 (8.53)	57.88 (9.83)	54.28 (6.53)	5.70	0.004	0.089	DBD > S-DBD > CONTR
Somatic complain	56.15 (6.55)	56.29 (5.17)	54.60 (5.39)	1.05	n.s.	0.018	
Social prob.	62.44 (6.36)	55.96 (5.86)	53.49 (4.68)	23.75	0.000	0.289	DBD > S-DBD > CONTR
Thought prob.	61.33 (7.30)	54.92 (5.63)	53.39 (5.24)	15.72	0.000	0.212	DBD > S-DBD > CONTR
Attention prob.	67.15 (8.07)	60.07 (8.49)	53.15 (3.75)	46.98	0.000	0.445	DBD > S-DBD > CONTR
Rules breaking	61.81 (8.11)	55.62 (4.87)	52.03 (3.37)	32.72	0.000	0.359	DBD > S-DBD > CONTR
Aggressive behavior	69.33 (10.84)	56.0 (6.63)	52.12 (3.17)	60.06	0.000	0.507	DBD > S-DBD > CONTR
DSM Affective prob.	65.04 (8.06)	58.85 (7.66)	54.18 (5.98)	21.23	0.000	0.266	DBD > S-DBD > CONTR
DSM anxiety prob.	63.74 (8.01)	58.40 (7.74)	55.27 (6.08)	11.03	0.000	0.159	DBD > S-DBD > CONTR
DSM somatic prob.	54.56 (7.98)	54.22 (4.79)	54.10 (4.92)	0.03	n.s.	0.001	
DSM ADHD prob.	67.93 (9.32)	58.44 (8.93)	52.03 (3.04)	52.16	0.000	0.471	DBD > S-DBD > CONTR
DSM ODT	65.33 (8.99)	55.70 (5.29)	52.63 (3.25)	44.20	0.000	0.430	DBD > S-DBD > CONTR
DSM conduct prob.	65.19 (8.72)	54.92 (4.92)	51.69 (2.97)	56.81	0.000	0.493	DBD > S-DBD > CONTR

Note. Prob.: Problem; ODT: Oppositional Defiant Problems.

A series of one-way ANCOVA inserting as dependent variables the APQ dimensions found no differences in positive parenting or corporal punishment among the three groups. On the contrary, a difference exists in negative parenting where DBD reported higher level of negative parenting than CONTR whilst adjusting for gender.

A series of one-way ANCOVA inserting as dependent variables the SRI dimensions showed that any difference exist in affection, conflict and rivalry between three groups whilst adjusting for gender. A series of one-way ANCOVAs inserting the CBCL dimensions as dependent variables showed that there were differences between the three groups in all scales and subscales of the CBCL questionnaire, except for somatic complaint, DSM somatic. DBD reported higher levels of disorder than S-DBD and CONTR children.

Results of ANCOVA are reported in Table 3.

3.4. DESR and DP Profile

The Chi-square test was performed using the distribution of DP among DBD, S-DBD and CONTR groups. Results showed that, among DBD children 9 (33.3%), presented DP, 11 (40.7%) DESR and 7 (26%) regular scores (above cut-off). Among S-DBD 2 children (7.4%) presented DP, 6 (22.2%) DESR and 19 (70.4%) regular score; in the CONTR group, none of children (0%) presented DP, one (1.5%) presented DESR and 67 (98.5%) regular scores. The difference of profile distribution among DBD and CONTR is significant (Chi^2 (4) = 58.95; p = 0.000). In fact, while DBD presented higher prevalence of DP and DESR, while CONTR presented higher prevalence of regular scores.

4. Discussion

Literature has widely shown the role of the family in shaping DBD in children and adolescents. However, studies mainly focus on the impact of parenting style on DBD children [25,69,70], neglecting the presence of siblings. A perspective that takes into consideration parenting style effect on sibling dyads (including non-clinical ones) may identify risk and protective factors for psychological adjustment of the offspring from the same family, in order to better address preventive interventions.

In this framework, this study aimed to explore the parenting style and sibling relationship reported in sibling dyads of clinical families (where one child had been diagnosed with DBD and the other had not received any psychiatric diagnosis) compared to control families (in which there were two non-clinical siblings).

This study also aimed to compare parenting style, sibling relationship, and emotional and behavior problems reported in clinical child (DBD), non-clinical sibling (S-DBD), and non-clinical child of control families (CONTR). To our knowledge, this observational study is the first to explore and compare the parenting style reported toward two children (clinical and non-clinical) in families with DBDs and control families.

Our results show that there is higher differential and negative parenting in clinical families compared to control group families. Specifically, negative parenting is reported more often toward the DBD child compared to his/her sibling. On the contrary, control families reported a similar style across offspring. Results seem to confirm that even when siblings live in the same family context, they can experience different relationships with the same parents [37,71], and be exposed to different levels of harsh and supportive parenting, thus resulting in different adjustments [70,72]. Our study therefore confirms the link between higher negative parenting, which includes harsh parenting, coercive, controlling and punitive methods, and DBDs [25]. However, in contrast with previous research [23,25], in our study, the level of parental corporal punishment towards DBD did not differ from that reported by S-DBD and control sibling.

However, when we compared parenting styles adopted toward DBD, S-DBD, and control child, it emerged that, although lower levels of negative parenting were reported towards S-DBDs than their DBD siblings, these levels of negative parenting were higher than toward non-clinical siblings of the control group. The post-hoc analysis revealed that the main difference concerned DBDs who reported more negative parenting than CONTR.

A possible explanation for this result may be the higher levels of parenting stress generated by the presence of a DBD child in clinical families [73,74], which induces parents to use negative parenting also toward the non-clinical sibling. Literature has widely shown an association between parenting stress and negative parenting [75–78], and between negative parenting and child difficulties, including externalizing behavior problems and adolescent deviance [79,80]. Thus, in line with the available literature [13,81–84], the use of negative parenting may be in part responsible for the severity of psychological disorders (as resulting from CBCL subscales scores). In our sample, DBD children, in a greater measure, and S-DBDs, in a lesser measure, reported higher externalizing problems (including rule-breaking behavior, aggressive behavior) than control siblings. It is possible that S-DBDs, despite being non-clinical siblings, could be at higher risk for externalizing disorders compared to non-clinical siblings growing up in non-clinical families, thus directly (personally) and/or indirectly (through observation of negative parenting style toward clinical sibling) exposed to negative parenting. In line with the literature, we could hypothesize that the clinical manifestation of DBDs (which includes irritability, aggression, and temper outburst) also constitutes a risk factor for the development of externalizing problems by siblings [81,82].

S-DBD children seem at higher risk for internalizing problems, such as anxious/depressed and withdrawn/depressed, compared to CONTR. In the case of internalizing problems and withdrawn/depressed scales, the level of problems reported by S-DBDs is not only higher than controls, but it is comparable to that reported by DBDs. A possible explanation is the parenting style. Several studies have reported an association between negative parenting (characterized by high levels of coercive control and negative emotionality) and internalizing more than externalizing symptoms [83]. In this case, it is possible that negative parenting reported toward DBDs and S-DBDs in clinical families increases the risk of internalizing problems in the offspring in general. Other explanations that must not be excluded are stressful life events, as well as negative and less supportive relationships with other family members, such as the father or other siblings, which may increase the possibility to develop internalizing problems. In literature, internalizing problems in DBDs have been described as predictors of persistence of externalizing problems in adolescents and/or of development of internalizing disorders over time [84,85]. Our research group has shown the efficacy of multimodal, CBT-based treatment involving DBD children and their parents, in improving internalizing problems in ODD patients by promoting effective and warm parenting, and supporting affect regulation and self–esteem in children [86]. We suppose that improvement in parenting style could have a positive effect in prevention of DBD sibling risk of internalizing problems.

Regarding emotional dysregulation profiles, the present study shows that about seven children in ten with DBDs manifest the clinical or severe profile of dysregulation (three in ten reported DP and four in ten reported DESR). This evidence is not surprising, because it is in line with the scientific literature that highlights the presence of poor emotional and behavioral self-regulation in children with DBDs alone or in comorbidity with ADHD and emotional problems [87–89].

An interesting result is the presence of a relevant percentage of DP in the S-DBD population; in fact, about three children in ten showed a clinical or severe profile (DESR and DP), while in the control group only 1.5% presented DESR and none reported DP. Our findings seem to suggest that not only clinical DBD children, but also non-clinical siblings of DBD families, show psychopathological vulnerability, being more prone to develop DESR and DP compared to the control group. The higher psychopathological vulnerability of S-DBD may be influenced by both environmental (such as parenting strategies) and genetic factors shared by the siblings in the clinical families. These data are worthy of attention, since the presence of DESR or DP could be considered both an indicator of clinical severity and a risk factor for developmental, emotional, or behavioral disorders from childhood to adulthood [63].

For this reason, during the diagnostic evaluation of the clinical child, the non-clinical sibling could also be involved, in order to identify or prevent the onset of emotional and behavioral problems early on. There is strong evidence that multimodal treatment programs for DBDs, usually including both youths and parents, have high efficacy in reducing externalizing behaviors and aggression in at-risk and clinic-referred youths [80,90–92]. Involvement of parents, aimed at reducing coercive strategies and promoting positive parenting styles, increases treatment efficacy [90,93], and could also have relevant positive effects for the siblings. It would be important to inform the families of children with DBDs about the potential psychopathological risks to the other children and provide intervention programs, such as parent training, to support positive parenting styles towards all offspring.

Regarding the sibling relationship, this study showed that there is no difference between sibling dyads for sibling relationship. In other words, both pairs of dyads reported the same sibling relationship. This is in line with the characteristics of the SRI. Moreover, no difference has been found for gender between DBD, S-DBD, and control children in affect, conflict, or rivalry. In other words, the sibling relationship in the clinical group is not characterized by more conflict compared to control group. It could be assumed that, due to the DBD clinical manifestation of disorder, the sibling relationship might be affected by greater levels of hostility; however, our results did not support this hypothesis.

Given the lack of difference between clinical and control groups, it seems that sibling relationship assumes a protective role in the clinical group. Thus, despite negative parenting reported toward DBDs and S-DBDs, the sibling relationship seems to be good enough for these children. This is a relevant aspect, because children spend more time with siblings than with parents, and within sibling dyads they develop social skills useful for future interactions with peers [94]. Like parent-child and peer relationships, sibling relationships provide an important socialization environment for children. Sibling relationships can be considered intense peer relationships, where children must learn to negotiate conflicts because they are unable to escape an aversive sibling relationship in the same manner as they would a peer [95].

According to our hypotheses, the results indicate a higher level of differential and negative parenting in clinical families, compared to control group families, confirming the link between higher negative parenting (i.e., harsh parenting, coercive, controlling and punitive methods), and DBDs and children with difficulties. Although negative parenting in clinical families is reported more often towards DBD children, DBD siblings showed higher levels than non-clinical siblings of the control group. The use of negative parenting seems to correlate with the severity of psychological disorders. In fact, in the clinical families, as resulting from CBCL subscale scores, higher externalizing problems (including rule-breaking behavior, aggressive behavior) were recorded not only in the DBD child, but also in the S-DBD, compared to control siblings (DBD > S-DBD > CONTR). Moreover, higher internalizing problems (including anxious/depressed and withdrawn/depressed) were recorded in DBD and S-DBD compared to control siblings (DBD = S-DBD > CONTR). In accordance with other studies [83], S-DBDs could be considered at higher risk for externalizing and internalizing problems than controls.

Contrary to our hypotheses, regarding sibling relationship, no differences between the two groups were found. In the clinical group, the sibling relationship seems to be good enough for these children, and in a preventive perspective, these data could highlight the importance of "protecting" the relationship between siblings in their growth path as a possible factor of resilience [50,95,96].

5. Strengths and Limitations of this Study

This is the first study that analyses the impact of parenting style on psychological disorders in DBD families (including both DBD clinical child and S-DBD non-clinical child) compared with non-clinical families. To this purpose, one of the main strengths of this study is the use of multiple source of information. In fact, we chose to include two siblings per family (who answered about sibling relationship), and one reference parent (who reported parenting style toward each child and psychological disorders shown by each child).

Although the sample size may appear quite small compared to other studies on sibling dyads [81], it must be noted that we chose to use strict inclusion criteria both for the clinical child (diagnosis of DBD according to DSM 5 instead of, for instance, the presence of externalizing behavior) and for sibling dyad (sibling dyads with maximum age spacing of four years in line with previous studies) [53]. The study presents a large effect size according to Cohen (1988) [97].

Second, we chose to consider only the mothers as reference parents, without involving fathers. We cannot exclude that paternal style may be different (i.e., more positive) than maternal, thus constituting a protective factor. The choice to consider the maternal report of parenting style comes from the consideration that Italian mothers play a major role both in and out of the home.

Finally, this is a cross sectional study. Thus, we cannot know if the parenting style changes over the time, including the level of psychological disorders expressed by the children.

6. Conclusions

In the developmental age, and more often in adolescence, there is physiological distancing in the sibling relationship, with a tendency to form their own groups of friends, who can often have interests in common and represent valid experiential contexts for prosocial purposes. In the case of families with DBDs, DBD children can dangerously tend to fit into groups of social marginalization that facilitate training in deviance with the adoption of highly antisocial values [98]. Maintaining a good sibling relationship could be a protective factor for DBDs against possible antisocial risks, and this aspect should be kept in mind, in cautionary and reinforcement messages to parents, and in therapeutic and preventive goals [99].

Finally, the involvement of parents in multimodal treatments to promote positive parenting could have positive effects not only for DBD children, but also for their siblings, in preventing internalizing and externalizing problems.

Author Contributions: Conceptualization A.M. and M.S.; Methodology, L.V. and E.I.; Formal Analysis, M.S.; Writing—Original Draft Preparation, M.S. and L.V.; Writing—Review and Editing, E.I., A.M.; Supervision, A.M. All authors have read and agreed to the published version of the manuscript.

Funding: This work has been supported by Ricerca Corrente (RC2763771), the 5 × 1000 voluntary contributions, Italian Ministry of Health.

Institutional Review Board Statement: The study conformed to the Declaration of Helsinki and the Regional Ethics Committee for Clinical Trials of Tuscany, Pediatric Ethics Committee section, approved the study (code 80/2018, data 7 June 2018; amendment code 62/2019 data 9 April 2019).

Informed Consent Statement: Written informed consent has been obtained from the patient(s) to publish this paper.

Data Availability Statement: Data are available by authors under reasonable request.

Acknowledgments: We wish to acknowledge the research staff from IRCCS Stella Maris Foundation involved in the study.

Conflicts of Interest: The authors declare no conflict of interest.

References

1. Coghill, D. Editorial: Do clinical services need to take conduct disorder more seriously? *J. Child Psychol. Psychiatry* **2013**, *54*, 921–923. [CrossRef] [PubMed]
2. Polanczyk, G.V.; Salum, G.A.; Sugaya, L.S.; Caye, A.; Rohde, L.A. Annual research review: A meta-analysis of the worldwide prevalence of mental disorders in children and adolescents. *J. Child Psychol. Psychiatry* **2015**, *56*, 345–365. [CrossRef]
3. Patalay, P.; Gage, S.H. Changes in millennial adolescent mental health and health-related behaviours over 10 years: A popula-tion cohort comparison study. *Int. J. Epidemiol.* **2019**, *48*, 1650–1664. [CrossRef] [PubMed]

4. American Psychiatric Association. *Diagnostic and Statistical Manual of Mental Disorders (DSM-5)*; American Psychiatric Asso-ciation: Philadelphia, PA, USA, 2013.
5. Moffitt, T.E.; Arseneault, L.; Jaffee, S.R.; Kim-Cohen, J.; Koenen, K.C.; Odgers, C.L.; Slutske, W.S.; Viding, E. Research review: DSM-V conduct disorder: Research needs for an evidence base. *J. Child Psychol. Psychiatry* **2008**, *49*, 3–33. [CrossRef] [PubMed]
6. Burke, J.D.; Hipwell, A.E.; Loeber, R. Dimensions of oppositional defiant disorder as predictors of depression and conduct disorder in preadolescent girls. *J. Am. Acad. Child Adolesc. Psychiatry* **2010**, *49*, 484–492. [CrossRef] [PubMed]
7. Fairchild, G.; Hawes, D.J.; Frick, P.J.; Copeland, W.E.; Odgers, C.L.; Franke, B.; Freitag, C.M.; De Brito, S.A. Conduct Disorder. *Nat. Rev.* **2019**, *5*, 43. [CrossRef]
8. Pardini, D.A.; Frick, P.J.; Moffitt, T.E. Building an evidence base for DSM-5 conceptualizations of oppositional defiant disorder and conduct disorder: Introduction to the special section. *J. Abnorm. Psychol.* **2010**, *119*, 683–688. [CrossRef]
9. Rivenbark, J.G.; Odgers, C.L.; Caspi, A.; Harrington, H.; Hogan, S.; Houts, R.M.; Poulton, R.; Moffitt, T.E. The high societal costs of childhood conduct problems: Evidence from administrative records up to age 38 in a longitudinal birth cohort. *J. Child Psychol. Psychiatry* **2018**, *59*, 703–710. [CrossRef]
10. Karwatowska, L.; Russell, S.; Solmi, F.; De Stavola, B.L.; Jaffee, S.; Pingault, J.-B.; Viding, E. Risk factors for disruptive behaviours: Protocol for a systematic review and meta-analysis of quasi-experimental evidence. *BMJ Open* **2020**, *10*, e038258. [CrossRef]
11. Jucksch, V.; Salbach-Andrae, H.; Lenz, K.; Goth, K.; Döpfner, M.; Poustka, F.; Holtmann, M. Severe affective and behavioural dysregulation is associated with significant psychosocial adversity and impairment. *Child Psychol. Psychiatry* **2011**, *52*, 686–695. [CrossRef]
12. Biederman, J.; Perry, C.R.; Day, H.; Goldin, R.L.; Spencer, T.; Faraone, S.V.; Surman, C.B.; Wozniak, J. Severity of the aggression/anxiety-depression/attention (A-A-A) CBCL profile discriminates between different levels of deficits in emotional regulation in youth with ADHD. *J. Dev. Behav. Pediatr.* **2012**, *33*, 236–243. [CrossRef]
13. Masi, G.; Muratori, P.; Manfredi, A.; Lenzi, F.; Polidori, L.; Ruglioni, L.; Muratori, F.; Milone, A. Response to treatments in youths with disruptive behavior disorders. *Compr. Psychiatry* **2013**, *54*, 1009–1015. [CrossRef]
14. Masi, G.; Pisano, S.; Milone, A.; Muratori, P. Child behavior checklist dysregulation profile in children with disruptive behavior disorders: A longitudinal study. *J. Affect. Disord.* **2015**, *186*, 249–253. [CrossRef] [PubMed]
15. Caspi, A. The child is father of the man: Personality continuities from childhood to adulthood. *J. Pers. Soc. Psychol.* **2000**, *78*, 158–172. [CrossRef] [PubMed]
16. Cavanagh, M.; Quinn, D.; Duncan, D.; Graham, T.; Balbuena, L.J. Oppositional Defiant Disorder Is Better Conceptualized as a Disorder of Emotional Regulation. *J. Atten. Disord.* **2017**, *21*, 381–389. [CrossRef] [PubMed]
17. Tremblay, R.E. Developmental origins of disruptive behaviour problems: The 'original sin' hypothesis, epigenetics and their consequences for prevention. *J. Child Psychol. Psychiatry* **2010**, *51*, 341–367. [CrossRef] [PubMed]
18. Pederson, C.A.; Fite, P.J. The impact of parenting on the associations between child aggression subtypes and oppositional defiant disorder symptoms. *Child Psychiatry Hum. Dev.* **2014**, *45*, 728–735. [CrossRef]
19. Bornovalova, M.A.; Hicks, B.M.; Iacono, W.G.; McGue, M. Familial transmission and heritability of childhood disruptive disorders. *Am. J. Psychiatry* **2010**, *167*, 1066–1074. [CrossRef] [PubMed]
20. Caspi, A.; McClay, J.; Moffitt, T.E.; Mill, J.; Martin, J.; Craig, I.W.; Taylor, A.; Poulton, R. Role of genotype in the cycle of violence in maltreated children. *Science* **2002**, *297*, 851–854. [CrossRef]
21. Rowe, R.; Costello, E.J.; Angold, A.; Copeland, W.E.; Maughan, B. Developmental pathways in oppositional defiant disorder and conduct disorder. *J. Abnorm. Psychol.* **2010**, *119*, 726–738. [CrossRef]
22. Tistarelli, N.; Fagnani, C.; Troianiello, M.; Stazi, M.A.; Adriani, W. The nature and nurture of ADHD and its comorbidities: A narrative review on twin studies. *Neurosci. Biobehav. Rev.* **2020**, *109*, 63–77. [CrossRef] [PubMed]
23. Malmberg, K.; Wargelius, H.L.; Lichtenstein, P.; Oreland, L.; Larsson, J.O. ADHD and Disruptive Behavior scores—Associations with MAO-A and 5-HTT genes and with platelet MAO-B activity in adolescents. *BMC Psychiatry* **2008**, *8*, 28. [CrossRef] [PubMed]
24. Stormshak, E.A.; Bierman, K.L.; McMahon, R.J.; Lengua, L.J. Parenting practices and child disruptive behavior problems in early elementary school. *J. Clin. Child Psychol.* **2000**, *29*, 17–29. [CrossRef] [PubMed]
25. Calkins, S.D.; Keane, S.P. Developmental origins of early antisocial behavior. *Dev. Psychopathol.* **2009**, *21*, 1095–1109. [CrossRef]
26. Muratori, P.; Milone, A.; Nocentini, A.; Manfredi, A.; Polidori, L.; Ruglioni, L.; Lambruschi, F.; Masi, G.; Lochmann, J.E. Maternal Depression and Parenting Practices Predict Treatment Outcome in Italian Children with Disruptive Behavior Disorder. *J. Child Fam. Stud.* **2015**, *24*, 2805–2816. [CrossRef]
27. Clark, J.E.; Frick, P.J. Positive parenting and callous-unemotional traits: Their association with school behavior problems in young children. *J. Clin. Child Adolesc. Psychol.* **2016**, *47*, S242–S254. [CrossRef]
28. Waller, R.; Gardner, F.; Hyde, L.W. What are the associations between parenting, callous–unemotional traits, and antisocial behavior in youth? A systematic review of evidence. *Clin. Psychol. Rev.* **2013**, *33*, 593–608. [CrossRef]
29. Waller, R.; Gardner, F.; Viding, E.; Shaw, D.S.; Dishion, T.J.; Wilson, M.N.; Hyde, L.W. Bidirectional associations between pa-rental warmth, callous unemotional behavior, and behavior problems in high-risk preschoolers. *J. Abnorm. Child Psychol.* **2014**, *42*, 1275–1285. [CrossRef]
30. Muratori, P.; Lochman, J.E.; Lai, E.; Milone, A.; Nocentini, A.; Pisano, S.; Righini, E.; Masi, G. Which dimension of parenting predicts the change of callous unemotional traits in children with disruptive behavior disorder? *Compr. Psychiatry* **2016**, *69*, 202–210. [CrossRef] [PubMed]

31. Patterson, G.R. The early development of coercive family process. In *Antisocial Behavior in Children and Adolescents: A Developmental Analysis and Model for Intervention*; Reid, J.B., Patterson, G.R., Snyder, J., Eds.; American Psychological Association: Washington, DC, USA, 2002.
32. Pettit, G.S.; Arsiwalla, D.D. Commentary on special section on "bidirectional parent–child relationships": The continuing evolution of dynamic, transactional models of parenting and youth behavior problems. *J. Child Psychol. Psychiatry* **2008**, *36*, 711–718. [CrossRef] [PubMed]
33. Deater-Deckard, K. Annotation: Recent research examining the role of peer relationships in the development of psychopathology. *J. Child Psychol. Psychiatry* **2001**, *42*, 565–579. [CrossRef]
34. Richmond, M.K.; Stocker, C.M.; Rienks, S.L. Longitudinal associations between sibling relationship quality, parental differential treatment, and children's adjustment. *J. Fam. Psychol.* **2005**, *19*, 550–559. [CrossRef]
35. Asbury, K.; Dunn, J.; Plomin, R. Birthweight-discordance and differences in early parenting relate to monozygotic twin differences in behaviour problems and academic achievement at age 7. *Dev. Sci.* **2006**, *9*, 22–31. [CrossRef]
36. Asbury, K.; Dunn, J.; Plomin, R. The use of discordant MZ twins to generate hypotheses regarding non-shared environmental influence on anxiety in middle childhood. *Soc. Dev.* **2006**, *15*, 564–570. [CrossRef]
37. Burt, S.A.; McGue, M.; Iacono, W.G.; Krueger, R.F. Differential Parent-child Relationships and Adolescent Externalizing Symptoms: Cross-Lagged Analyses within a Twin Differences Design. *Dev. Psychol.* **2006**, *42*, 1289–1298. [CrossRef]
38. Mullineaux, P.Y.; Deater-Deckard, K.; Petrill, S.A.; Thompson, L.A. Parenting and child behaviour problems: A longitudinal analysis of non-shared environment. *Infant Child Dev.* **2009**, *18*, 133–148. [CrossRef]
39. Ilomäki, E.; Viilo, K.; Hakko, H.; Marttunen, M.; Mäkikyrö, T.; Räsänen, P. Familial risks, conduct disorder and violence: A Finnish study of 278 adolescent boys and girls. *Eur. Child Adolesc. Psychiatry* **2006**, *15*, 46–51. [CrossRef] [PubMed]
40. Feinberg, M.E.; Hetherington, E.M. Differential parenting as a within-family variable. *J. Fam. Psychol.* **2001**, *15*, 22–37. [CrossRef] [PubMed]
41. Stocker, C.M.; McHale, S. The nature and family correlates of preadolescents' perceptions of their sibling relationships. *J. Soc. Pers. Relat.* **1992**, *9*, 179–185. [CrossRef]
42. Dalsgaard, S.; Ostergaard, S.D.; Leckman, J.F.; Mortensen, P.B.; Pedersen, M.G. Mortality in children, adolescents, and adults with attention deficit hyperactivity disorder: A nationwide cohort study. *Lancet* **2015**, *385*, 2190–2196. [CrossRef]
43. Maibing, C.F.; Pedersen, C.B.; Benros, M.E.; Mortensen, P.B.; Dalsgaard, S.; Nordentoft, M. Risk of schizophrenia increases after all child and adolescent psychiatric disorders: A nationwide study. *Schizophr. Bull.* **2015**, *41*, 963–970. [CrossRef]
44. Erskine, H.E.; Ferrari, A.J.; Polanczyk, G.V.; Moffitt, T.E.; Murray, C.J.; Vos, T.; Whiteford, H.A.; Scott, J.G. The global burden of conduct disorder and attention-deficit/hyperactivity disorder in 2010. *J. Child Psychol. Psychiatry* **2014**, *55*, 328–336. [CrossRef]
45. Carrà, E.; Marta, E. *Relazioni Familiari e Adolescenza [Family Relationships and Adolescence]*; Franco Angeli: Milano, Italy, 1995.
46. Scabini, E. Parent–child relationships in Italian families: Connectedness and autonomy in the transition to adulthood. *Psicol. Teor. Pesqui.* **2000**, *16*, 023–030. [CrossRef]
47. McArdle, P.; Wiegersma, A.; Gilvarry, E.; Kolte, B.; McCarthy, S.; Fitzgerald, M.; Brinkley, A.; Blom, M.; Stoeckel, I.; Pierolini, A.; et al. European adolescent substance use: The roles of family structure, function and gender. *Addiction* **2002**, *97*, 329–336. [CrossRef]
48. Smorti, M.; Guarnieri, S.; Ingoglia, S. The parental bond, resistance to peer influence, and risky driving in adolescence. *Transp. Res. Part F Traffic Psychol. Behav.* **2014**, *22*, 184–195. [CrossRef]
49. Brody, G.H.; Stoneman, Z.; McCoy, J.K. Associations of maternal and paternal direct and differential behavior with sibling relationships: Contemporaneous and longitudinal analyses. *Child Dev.* **1992**, *63*, 82–92. [CrossRef] [PubMed]
50. McHale, S.M.; Updegraff, K.A.; Whiteman, S.D. Sibling Relationships and Influences in Childhood and Adolescence. *J. Marriage Fam.* **2012**, *74*, 913–930. [CrossRef] [PubMed]
51. Singer, A.T.; Weinstein, R.S. Differential parental treatment predicts achievement and self-perceptions in two cultural contexts. *J. Fam. Psychol.* **2000**, *14*, 491–509. [CrossRef]
52. Shanahan, L.; McHale, S.M.; Crouter, A.C.; Osgood, D. Linkages between parents' differential treatment, youth depressive symptoms, and sibling relationships. *J. Marriage Fam.* **2008**, *70*, 480–494. [CrossRef]
53. Tamrouti-Makkink, I.D.; Dubas, J.S.; Gerris, J.R.; van Aken, M.A. The relation between the absolute level of parenting and differential parental treatment with adolescent siblings' adjustment. *J. Child Psychol. Psychiatry* **2004**, *45*, 1397–1406. [CrossRef]
54. Kaufman, J.; Birmaher, B.; Brent, D.; Rao, U.; Flynn, C.; Moreci, P.; Williamson, D.; Ryan, N. Schedule for affective disorders and schizophrenia for school-age children-present and lifetime version (K-SADS-PL): Initial reliability and validity data. *J. Am. Acad. Child Adolesc. Psychiatry* **1997**, *36*, 980–988. [CrossRef] [PubMed]
55. Wechsler, D. *WISC-IV Technical and Interpretive Manual*; The Psychological Association: San Antonio, TX, USA, 2003.
56. Achenbach, T.; Rescorla, L. *Manual for the ASEBA School-Age Forms & Profiles*; University of Vermont: Burlington, VT, USA, 2001.
57. Achenbach, T.M.; Dumenci, L.; Rescorla, L.A. DSM-oriented and empirically based approaches to constructing scales from the same item pools. *J. Clin. Child Adolesc. Psychol.* **2003**, *32*, 328–340. [CrossRef] [PubMed]
58. Frigerio, A.; Vanzin, L.; Pastore, V.; Nobile, M.; Giorda, R.; Marino, C.; Molteni, M.; Rucci, P.; Ammaniti, M.; Lucarelli, L.; et al. The Italian preadolescent mental health project (PrISMA): Rationale and methods. *Int. J. Methods Psychiatr. Res.* **2006**, *5*, 22–35. [CrossRef] [PubMed]

59. Masi, G.; Muratori, P.; Manfredi, A.; Pisano, S.; Milone, A. Child Behaviour Checklist emotional dysregulation profiles in youth with disruptive behaviour disorders: Clinical correlates and treatment implications. *Psychiatry Res.* **2015**, *225*, 191–196. [CrossRef]
60. Muratori, P.; Pisano, S.; Milone, A.; Masi, G. Is emotional dysregulation a risk indicator for auto-aggression behaviors in adolescents with oppositional defiant disorder? *J. Affect. Disord.* **2017**, *208*, 110–112. [CrossRef]
61. Biederman, J.; Petty, C.R.; Monuteaux, M.C.; Evans, M.; Parcell, T.; Faraone, S.V.; Wozniak, J. The child behavior checklist-pediatric bipolar disorder profile predicts a subsequent diagnosis of bipolar disorder and associated impairments in ADHD youth growing up: A longitudinal analysis. *J. Clin. Psychiatry* **2009**, *70*, 732–740. [CrossRef]
62. Ayer, L.; Althoff, R.; Ivanova, M.; Rettew, D.; Waxler, E.; Sulman, J.; Hudziak, J. Child Behavior Checklist Juvenile Bipolar Disorder (CBCL-JBD) and CBCL Posttraumatic Stress Problems (CBCL-PTSP) scales are measures of a single dysregulatory syndrome. *J. Child Psychol. Psychiatry* **2009**, *50*, 1291–1300. [CrossRef]
63. Holtmann, M.; Buchmann, A.F.; Esser, G.; Schmidt, M.H.; Banaschewski, T.; Laucht, M. The Child Behavior Checklist-Dysregulation Profile predicts substance use, suicidality, and functional impairment: A longitudinal analysis. *J. Child Psychol. Psychiatry* **2011**, *52*, 139–147. [CrossRef]
64. Sheldon, K.K.; Frick, P.J.; Wootton, J. Assessment of parenting practices in families of elementary school-age children. *J. Clin. Child Psychol* **1996**, *25*, 317–329. [CrossRef]
65. Esposito, A.; Servera, M.; Garcia-Banda, G.; Del Giudice, E. Factor analysis of the Italian version of the Alabama Parenting Questionnaire in a community sample. *J. Child. Fam. Stud.* **2016**, *25*, 1208–1217. [CrossRef]
66. Stocker, C.M.; Lanthier, R.P.; Furman, W. Sibling relationships in early adulthood. *J. Fam. Psychol.* **1997**, *11*, 210–221. [CrossRef]
67. Lecce, S.; De Bernart, D.; Vezzani, C.; Pinto, G.; Primi, C. Measuring the quality of the sibling relationship during middle childhood: The psychometric properties of the Sibling Relationship Inventory. *Eur. J. Dev. Psychol.* **2011**, *8*, 423–436. [CrossRef]
68. Curran, P.J.; West, S.G.; Finch, J.F. The robustness of test statistics to non normality and specification error in confirmatory factor analysis. *Psychol. Methods* **1996**, *1*, 16–29. [CrossRef]
69. Burke, J.D.; Pardini, D.A.; Loeber, R. Reciprocal relationships between parenting behavior and disruptive psychopathology from childhood through adolescence. *J. Abnorm. Child Psychol.* **2008**, *36*, 679–692. [CrossRef] [PubMed]
70. Tung, I.; Lee, S.S. Negative parenting behavior and childhood oppositional defiant disorder: Differential moderation by positive and negative peer regard. *Aggress. Behav.* **2014**, *40*, 79–90. [CrossRef]
71. Dunn, J.F.; Stocker, C.; Plomin, R. Nonshared experiences within the family: Correlates of behavioral problems in middle childhood. *Dev. Psychopathol.* **1990**, *2*, 113–125. [CrossRef]
72. Jeannin, R.; Van Leeuwen, K. Associations between direct and indirect perceptions of parental differential treatment and child socio-emotional adaptation. *J. Child Fam. Stud.* **2015**, *24*, 1838–1855. [CrossRef]
73. Hart, M.S.; Kelley, M.L. Fathers' and mothers' work and family issues as related to internalizing and externalizing behavior of children attending day care. *J. Fam. Stress* **2006**, *27*, 252–270. [CrossRef]
74. Spratt, E.G.; Saylor, C.F.; Macias, M.M. Assessing parenting stress in multiple samples of children with special needs (CSN). *Fam. Syst. Health* **2007**, *25*, 435–449. [CrossRef]
75. Abidin, R.R. *Parenting Stress Index*, 2nd ed.; Pediatric Psychology Press: Charlottesville, VA, USA, 1986.
76. Deater-Deckard, K.; Scarr, S. Parenting stress among dual-earner mothers and fathers: Are there gender differences? *J. Fam. Psychol.* **1996**, *1*, 45–59. [CrossRef]
77. Le, Y.; Fredman, S.J.; Feinberg, M.E. Parenting stress mediates the association between negative affectivity and harsh parenting: A longitudinal dyadic analysis. *J. Fam. Psychol.* **2017**, *31*, 679–688. [CrossRef]
78. Mak, M.C.K.; Yin, L.; Li, M.; Cheung, R.Y.-H.; Oon, P.-T. The Relation between Parenting Stress and Child Behavior Problems: Negative Parenting Styles as Mediator. *J. Child Fam. Stud.* **2020**, *29*, 2993–3003. [CrossRef]
79. Qi, C.H.; Kaiser, A.P. Behavior problems of preschool children from low-income families: Review of the literature. *Top. Early Child. Spec. Educ.* **2003**, *23*, 188–216. [CrossRef]
80. Bradley, R.H.; Corwyn, R.F. Externalizing problems in fifth grade: Relations with productive activity, maternal sensitivity, and harsh parenting from infancy through middle childhood. *Dev. Psychol.* **2007**, *43*, 1390–1401. [CrossRef]
81. Craine, J.L.; Tanaka, T.A.; Nishina, A.; Conger, K.J. Understanding adolescent delinquency: The role of older siblings' delinquency and popularity with peers. *Merrill-Palmer Q.* **2009**, *55*, 436. [CrossRef] [PubMed]
82. Defoe, I.N.; Keijsers, L.; Hawk, S.T.; Branje, S.; Dubas, J.S.; Buist, K.; Frijns, T.; van Aken, M.A.; Koot, H.M.; van Lier, P.A.; et al. Siblings versus parents and friends: Longitudinal linkages to adolescent externalizing problems. *J. Child Psychol. Psychiatry* **2013**, *54*, 881–889. [CrossRef] [PubMed]
83. Pinquart, M. Associations of parenting dimensions and styles with externalizing problems of children and adolescents: An updated meta-analysis. *Dev. Psychol.* **2017**, *53*, 873. [CrossRef]
84. Jacobs, R.H.; Becker-Weidman, E.G.; Reinecke, M.A.; Jordan, N.; Silva, S.G.; Rohde, P.; March, J.S. Treating depression and oppositional behavior in adolescents. *J Clin. Child Adolesc. Psychol.* **2010**, *39*, 559–567. [CrossRef] [PubMed]
85. Nock, M.K.; Kazdin, A.E.; Hiripi, E.; Kessler, R.C. Lifetime prevalence, correlates and persistence of oppositional defiant dis-order: Results from the National Comorbidity Survey Replication. *J. Child Psychol. Psychiatry* **2007**, *48*, 703–713. [CrossRef] [PubMed]
86. Masi, G.; Milone, A.; Paciello, M.; Lenzi, F.; Muratori, P.; Manfredi, A.; Polidoi, L.; Ruglioni, L.; Lochman, J.E.; Muratori, F. Effi-cacy of a multimodal treatment for disruptive behavior disorders in children and adolescents: Focus on internalizing problems. *Psychiatry Res.* **2014**, *219*, 617–624. [CrossRef] [PubMed]

87. Muratori, P.; Milone, A.; Manfredi, A.; Polidori, L.; Ruglioni, L.; Lambruschi, F.; Masi, G.; Lochman, J.E. Evaluation of Improvement in Externalizing Behaviors and Callous-Unemotional Traits in Children with Disruptive Behavior Disorder: A 1-Year Follow Up Clinic-Based Study. *Adm. Policy Ment. Health Ment. Health Serv. Res.* **2017**, *44*, 452–462. [CrossRef] [PubMed]
88. Aitken, M.; Battaglia, M.; Marino, C.; Mahendran, N.; Andrade, B.F. Clinical utility of the CBCL Dysregulation Profile in children with disruptive behavior. *J. Affect. Disord.* **2019**, *15*, 87–95. [CrossRef] [PubMed]
89. Spencer, T.J.; Faraone, S.V.; Surman, C.B.H.; Petty, C.; Clarke, A.; Batchelder, H.; Wozniak, J. Towards defining deficient emo-tional self-regulation in youth with attention deficit hyperactivity disorder using the Child Behavior Checklist: A controlled study. *Postgrad. Med. J.* **2011**, *123*, 50–59. [CrossRef] [PubMed]
90. Eyberg, S.M.; Nelson, M.M.; Boggs, S.R. Evidence-based psychosocial treatments for children and adolescents with disruptive behavior. *J. Clin. Child Adolesc. Psychol.* **2008**, *37*, 215–237. [CrossRef] [PubMed]
91. Lochman, J.E.; Powell, N.P.; Boxmeyer, C.L.; Jimenez-Camargo, L. Cognitive behavioral therapy for externalizing disorders in children and adolescents. *Child Adolesc. Psychiatr. Clin. N. Am.* **2011**, *20*, 305–318. [CrossRef] [PubMed]
92. Kochanska, G.; Kim, S.; Boldt, L.J.; Yoon, J.E. Children's callous-unemotional traits moderate links between their positive relationships with parents at preschool age and externalizing behavior problems at early school age. *J. Child Psychol. Psychiatry Allied Discip.* **2013**, *54*, 1251–1260. [CrossRef] [PubMed]
93. Garland, A.F.; Hawley, K.M.; Brookman-Frazee, L.; Hurlburt, M.S. Identifying common elements of evidence-based psycho-social treatments for children's disruptive behaviour problems. *J. Am. Acad. Child Adolesc. Psychiatry* **2008**, *47*, 5–15. [CrossRef]
94. Smorti, M.; Ponti, L. How Does Sibling Relationship Affect Children's Prosocial Behaviors and Best Friend Relationship Quality? *J. Fam. Issues* **2018**, *39*, 2413–2436. [CrossRef]
95. Newman, J. Conflict and friendship in sibling relationships: A review. *Child Study J.* **1994**, *24*, 119–152.
96. Gass, K.; Jenkins, J.; Dunn, J. Are sibling relationships protective? A longitudinal study. *J. Child Psychol. Psychiatry* **2007**, *48*, 167–175. [CrossRef]
97. Cohen, J. *Statistical Power Analysis for the Behavioral Sciences*; Erlbaum: Hillsdale, NJ, USA, 1988.
98. Chen, D.; Drabick, D.A.G.; Burgers, D.E. A Developmental Perspective on Peer Rejection, Deviant Peer Affiliation, and Conduct Problems among Youth. *Child Psychiatry Hum. Dev.* **2015**, *46*, 823–838. [CrossRef] [PubMed]
99. Feinberg, M.E.; Solmeyer, A.R.; McHale, S.M. The Third Rail of Family Systems: Sibling Relationships, Mental and Behavioral Health, and Preventive Intervention in Childhood and Adolescence. *Clin. Child Fam. Psychol. Rev.* **2012**, *15*, 43–57. [CrossRef] [PubMed]

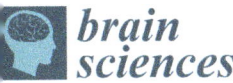

Article

Antisocial Personality Problems in Emerging Adulthood: The Role of Family Functioning, Impulsivity, and Empathy

Eleonora Marzilli [1], Luca Cerniglia [2] and Silvia Cimino [1,*]

1 Department of Dynamic and Clinical Psychology, Sapienza, University of Rome, Via degli Apuli, 1, 00185 Rome, Italy; eleonora.marzilli@uniroma1.it
2 Faculty of Psychology, International Telematic University Uninettuno, 00186 Rome, Italy; l.cerniglia@uninettunouniversity.net
* Correspondence: silvia.cimino@uniroma1.it; Tel.: +39-06-444-2794

Abstract: International research has evidenced the key role played by adults' and adolescents' family functioning, impulsivity, and empathy in antisocial personality problems. To date, no study has assessed the complex interaction between these variables during emerging adulthood. This study aimed to explore the possible interplay between antisocial personality problems, the quality of family functioning, impulsivity, and empathetic problems in a community sample of 350 emerging adults. Descriptive, correlational, hierarchical regression, and mediation analyses were performed, controlling relevant socio-demographic variables. Results showed a predictive effect of parental behavioral control, motor impulsivity, and empathetic concern in antisocial personality problems. Moreover, motor impulsivity and empathetic concern partially mediated the relationship between parental behavioral control and emerging adults' antisocial personality problems. This study supports the recent evidence on the complex relationship between individual and relational protective and risk factors involved in antisocial personality problems during emerging adulthood, with important implications for their intervention treatments.

Keywords: antisocial personality problems; emerging adulthood; family functioning; impulsivity; empathy

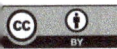

1. Introduction

Antisocial personality disorder (ASPD) is a severe personality disorder characterized by a pervasive pattern of disregarding or violating others' rights, often without showing interest in the feelings of others [1]. Specifically, according to the Diagnostic and Statistical Manual (DSM-5) [2], diagnostic criteria for ASPD include a set of seven criteria referring to both personality-oriented and behavior-focused indicators, including failure to conform to social norms; impulsivity; consistent irresponsibility; irritability and aggressiveness; and lack of remorse for having hurt, mistreated, or stolen from another. Moreover, to be diagnosed with ASPD, the subject must be at least 18 years old and must have had conduct disorder since at least the age of 15 [2]. However, personality and behavioral symptoms of ASPD are not uncommon in the general population [3], especially during adolescence and young adulthood, occurring in subclinical forms that do not satisfy the criteria to pose a diagnosis of ASPD [4]. This phenomenon represents a major public policy and health concern [5], due to its high rates of prevalence (more than 10% among youths) [6–8], and the recent increase in its global incidence [9]. In this field, although there is a wide range of studies that have examined antisocial personality problems among the adolescent population [10–13], far fewer studies have focused on this topic in the transition from adolescence to adulthood [14–17].

The developmental period of "emerging adulthood" (between the ages of 18 and 25) [18] is a developmental stage characterized by multiple challenges related to identity explorations and transitions in social roles; behavioral styles and personality traits emerge in this stage, with stability over time [19]. Thus, this critical window of maturation represents a key stage for studying personality difficulties involving antisocial personality problems. Indeed, although it has been underlined that antisocial behaviors generally have a peak of increase during late adolescence, with a decline in the course of emerging adulthood [20], there are individual differences in trajectories of antisocial personality problems [21–23]. Some youths, defined as "adolescence-limited" antisocials, show antisocial behaviors and callous–unemotional traits in late adolescence but tend to desist during emerging adulthood. In other cases, individuals may show persistent antisocial problems from adolescence to adulthood, a subtype of antisocials named "life-course persistent". Finally, the presence of "late-onset" antisocials has also been evidenced, which manifest antisocial tendencies from emerging adulthood [17,21–23]. Consequently, it is important to identify risk and protective factors associated with antisocial personality problems in emerging adulthood, to implement the knowledge of underpinning mechanisms related to their persistent and/or late onset and to guide preventive programs and post-onset interventions [24]. The Developmental Psychopathology theoretical framework suggests considering the role played by multiple levels of analyses [25], from personality traits of vulnerability to environmental factors which may promote or mitigate antisocial personality problems in this developmental stage [26].

In this field, some studies have shown that social role changes occurring during emerging adulthood, including the presence of romantic relationships and employment, may exert a protective role on desistance from problem behaviors [27,28], with a significant increase in prosocial activities and a decrease in antisocial attitudes [29]. Despite these potential benefits, in the last decade, social and economic changes have resulted in a delay in the acquisition of these traditional adult social roles to which emerging adults increasingly tend to have access around age 30 [30], with a consequent increase in staying in the family home [31–33]. Moreover, some authors have suggested that previous parental influence could be internalized and continue to affect emerging adults' psychological well-being even if the youth lives outside the family home [15,34]. Consequently, parental support and the quality of family functioning continue to assume a central source of reference and influence for early adults [30] and may represent a key protective and/or risk factor for the involvement in antisocial behaviors and personality problems [14,16]. In particular, international research has shown that the lack of parental warmth, emotional support, and behavioral control are associated with a wide range of youth's externalizing problems, including aggression [35,36], addictive behaviors [37–39], and risk-taking [40,41]. Recently, the same associations have been reported also with antisocial traits and delinquency [42–45], but focusing almost exclusively on adolescent samples. Only a few studies have explored the association between family functioning and ASPD symptoms among the emerging adulthood population [14–17,46], although the important role played by emerging adults' family functioning for their psychological well-being has been widely shown [33,47]. Regarding individual vulnerability factors, the presence of specific personality traits can further promote the onset or maintenance of youths' antisocial personality problems [48,49]. Impulsivity and low empathy are two of the main personality dimensions most frequently associated with ASPD symptoms among emerging adults, both in clinical samples and in the general population [48–56]. Impulsivity traits may be defined as a predisposition to rapid, unplanned reactions to internal or external stimuli without considering the negative consequences of these reactions for the individual or others [57]. On the other hand, an emerging adult who manifests low empathy may have difficulties in understanding other's feelings and disapproval, as well as the impact of their negative behaviors on others [58]. Although these personality characteristics are part of the DSM-5 diagnostic criteria for ASPD [2], a key role of impulsivity and low empathy in predicting personality disorder symptoms [48,49,54,59], including ASPD symptoms [48,49,54–56], has been shown. However, impulsivity and empathy are multidimensional constructs, but only a few studies have explored which specific dimension of these personality traits may be more predictive of antisocial personality problems during emerging adulthood [60–63].

Overall, a growing body of research has evidenced that young adults' perception of a poor family functioning, low levels of empathy, and high impulsivity traits may exert a significant contribution to antisocial personality problems [14–17,46,48,54–56]. Interestingly, on the relationship between these risk factors, a predictive role of worse family functioning on both impulsivity problems [64–66] and low empathy [42,67] has been evidenced. Moreover, recent findings have shown that these personality traits mediated the relationship between a poor quality of family functioning and both psychological difficulties [39,68] and personality disorder symptoms [66]. In the field of antisocial personality problems, a recent study by Álvarez-García et al. [44] has found that impulsivity and empathy mediated the relationship between family functioning and antisocial behaviors among the adolescent population. However, despite this emerging evidence, to our best knowledge, no study has yet explored the possible mediation role played by empathy and impulsivity problems on the relationship between emerging adults' perception of their family functioning and antisocial personality problems.

Based on these premises and literature gaps, the present study aimed to explore, in a community sample of male and female emerging adults, the complex relationship between antisocial personality problems and family functioning, impulsivity, and empathy. Specifically, we hypothesized that good quality of emerging adult's family functioning and an adequate level of empathy had a protective effect on antisocial personality problems, whereas impulsivity problems had a risk effect. Moreover, we hypothesized that the relationship between family functioning and antisocial personality problems could be mediated by impulsivity and empathy. Figure 1 shows the conceptual model.

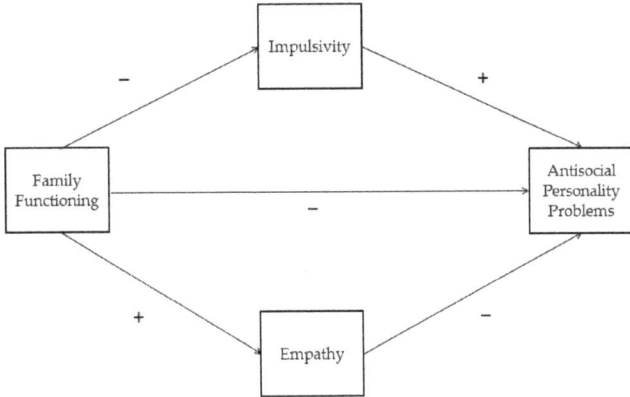

Figure 1. Conceptual model. + indicates positive statistical relationships; − indicates negative statistical relationships.

2. Materials and Methods

2.1. Sample Recruitment and Procedure

Over a period of 1 year, 443 emerging adults ranging in age from 18 to 25 years were recruited via notices posted on online psychology research websites and on social media. Prior to taking part in the study, all youths completed the written informed consent and gave their agreement to participate. The study was approved by the Ethical Committee of the Department of Dynamic and Clinical Psychology at Sapienza University of Rome (protocol N. 142/2019), in accordance with the Declaration of Helsinki. All participants who accepted to take part in the study filled out an anonymous self-completed online survey. First, participants completed an ad hoc questionnaire regarding sociodemographic data (i.e., age, gender, relationship status, living setup, educational level, and employment status). Then, self-report questionnaires for the assessment of antisocial personality traits, family functioning, impulsivity, and empathy (described below) were administered.

2.2. Measures

2.2.1. Assessment of Antisocial Personality Problems of Emerging Adults

The Adult Self-Report (ASR) [69] is a 126-item self-report questionnaire assessing the psychological functioning of adults (ages 18–59). Items are rated on a 3-point Likert scale (from 0 = "not true" to 2 = "very true"). The ASR provides scores for eight syndrome scales (anxious/depressed, withdrawn, somatic complaints, thought problems, attention problems, aggressive behavior, rule-breaking behavior, and intrusive behavior) and six DSM-oriented scales (depressive problems, anxiety problems, somatic problems, avoidant personality problems, attention-deficit/hyperactivity problems, and antisocial personality problems). For the aim of this study, we used the scores of antisocial personality problems of the DSM-oriented scales. Specifically, the 20 items of the Antisocial Personality Problems scale refer to the symptoms of ASPD described in the DSM-5 [2]. Coherently, some items evaluate personality features of ASPD (e.g., "I blame others for my problems ", "I don't feel guilty after doing something I shouldn't have done", "I have a hot temper"), while others explore behavioral aspects of the disorder (e.g., "I damage or destroy things of others", "I lie or cheat", "I physically attack people"). The scores of the 20 items were summed to compute the ASR Antisocial Personality Behavior. Achenbach and Rescorla [69] recommended using raw scores for analyses to avoid problems associated with censored measures. Consequently, as also suggested by other studies in the field [70], raw scores were used in the statistical analyses. The ASR showed good reliability and validity [69]. In the current sample, the ASR showed good internal coherence (Cronbach alpha = 0.82).

2.2.2. Assessment of Family Functioning of Emerging Adults

The Family Assessment Device (FAD) [71,72] is a 60-item self-report questionnaire that was developed to measure various aspects of family functioning. Items are evaluated on a 4-point scale (from 1 = "strongly agree" to 4 = "strongly disagree") and allow measuring six dimensions of the McMaster Model of Family Functioning: (1) Problem Solving (PS), which addresses the family's ability to solve problems (e.g., "We resolve most emotional upsets that come up"); (2) Communication (COM), which evaluates whether communication between the family members is clear and direct or vague and indirect (e.g., "We are frank with each other"); (3) Roles, which addresses the issue of how roles and responsibilities are allocated among the family members (e.g., "We discuss who is to do household jobs"); (4) Affective Responsiveness (AR), which addresses ability of the family members to respond to a range of situations with appropriate quality and amount of emotion (e.g., "We do not show our love for each other"); (5) Affective Involvement (AI), which assesses how family members experience interest and involvement with each other (e.g., "If someone is in trouble, the others become involved too"); and (6) Behavioral Control (BC), which evaluates whether the family has norms or standards governing individual behavior and responses to emergency situations (e.g., "We have rules about hitting people"). Psychometric properties showed a good validity, reliability, and internal consistency [71,72]. In this study, the internal consistency of the six subscales was also adequate (Cronbach α = 0.78–0.92).

2.2.3. Assessment of Impulsivity of Emerging Adults

The Barratt Impulsiveness Scale 11 (BIS-11) [73], is a self-report questionnaire for the assessment of impulsive behaviors. It is composed of 30 items that are assessed on a 4-point scale (from 1 = "never–rarely" to 4 = "almost always–always"). The BIS-11 allows obtaining a score on three main scales: (a) Attentional Impulsivity (inability to focus attention or concentrate, e.g., "Am a steady thinker"); (b) Motor Impulsivity (acting without thinking, e.g., "spend more than earn"); (c) Non-planning Impulsivity (lack of future orientation or forethought, e.g., "plan for job security"). Higher scores (i.e., >75) indicate an impulse-control disorder, while scores between 70 and 75 points indicate pathological impulsivity. Psychometric proprieties of the Italian version [74] showed good qualities (Cronbach's alpha = 0.79 and test–retest reliability r = 0.88). Reliability values in the current sample were as follows: Attentional Impulsivity = 0.79, Motor Impulsivity = 0.88, and Non-planning Impulsivity = 0.89.

2.2.4. Assessment of Empathy of Emerging Adults

The Interpersonal Reactivity Index (IRI) [75–77] is a 28-item self-report measuring separate but intercorrelated components of empathy. Items are rated on a 5-point scale (from 1 = "Does not describe me well" to 5 = "Describes me very well") which allows obtaining a score of four dimensions of empathy: (1) Perspective Taking (PT), which refers to the reported tendency to spontaneously adopt the psychological point of view of others in everyday life (e.g., "I try to look at everybody's side of a disagreement before I make a decision"); (2) Empathic Concern (EC), which refers the tendency to experience feelings of sympathy and compassion for unfortunate others (e.g., "I often have tender, concerned feelings for people less fortunate than me"); (3) Personal Distress (PD), which assesses the tendency to experience severe discomfort in response to extreme distress in others during a tense emotional situation (e.g., "In emergency situations, I feel apprehensive and ill-at-ease"); (4) Fantasy (FS), which measures the tendency to imaginatively transpose oneself into fictional situations (e.g., "I daydream and fantasize, with some regularity, about things that might happen to me"). The IRI showed good psychometric properties [78], as did the Italian version [77]. In the present study, the internal consistency of the four dimensions was also adequate (Cronbach α = 0.81–0.89).

2.3. Statistical Analyses

Preliminary statistical analyses were conducted using descriptive statistics (reliability of the measures, frequencies, and mean scores). Then, Pearson's correlation analyses were carried out to determine initial correlations between study variables. Based on significant correlations, we conducted hierarchical multiple regression analyses to identify the main effects of family functioning, impulsivity, and empathy on emerging adults' antisocial problems, controlling for relevant demographic factors (i.e., age, gender, romantic relationship status, living status, level of education, and employment status). Finally, parallel mediation analyses were conducted to test whether impulsivity and empathy mediated the effect of family functioning on emerging adults' antisocial personality problems. The covariates that showed a significant effect in regression analyses were also inserted as covariates in the mediation analyses. To this end, we used Hayes's PROCESS macro [79] (Model 4), which provides coefficient estimates for total, direct, and indirect effects of variables using ordinary least squares regression. Indirect (i.e., mediating) effects were evaluated with 95% bias-corrected confidence intervals (CIs) based on 10.000 bootstrap samples. When a CI does not include zero, it indicates that the effect is significant at α = 0.05. All analyses were performed using IBM SPSS software 25.0.

3. Results

3.1. Sample Characteristics

From the total sample, emerging adults that did not complete the assessment procedure (N = 46), reported a psychopathological diagnosis and/or physical disabilities (N = 24), or were following psychological and/or psychiatric treatment (N = 23) were excluded. The final sample consisted of N = 350 emerging adults (52.6% females) with average age of 22.16 years (DS = 2.18). The minority (38%) was single and 60% lived within the family. Participants most often reported their highest level of education being high school (44.3%) or more than high school (47.1%), and the vast majority were students without a job (30.6%) or part-time employed (24.9%). Table 1 shows the complete description of the sample demographic characteristics.

3.2. Bivariate Associations between Study Variables

Results of Pearson's correlation analyses showed that the score of antisocial personality problems was significantly associated with all dimensions of FAD, except for problem solving and communication; with all dimensions of IRI, except for PD; and with all dimensions of BIS-11. Moreover, impulsivity and empathy were related to many of the FAD dimensions, allowing for the possibility that the relationship between family functioning and antisocial personality problems may be mediated by impulsivity and empathy (Table 2).

Table 1. Sample demographic characteristics.

Age in years, M (SD)		22.16 (2.18)
Gender, n (%)		
	Male	166 (47.4)
	Female	184 (52.6)
Romantic relationship status, n (%)		
	Single	133 (38)
	Partnered	137 (39.1)
	Cohabitant	62 (17.7)
	Married	18 (5.1)
Living status, n (%)		
	Living with family members	245 (60)
	Not living with family members	105 (30)
Level of education, n (%)		
	Less than high school	30 (8.6)
	High school	155 (44.3)
	More than high school	165 (47.1)
Employment status, n (%)		
	Unemployed	57 (16.3)
	Unemployed student	107 (30.6)
	Employed student	30 (8.6)
	Part-time employment	87 (24.9)
	Full-time employment	69 (19.7)

3.3. Main Effects of Family Functioning, Impulsivity, and Empathy on Antisocial Personality Problems

Based on significant correlations, hierarchical multiple regression analyses were conducted to investigate whether family functioning, impulsivity, and empathy were predictive of levels of antisocial personality problems. After controlling for covariates, a significant negative effect of the dimension of behavioral control of FAD was found for early adults' antisocial personality problems. Moreover, empathic concern was significantly negatively associated with antisocial personality problems, and a significant positive effect of motor impulsivity was also found. This model explained 64% of the variance (Table 3).

Table 2. Descriptive statistics and Pearson correlation coefficients between the starting theoretical model variables.

	1	2	3	4	5	6	7	8	9	10	11	12	13	14
1.ASR_Antis	1													
2. FAD_PS	−0.05	1												
3.FAD_Com	−0.05	0.46 **	1											
4.FAD_Rol	−0.34 **	0.30 **	−0.09	1										
5.FAD_AI	−0.49 **	0.31 **	−0.20 **	0.53 **	1									
6.FAD_AR	−0.36 **	0.08	−0.08	0.38 *	0.42 **	1								
7.FAD_BC	−0.63 **	0.06	0.12 *	0.34 *	0.53 **	0.41 **	1							
8.IRI_PT	−0.49 **	−0.04	0.04	0.13 *	0.27 **	0.14 **	0.37 **	1						
9.IRI_FS	−0.23 **	0.04	0.11 *	0.02	0.10 *	0.08	0.26 **	0.36 **	1					
10.IRI_PD	0.06	0.15 **	0.04	−0.16 **	−0.15 **	−0.15 **	−0.10	0.01	0.31 **	1				
11.IRI_EC	−0.53 **	−0.04	−0.02	0.15 **	0.28 **	0.16 **	0.34 **	0.59 **	0.44 **	0.10	1			
12.BIS_Att	0.43 **	0.01	−0.01	−0.19 **	−0.23 **	−0.20 **	−0.26 **	−0.28 **	−0.04	0.10	−0.28 **	1		
13.BIS_Mot	0.59 **	−0.01	0.01	−0.23 **	−0.39 **	−0.26 **	−0.43 **	−0.41 **	−0.12 *	0.01	−0.40 **	0.56 **	1	
14.BIS_NP	0.44 **	0.04	−0.02	−0.17 **	−0.24 **	−0.15 **	−0.31 **	−0.43 **	−0.24 **	0.03	−0.36 **	0.43 **	0.56 **	1
M	6.63	14.28	19.22	24.94	19.32	15.56	24.38	18.82	16.42	12.24	19.36	16.26	20.14	24.26
DS	6.62	3.01	2.79	3.39	3.52	2.70	3.36	4.46	4.56	4.42	4.29	3.33	4.51	4.29

Note. ASR = Adult Self Report; FAD = Family Assessment Device; IRI = Interpersonal Reactivity Index; BIS-11 = Barratt Impulsiveness Scale; Antisoc: Antisocial Personality Problem; PS = Problem Solving, Com = Communication, Rol = Roles, AI = Affective Involvement; AR = Affective Responsiveness, PT = Perspective Taking, FS = Fantasy, EC = Empathic Concern, PD = Personal Distress, BC = Behavioral Control, Att = Attentional Impulsivity, Mot = Motor Impulsivity, NP = Non-planning Impulsivity. * $p < 0.05$, ** $p < 0.01$.

3.4. Emerging Adults' Impulsivity and Empathy as Mediators of the Relationship between Family Functioning and Antisocial Personality Problems

Finally, based on significant predictive relationships that emerged in regression analyses, parallel mediation analyses were conducted to verify whether the relationship between behavioral control perceived by early adults in their family functioning and their own levels of antisocial personality problems was mediated by their motor impulsivity and empathic concern problems. Mediation analyses were adjusted for covariates that we found significantly related to antisocial personality problems in previous analyses (i.e., relationship status and occupation). Results of parallel mediation analyses showed that the total effect of behavioral control on emerging adults' antisocial personality problems was significant. Moreover, behavioral control was negatively associated with motor impulsivity, which in turn was positively related to antisocial personality problems. On the other hand, behavioral control was positively related to empathic concern, which in turn was negatively associated with antisocial personality problems. When considering the effects of mediators, the direct effect of behavioral control on antisocial personality problems remained significant. Overall, the model explained 65% of the variance in emerging adults' antisocial personality problems (Figure 2).

Regarding indirect effects, as possible to see in Table 4, the indirect paths via empathetic concern and motor impulsivity were significant. However, the coefficient of direct effect was larger than indirect effects, indicating a partial mediation.

Table 3. Results of hierarchical regression analyses predicting emerging adults' antisocial personality problems.

			Adjusted Coefficients		
			B (SE)	t	p
Covariates					
	Gender [a]		0.05 (0.45)	0.18	0.90
	Age		0.12 (0.10)	1.19	0.23
	Relationship status [b]				
		Partnered	−1.36 (0.52)	−2.61	0.009 **
		Cohabit	−1.29 (1.00)	−1.28	0.20
		Married	−0.75 (1.30)	−0.57	0.56
	Living setup [c]		−0.28 (0.96)	−0.29	0.71
	Level of education [d]				
		High school	−0.29 (0.81)	−0.36	0.71
		More than high school	−0.89 (0.86)	−1.04	0.29
	Occupation [e]				
		Unemployed student	−1.34 (0.69)	−1.94	0.06
		Employed student	−1.15 (0.96)	−1.19	0.23
		Employed part time	−1.83 (0.83)	−2.20	0.03 *
		Employed full time	−2.74 (0.90)	−3.02	0.003 **
Predictors					
	FAD	Roles	−0.07 (0.07)	−1.03	0.30
		Affective Involvement	−0.11 (0.08)	−1.34	0.18
		Affective Responsiveness	−0.14 (0.09)	−1.51	0.13
		Behavioral Control	−0.54 (0.08)	−6.27	0.000 ***
	IRI	Perspective Taking	−0.11 (0.06)	−1.77	0.08
		Fantasy	0.06 (0.05)	1.27	0.20
		Empathic Concern	−0.34 (0.06)	−5.07	0.000 ***
	BIS-11	Attentional Impulsivity	0.14 (0.08)	1.79	0.07
		Motor Impulsivity	0.26 (0.07)	3.73	0.000 ***
		Non-planning Impulsivity	0.06 (0.06)	1.02	0.30
Adjusted R^2					0.64

Note. [a] Female is the reference group, [b] single is the reference group, [c] living with family members is the reference group, [d] less than high school is the reference group, [e] unemployed is the reference group; SE = Standard error. * $p < 0.05$, ** $p < 0.01$, *** $p < 0.001$.

Table 4. Indirect effects of behavioral control on antisocial personality problems through motor impulsivity and empathic concern.

Indirect Effect	Effect (BootSE)	LLCI	ULCI
Total	−0.37 (0.05)	−0.49	−0.27
Behavioral Control→Empathic Concern→Antisocial Personality Problems	−0.15 (0.03)	−0.23	−0.09
Behavioral Control→Motor Impulsivity→Antisocial Personality Problems	−0.22 (0.04)	−0.31	−0.14

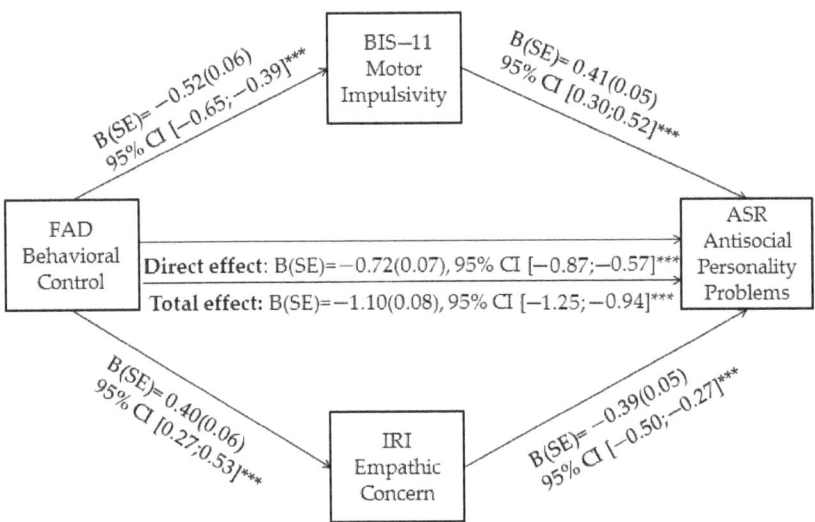

Figure 2. Parallel mediation of motor impulsivity and empathic concern on the relationship between parental behavioral control and emerging adults' antisocial personality problems. *** $p < 0.001$.

4. Discussion

This study aimed to further increase the knowledge on protective and risk factors involved in antisocial personality problems in emerging adulthood. To this end, we have chosen to focus on relational and individual variables (i.e., family functioning, impulsivity, and empathy) that previous literature on adolescent and adult populations has indicated as significant predictors of both personality [48,49,54–56] and behavior features [44,45,52,80,81] of antisociality. In addition, we tested a conceptual framework that took into consideration the complex relationships between these variables, considering both the direct effect of family functioning and indirect effects via emerging adults' impulsivity and empathy. Overall, our results are in accordance with our hypothesized model (Figure 1).

In particular, hierarchical regression analyses confirmed a significant role of some specific dimensions of the emerging adult's family functioning, impulsivity, and empathy on his/her antisocial personality problems. Specifically, after controlling relevant sociodemographic factors, the results showed a predictive effect of parental behavioral control, motor impulsivity, and empathetic concern, accounting for 64% of the variance in antisocial personality problems. High levels of parental behavioral control and empathetic concern were associated with low levels of antisocial problems, whereas high motor impulsivity problems had a positive effect. These results are in line with previous studies on individual personality traits, which have shown the central role played by impulsivity and empathy on the development of ASPD symptoms [48,54–56]. The association between impulsivity and antisocial personality problems is not surprising given that the Diagnostic and Statistical Manual of Mental Disorders (DSM-5) [2] also indicates the presence of impulsivity as one of the main criteria of ASPD. However, recent evidence has shown the importance of investigating which specific dimension of impulsivity can place the individual at a greater risk of antisocial personality problems [60–63]. Our results showed that only the motor dimension of impulsivity (defined as acting on the spur of the moment) was positively associated with antisocial personality problems. These findings are in line with the studies by Umut et al. [61] and Urben et al. [62] that found higher levels of motor impulsivity among individuals at risk and/or with a diagnosis of ASPD than in those without it. Interestingly, it has been recently evidenced that motor impulsivity may be implicated in the recidivism of antisocial behaviors [63]. In accordance with previous studies, our findings suggested that the behavioral aspect of impulsivity may be more predictive of antisocial personality problems in emerging adulthood.

Moreover, our results showed that emerging adults' antisocial personality problems were negatively predicted by high levels of empathetic concern, an affective dimension of empathy which refers to the ability to experience another's feelings. These findings are in line with previous studies that have evidenced a close relationship between empathy and prosocial behaviors [82,83], suggesting a protective effect on behavioral aspects of antisocial personality problems. Conversely, empathy impairment, especially of the affective component, was be found in association with a higher risk of ASDP symptoms [84–86]. At the same time, experimental studies have revealed lower levels of physiological reactivity responses to social distress cues [87], as well as lower levels of neural response to viewing other's pain compared to healthy controls [88,89].

Finally, regarding family functioning, previous studies have evidenced that a parent–child relationship characterized by warmth and emotional support and in which parents set limits and supervise children's behaviors exerts a protective role on adolescents' externalizing problems, addictive behaviors, and antisocial behaviors [35,37,67]. The research examining these associations in emerging adulthood is scarce but, in line with our study, has evidenced a protective effect on the emerging adult's antisocial personality problems [14,19]. Indeed, although social influences from peer and romantic relationships exert increasing weight during this developmental stage, parents continue to assume, for better or worse, a significant role in children's lives, remaining a key source of social and material support [18,30]. Moreover, even when the emerging adult is no longer living in the family and under direct parental behavioral control, the messages of parental control experienced during adolescence may, in turn, be internalized, still exerting effects on young adults and preventing antisocial personality problems [15].

The protective role of parental behavioral control on emerging adults' antisocial personality problems was also confirmed by our parallel mediation model. Indeed, both direct and total effects were significant. Moreover, as expected, parental behavioral control predicted low levels of motor impulsivity (that in turn predicted high antisocial personality problems) and high levels of empathic concern (that in turn predicted low antisocial personality problems). The relationships between parental behavioral control and antisocial personality problems via motor impulsivity and empathic concern were also significant. These findings have supported the recent evidence on the complex relationship between emerging adults' perception of their family functioning, impulsivity problems, empathy functioning, and psychological difficulties [39,68], including personality disorder symptoms [66]. Recently [44], the same findings were also shown in relation to adolescent's antisocial behaviors. However, to our best knowledge, this is the first study that has explored the possible role played by these associations on emerging adults' ASPD symptoms. In line with our results, previous studies have shown that the lack of parental behavioral control is prospectively associated with children's antisocial personality problems [14–17], impulsivity [90,91], and empathetic impairment [35,67], which international literature has widely shown to be risk factors for antisocial personality problems [48–56]. Beyond the direct effect of parental behavioral control on antisocial personality problems, our findings have also supported the recent evidence on indirect effects through its protective influence on impulsivity and empathy [44]. However, the direct effect was greater than indirect effects, suggesting that emerging adults' motor impulsivity and empathic concern only partially mediate the impact of parental behavior on antisocial personality problems.

Limitation, Strength, and Implications

There are some limitations to the current study. We conducted an online convenience sampling to collect the data, which does not produce representative results generalizable to the population as a whole. Further studies should use probability sampling techniques. In addition, we evaluated emerging adults' antisocial personality problems, family functioning, impulsivity, and empathy through self-report instruments. Although these tools are widely validated and extensively used in the field of developmental psychopathology research, further studies should assess these variables using more robust and objective measures (e.g., clinical interviews). Moreover, the instrument we used for the assessment of emerging adults' family functioning allows obtaining a measure of perceived family functioning. Consequently, information provided may be influenced by emerging adult's perception biases and should be interpreted with caution. Furthermore, this was a cross-sectional study, which implies considering the causal nature of the relationships that emerged with caution. Subsequent longitudinal studies are needed to confirm our findings. Moreover, although many relevant variables have been included, we have not considered the possible role played by other individual and relational variables that studies have shown to be associated with antisocial personality problems in emerging adulthood (e.g., genetic vulnerabilities, alexithymic characteristics, childhood traumatic experiences, peer influence) [54,92,93]. Notwithstanding the above limitations, the present study has several strengths. This study was the first study to explore the complex relationship between emerging adults' antisocial personality problems, family functioning, impulsivity, and empathy. Moreover, our sample included both male and female emerging adults, evidencing no significant sex differences in antisocial personality problems. Conversely, historically, the majority of studies have focused almost exclusively on male samples, given that a higher rate of ASPD is generally reported among males than females. However, recent evidence has increasingly shown an increment in antisocial personality problems also among females, suggesting the importance of focusing on both sexes for a better understanding of the phenomenon.

5. Conclusions

Overall, this study has supported the importance of considering the complex relationship between the quality of family functioning, empathy, and impulsivity traits in studying antisocial personality problems in emerging adulthood. Specifically, our results suggested a key role played by parental behavioral control that exerted its protective influence on antisocial personality problems both directly and via motor impulsivity and empathic concern. Although further longitudinal studies using probability sampling techniques are needed to provide higher statistical power and support our preliminary results, our findings have various clinical and public health implications. Indeed, our findings could be informative for the planning of more targeted and effective intervention treatments, supporting the recent evidence that parental involvement in prevention and treatment programs is a critical factor in ensuring success in people of this stage [14]. Moreover, this study has also suggested that the planning of interventions focused on the improvement of self-control and affective empathy should be promoted [94,95].

Author Contributions: Conceptualization, E.M. and L.C.; methodology, E.M.; writing—original draft preparation, S.C., E.M., and L.C.; writing—review and editing, L.C.; supervision, S.C. All authors have read and agreed to the published version of the manuscript.

Funding: This research received no external funding.

Institutional Review Board Statement: The study was conducted according to the guidelines of the Declaration of Helsinki and approved by the Ethics Committee of the Department of Dynamic and Clinical Psychology at Sapienza University of Rome (protocol code N. 142/2019, date of approval: 07/02/2019).

Informed Consent Statement: Informed consent was obtained from all subjects involved in the study.

Data Availability Statement: Data available on request to the authors.

Acknowledgments: We thank all emerging adults who agreed to participate in this study.

Conflicts of Interest: The authors declare no conflict of interest.

References

1. Raine, A. Antisocial Personality as a Neurodevelopmental Disorder. *Annu. Rev. Clin. Psychol.* **2018**, *14*, 259–289. [CrossRef] [PubMed]
2. American Psychiatric Association. *Diagnostic and Statistical Manual of Mental Disorders (DSM-5)*; American Psychiatric Publishing: Washington, DC, USA, 2013.
3. Delk, L.A.; Spangler, D.P.; Guerra, R.; Ly, V.; White, B.A. Antisocial Behavior: The Impact of Psychopathic Traits, Heart Rate Variability, and Gender. *J. Psychopathol. Behav. Assess.* **2020**, *42*, 637–646. [CrossRef]
4. Rafiey, H.; Alipour, F.; Lebeau, R.; Salimi, Y. Development and Validation of the Antisocial Traits Scale in the General Population. *Crim. Justice Behav.* **2020**, *47*, 369–380. [CrossRef]
5. Hammerton, G.; Mahedy, L.; Murray, J.; Maughan, B.; Edwards, A.C.; Kendler, K.S.; Hickman, M.; Heron, J. Effects of Excessive Alcohol Use on Antisocial Behavior Across Adolescence and Early Adulthood. *J. Am. Acad. Child Adolesc. Psychiatry* **2017**, *56*, 857–865. [CrossRef]
6. Foster, E.M.; Jones, D.E. The high costs of aggression: Public expenditures resulting from conduct disorder. *J. Public Health* **2005**, *95*, 1767–1772. [CrossRef]
7. Nock, M.K.; Kazdin, A.E.; Hiripi, E.; Kessler, R.C. Prevalence, subtypes, and correlates of DSM-IV conduct disorder in the National Comorbidity Survey Replication. *Psychol. Med.* **2006**, *36*, 699–710. [CrossRef] [PubMed]
8. Werner, K.B.; Few, L.R.; Bucholz, K.K. Epidemiology, comorbidity, and behavioral genetics of antisocial personality disorder and psychopathy. *Psychiat. Ann.* **2015**, *45*, 195–199. [CrossRef] [PubMed]
9. Livesley, W.J.; Larstone, R. *Handbook of Personality Disorders: Theory, Research, and Treatment*; Guilford Press: New York, NY, USA, 2018.
10. Wallace, G.L.; Shaw, P.; Lee, N.R.; Clasen, L.S.; Raznahan, A.; Lenroot, R.K.; Martin, A.; Giedd, J.N. Distinct cortical correlates of autistic versus antisocial traits in a longitudinal sample of typically developing youth. *J. Neurosci.* **2012**, *32*, 4856–4860. [CrossRef] [PubMed]
11. Morgado, A.M.; da Luz Vale-Dias, M. The antisocial phenomenon in adolescence: What is literature telling us? *Aggress. Violent Behav.* **2013**, *18*, 436–443. [CrossRef]
12. Moffitt, T.E. Male antisocial behaviour in adolescence and beyond. *Nat. Hum. Behav.* **2018**, *2*, 177–186. [CrossRef]
13. Nasaescu, E.; Zych, I.; Ortega-Ruiz, R.; Farrington, D.P.; Llorent, V.J. Longitudinal patterns of antisocial behaviors in early adolescence: A latent class and latent transition analysis. *Eur. J. Psychol. Appl. Leg. Context* **2020**, *12*, 85–92. [CrossRef]
14. Johnson, J.G.; Cohen, P.; Chen, H.; Kasen, S.; Brook, J.S. Parenting behaviors associated with risk for offspring personality disorder during adulthood. *Arch. Gen. Psychiatry* **2006**, *63*, 579–587. [CrossRef]
15. Harris-McKoy, D.; Cui, M. Parental control, adolescent delinquency, and young adult criminal behavior. *J. Child Fam. Stud.* **2013**, *22*, 836–843. [CrossRef]
16. Johnson, W.L.; Giordano, P.C.; Longmore, M.A.; Manning, W.D. Parents, identities, and trajectories of antisocial behavior from adolescence to young adulthood. *J. Dev. Life Course Criminol.* **2016**, *2*, 442–465. [CrossRef] [PubMed]
17. Blonigen, D.M.; Littlefield, A.K.; Hicks, B.M.; Sher, K.J. Course of Antisocial Behavior during Emerging Adulthood: Developmental Differences in Personality. *J. Res. Pers.* **2010**, *44*, 729–733. [CrossRef]
18. Arnett, J.J. Emerging adulthood. A theory of development from the late teens through the twenties. *Am. Psychol.* **2000**, *55*, 469–480. [CrossRef]
19. Polek, E.; Jones, P.B.; Fearon, P.; Brodbeck, J.; Moutoussis, M.; Dolan, R.; Fonagy, P.; Bullmore, E.T.; Goodyer, I.M. Personality dimensions emerging during adolescence and young adulthood are underpinned by a single latent trait indexing impairment in social functioning. *BMC Psychiatry* **2018**, *26*, 18–23. [CrossRef]
20. Hyde, L.W.; Waller, R.; Shaw, D.S.; Murray, L.; Forbes, E.E. Deflections from adolescent trajectories of antisocial behavior: Contextual and neural moderators of antisocial behavior stability into emerging adulthood. *J. Child Psychol. Psychiatry* **2018**, *59*, 1073–1082. [CrossRef] [PubMed]
21. Moffitt, T.E. Adolescence-limited and life-course-persistent antisocial behavior: A developmental taxonomy. *Psychol. Rev.* **1993**, *100*, 674–701. [CrossRef] [PubMed]
22. Diamantopoulou, S.; Verhulst, F.C.; van der Ende, J. Testing developmental pathways to antisocial personality problems. *J. Abnorm. Child Psychol.* **2010**, *38*, 91–103. [CrossRef] [PubMed]
23. Mikolajewski, A.J.; Bobadilla, L.; Taylor, J. Antisocial Personality Disorder. In *Encyclopedia of Adolescence*; Levesque, R.J.R., Ed.; Springer: New York, NY, USA, 2016; pp. 1–13.
24. Kazemian, L. Desistence from crime: Theoretical, empirical, methodological, and policy considerations. *J. Contemp. Crim. Justice* **2007**, *23*, 5–27. [CrossRef]
25. Wood, D.; Crapnell, T.; Lau, L.; Bennett, A.; Lotstein, D.; Ferris, M.; Kuo, A. Emerging adulthood as a critical stage in the life course. In *Handbook of Life Course Health Development*; Halfon, N., Forrest, C.B., Lerner, R.M., Faustman, E.M., Eds.; Springer: Cham, Switzerland, 2018; pp. 123–143.
26. Frick, P.J.; Viding, E. Antisocial behavior from a developmental psychopathology perspective. *Dev. Psychopathol.* **2009**, *21*, 1111–1131. [CrossRef]

37. Rhule-Louie, D.M.; McMahon, R.J. Problem behavior and romantic relationships: Assortative mating, behavior contagion, and desistance. *Clin. Child Fam. Psychol. Rev.* **2007**, *10*, 53–100. [CrossRef]
38. Monahan, K.C.; Steinberg, L.; Cauffman, E. Age differences in the impact of employment on antisocial behavior. *Child Dev.* **2013**, *84*, 791–801. [CrossRef] [PubMed]
39. Burt, S.A.; Donnellan, M.B.; Humbad, M.N.; Hicks, B.M.; McGue, M.; Iacono, W.G. Does marriage inhibit antisocial behavior? An examination of selection vs causation via a longitudinal twin design. *Arch. Gen. Psychiatry* **2010**, *67*, 1309–1315. [CrossRef] [PubMed]
40. Arnett, J.J. *The Oxford Handbook of Emerging Adulthood*; Oxford University Press: New York, NY, USA, 2016.
41. Fingerman, K.L.; Yahirun, J.J. Emerging adulthood in the context of family. In *The Oxford Handbook of Emerging Adulthood*; Arnett, J.J., Ed.; Oxford University Press: New York, NY, USA, 2016; pp. 163–176.
42. Lee, C.Y.S.; Goldstein, S.E. Loneliness, stress, and social support in young adulthood: Does the source of support matter? *J. Youth Adolesc.* **2016**, *45*, 568–580. [CrossRef] [PubMed]
43. Parra, Á.; Sánchez-Queija, I.; García-Mendoza, M.D.C.; Coimbra, S.; Egídio Oliveira, J.; Díez, M. Perceived parenting styles and adjustment during emerging adulthood: A cross-national perspective. *Int. J. Environ. Res. Public Health* **2019**, *16*, 2757. [CrossRef]
44. Hassan, T.; Alam, M.M.; Wahab, A.; Hawlader, M.D. Prevalence and associated factors of internet addiction among young adults in Bangladesh. *J. Egypt Public Health Assoc.* **2020**, *95*, 3. [CrossRef]
45. Hoskins, D.H. Consequences of parenting on adolescent outcomes. *Societie* **2014**, *4*, 506–531. [CrossRef]
46. Pérez-Fuentes, M.D.C.; Molero Jurado, M.D.M.; Barragán Martín, A.B.; Gázquez Linares, J.J. Family functioning, emotional intelligence, and values: Analysis of the relationship with aggressive behavior in adolescents. *Int. J. Environ. Res. Public Health* **2019**, *16*, 478. [CrossRef]
47. Hawi, N.S.; Samaha, M. Relationships among smartphone addiction, anxiety, and family relations. *Behav. Inf. Technol.* **2017**, *36*, 1046–1052. [CrossRef]
48. Pereira-Morales, A.J.; Adan, A.; Camargo, A.; Forero, D.A. Substance use and suicide risk in a sample of young Colombian adults: An exploration of psychosocial factors. *Am. J. Addict.* **2017**, *26*, 388–394. [CrossRef]
49. Marzilli, E.; Cerniglia, L.; Ballarotto, G.; Cimino, S. Internet Addiction among Young Adult University Students: The Complex Interplay between Family Functioning, Impulsivity, Depression, and Anxiety. *Int. J. Environ. Res. Public Health* **2020**, *17*, 8231. [CrossRef]
50. Ju, C.; Wu, R.; Zhang, B.; You, X.; Luo, Y. Parenting style, coping efficacy, and risk-taking behavior in Chinese young adults. *J. Pacific. Rim. Psychol.* **2020**, *14*, E3. [CrossRef]
51. Marzilli, E.; Ballarotto, G.; Cimino, S.; Cerniglia, L. Motor vehicle collisions in adolescence: The role of family support. [Incidenti stradali in adolescenza: Il ruolo del supporto genitoriale]. *Rass. Psicol.* **2018**, *34*, 17–28.
52. Asano, R.; Yoshizawa, H.; Yoshida, T.; Harada, C.; Tamai, R.; Yoshida, T. Effects of parental parenting attitudes on adolescents' socialization via adolescents' perceived parenting. *Jpn. J. Psychol.* **2016**, *87*, 284–293. [CrossRef]
53. Pinquart, M. Associations of parenting dimensions and styles with externalizing problems of children and adolescents: An updated meta-analysis. *Dev. Psychol.* **2017**, *53*, 873–932. [CrossRef] [PubMed]
54. Álvarez-García, D.; González-Castro, P.; Núñez, J.C.; Rodríguez, C.; Cerezo, R. Impact of family and friends on antisocial adolescent behavior: The mediating role of impulsivity and empathy. *Front. Psychol.* **2019**, *10*, 2071. [CrossRef] [PubMed]
55. Inguglia, C.; Costa, S.; Ingoglia, S.; Cuzzocrea, F.; Liga, F. The role of parental control and coping strategies on adolescents' problem behaviors. *Curr. Psychol.* **2020**, 1–14. [CrossRef]
56. Lee, J.Y.; Brook, J.S.; Finch, S.J.; Brook, D.W. An adverse family environment during adolescence predicts marijuana use and antisocial personality disorder in adulthood. *J. Child Fam. Stud.* **2016**, *25*, 661–668. [CrossRef]
57. Shen, J.J.; Cheah, C.S.L.; Yu, J. Asian American and European American emerging adults' perceived parenting styles and self-regulation ability. *Asian Am. J. Psychol.* **2018**, *9*, 140–148. [CrossRef]
58. Fossati, A.; Barratt, E.S.; Carretta, I.; Leonardi, B.; Grazioli, F.; Maffei, C. Predicting borderline and antisocial personality disorder features in nonclinical subjects using measures of impulsivity and aggressiveness. *Psychiatry Res.* **2004**, *125*, 161–170. [CrossRef] [PubMed]
59. Fossati, A.; Barratt, E.S.; Borroni, S.; Villa, D.; Grazioli, F.; Maffei, C. Impulsivity, aggressiveness, and DSM-IV personality disorders. *Psychiatry Res.* **2007**, *149*, 157–167. [CrossRef]
60. Jones, S.E.; Miller, J.D.; Lynam, D.R. Personality, antisocial behavior, and aggression: A meta-analytic review. *J. Crim. Justice* **2011**, *39*, 329–337. [CrossRef]
61. Maneiro, L.; Gómez-Fraguela, J.A.; Cutrín, O.; Romero, E. Impulsivity traits as correlates of antisocial behaviour in adolescents. *Pers. Individ. Dif.* **2017**, *104*, 417–422. [CrossRef]
62. Schmits, E.; Glowacz, F. Delinquency and drug use among adolescents and emerging adults: The role of aggression, impulsivity, empathy, and cognitive distortions. *J. Subst. Use* **2019**, *24*, 162–169. [CrossRef]
63. Van Langen, M.A.; Wissink, I.B.; Van Vugt, E.S.; Van der Stouwe, T.; Stams, G.J.J.M. The relation between empathy and offending: A meta-analysis. *Aggress. Violent Behav.* **2014**, *19*, 179–189. [CrossRef]
64. Velotti, P.; Garofalo, C.; Dimaggio, G.; Fonagy, P. Mindfulness, alexithymia, and empathy moderate relations between trait aggression and antisocial personality disorder traits. *Mindfulness* **2019**, *10*, 1082–1090. [CrossRef]

55. Garofalo, C.; Velotti, P.; Callea, A.; Popolo, R.; Salvatore, G.; Cavallo, F.; Dimaggio, G. Emotion dysregulation, impulsivity and personality disorder traits: A community sample study. *Psychiatry Res.* **2018**, *266*, 186–192. [CrossRef]
56. Rhee, S.H.; Woodward, K.; Corley, R.P.; du Pont, A.; Friedman, N.P.; Hewitt, J.K.; Hink, L.K.; Robinson, J.; Zahn-Waxler, C. The association between toddlerhood empathy deficits and antisocial personality disorder symptoms and psychopathy in adulthood. *Dev. Psychopathol.* **2021**, *33*, 173–183. [CrossRef]
57. Moeller, F.G.; Barratt, E.S.; Dougherty, D.M.; Schmitz, J.M.; Swann, A.C. Psychiatric aspects of impulsivity. *Am. J. Psychiatry* **2001**, *158*, 1783–1793. [CrossRef] [PubMed]
58. Massey, S.H.; Newmark, R.L.; Wakschlag, L.S. Explicating the role of empathic processes in substance use disorders: A conceptual framework and research agenda. *Drug Alcohol. Rev.* **2018**, *37*, 316–332. [CrossRef] [PubMed]
59. Fossati, A.; Gratz, K.L.; Maffei, C.; Borroni, S. Emotion dysregulation and impulsivity additively predict borderline personality disorder features in Italian nonclinical adolescents. *Pers. Ment. Health* **2013**, *7*, 320–333. [CrossRef] [PubMed]
60. Komarovskaya, I.; Loper, A.B.; Warren, J. The role of impulsivity in antisocial and violent behavior and personality disorders among incarcerated women. *Crim. Justice Behav.* **2007**, *34*, 1499–1515. [CrossRef]
61. Umut, G.; Evren, C.; Alniak, I.; Karabulut, V.; Cetin, T.; Agachanli, R.; Evren, B. Relationship between impulsivity and antisocial personality disorder, severity of psychopathology and novelty seeking in a sample of inpatients with heroin use disorder. *Heroin Addict. Relat. Clin. Probl.* **2017**, *19*, 65–72.
62. Urben, S.; Habersaat, S.; Suter, M.; Pihet, S.; De Ridder, J.; Stéphan, P. Gender differences in at risk versus offender adolescents: A dimensional approach of antisocial behavior. *Psychiatr. Q* **2016**, *87*, 619–631. [CrossRef]
63. Martin, S.; Zabala, C.; Del-Monte, J.; Graziani, P.; Aizpurua, E.; Barry, T.J.; Ricarte, J. Examining the relationships between impulsivity, aggression, and recidivism for prisoners with antisocial personality disorder. *Aggress. Violent Behav.* **2019**, *49*, 101314. [CrossRef]
64. Grant, J.E.; Chamberlain, S.R. Obsessive compulsive personality traits: Understanding the chain of pathogenesis from health to disease. *J. Psychiatr. Res.* **2019**, *116*, 69–73. [CrossRef]
65. Ryan, S.R.; Friedman, C.K.; Liang, Y.; Lake, S.L.; Mathias, C.W.; Charles, N.E.; Acheson, A.; Dougherty, D.M. Family Functioning as a Mediator of Relations between Family History of Substance Use Disorder and Impulsivity. *Addict. Disord. Their. Treat.* **2016**, *15*, 17–24. [CrossRef]
66. Khan, S.; Kamal, A. Adaptive family functioning and borderline personality disorder: Mediating role of impulsivity. *J. Pak. Med. Assoc.* **2020**, *70*, 86–89. [CrossRef]
67. Boele, S.; Van der Graaff, J.; De Wied, M.; Van der Valk, I.E.; Crocetti, E.; Branje, S. Linking parent–child and peer relationship quality to empathy in adolescence: A multilevel meta-analysis. *J. Youth Adolesc.* **2019**, *48*, 1033–1055. [CrossRef]
68. Asghari Sharabiani, A.; Basharpoor, S. The mediating role of empathy in the relationship between family functioning and bullying in students. *J. Fam. Psychol.* **2019**, *5*, 15–26.
69. Achenbach, T.M.; Rescorla, L.A. *Manual for the ASEBA Adult Forms & Profiles*; Research Center for Children, Youth & Families: Burlington, VT, USA, 2003.
70. Paquette Boots, D.; Wareham, J. An exploration of DSM-oriented scales in the prediction of criminal offending among urban American youths. *Crim. Justice Behav.* **2009**, *36*, 840–860. [CrossRef]
71. Epstein, N.B.; Baldwin, L.M.; Bishop, D.S. The McMaster family assessment device. *J. Marital Fam. Ther.* **1983**, *9*, 171–180. [CrossRef]
72. Grandi, S.; Fabbri, S.; Scortichini, S.; Bolzani, R. Validazione italiana del Family Assessment Device (FAD). *Riv. Psichiatr.* **2007**, *42*, 114–122. [CrossRef]
73. Patton, J.H.; Stanford, M.S.; Barratt, E.S. Factor structure of the Barratt impulsiveness scale. *J. Clin. Psychol.* **1995**, *51*, 768–774. [CrossRef]
74. Fossati, A.; Di Ceglie, A.; Acquarini, E.; Barratt, E.S. Psychometric properties of an Italian version of the Barratt Impulsiveness Scale-11 (BIS-11) in nonclinical subjects. *J. Clin. Psychol.* **2001**, *57*, 815–828. [CrossRef]
75. Davis, M.H. A multidimensional approach to individual differences in empathy. *JSAS Cat. Sel. Doc. Psychol.* **1980**, *10*, 85.
76. Davis, M.H. Measuring individual differences in empathy: Evidence for a multidimensional approach. *J. Pers. Soc. Psychol.* **1983**, *44*, 113–126. [CrossRef]
77. Albiero, P.; Ingoglia, S.; Lo Coco, A. Contributo all'adattamento italiano dell'Interpersonal Reactivity Index. *TPM Test. Psychom. Method Appl. Psychol.* **2006**, *13*, 107–125.
78. Pulos, S.; Elison, J.; Lennon, R. Hierarchical structure of the Interpersonal Reactivity Index. *Soc. Behav. Personal.* **2004**, *32*, 355–360. [CrossRef]
79. Hayes, A.F. *Introduction to Mediation, Moderation, and Conditional Process Analysis: A Regression-Based Approach*, 2nd ed.; Guilford Publications: New York, NY, USA, 2017.
80. Marsden, J.; Glazebrook, C.; Tully, R.; Völlm, B. Do adult males with antisocial personality disorder (with and without co-morbid psychopathy) have deficits in emotion processing and empathy? A systematic review. *Aggress. Violent Behav.* **2019**, *48*, 197–217. [CrossRef]
81. Azevedo, J.; Vieira-Coelho, M.; Castelo-Branco, M.; Coelho, R.; Figueiredo-Braga, M. Impulsive and premeditated aggression in male offenders with antisocial personality disorder. *PLoS ONE* **2020**, *15*, e0229876. [CrossRef] [PubMed]

82. Luberto, C.M.; Shinday, N.; Song, R.; Philpotts, L.L.; Park, E.R.; Fricchione, G.L.; Yeh, G.Y. A systematic review and meta-analysis of the effects of meditation on empathy, compassion, and prosocial behaviors. *Mindfulness* **2018**, *9*, 708–724. [CrossRef] [PubMed]
83. Mayer, S.V.; Jusyte, A.; Klimecki-Lenz, O.M.; Schönenberg, M. Empathy and altruistic behavior in antisocial violent offenders with psychopathic traits. *Psychiatry Res.* **2018**, *269*, 625–632. [CrossRef]
84. Pfabigan, D.M.; Seidel, E.M.; Wucherer, A.M.; Keckeis, K.; Derntl, B.; Lamm, C. Affective empathy differs in male violent offenders with high-and low-trait psychopathy. *J. Pers. Disord.* **2015**, *29*, 42–61. [CrossRef] [PubMed]
85. Sezen-Balcikanli, G.; Sezen, M. The relationship between empathy and antisocial-prosocial behaviours in youth field hockey players. *Int. J. Learn. Chang.* **2019**, *11*, 57–65. [CrossRef]
86. Seidel, E.M.; Pfabigan, D.M.; Keckeis, K.; Wucherer, A.M.; Jahn, T.; Lamm, C.; Derntl, B. Empathic competencies in violent offenders. *Psychiatry Res.* **2013**, *210*, 1168–1175. [CrossRef] [PubMed]
87. Verona, E.; Bresin, K.; Patrick, C.J. Revisiting psychopathy in women: Cleckley/Hare conceptions and affective response. *J. Abnorm. Psychol.* **2013**, *122*, 1088–1093. [CrossRef]
88. Decety, J.; Chen, C.; Harenski, C.; Kiehl, K.A. An fMRI study of affective perspective taking in individuals with psychopathy: Imagining another in pain does not evoke empathy. *Front. Hum. Neurosci.* **2013**, *7*, 489. [CrossRef]
89. Marsh, A.A.; Finger, E.C.; Fowler, K.A.; Adalio, C.J.; Jurkowitz, I.T.; Schechter, J.C.; Pine, D.S.; Decety, J.; Blair, R.J. Empathic responsiveness in amygdala and anterior cingulate cortex in youths with psychopathic traits. *J. Child. Psychol. Psychiatry* **2013**, *54*, 900–910. [CrossRef]
90. Li, D.; Zhang, W.; Wang, Y. Parental behavioral control, psychological control and chinese adolescents' peer victimization: The mediating role of self-control. *J. Child Fam. Stud.* **2015**, *24*, 628–637. [CrossRef]
91. Chamberlain, S.R.; Tiego, J.; Fontenelle, L.F.; Hook, R.; Parkes, L.; Segrave, R.; Hauser, T.U.; Dolan, R.J.; Goodyer, I.M.; Bullmore, E.; et al. Fractionation of impulsive and compulsive trans-diagnostic phenotypes and their longitudinal associations. *Aust. N. Z. J. Psychiatry* **2019**, *53*, 896–907. [CrossRef] [PubMed]
92. Friedman, N.P.; Rhee, S.H.; Ross, J.M.; Corley, R.P.; Hewitt, J.K. Genetic and environmental relations of executive functions to antisocial personality disorder symptoms and psychopathy. *Int. J. Psychophysiol.* **2018**, *18*, 30331–30333. [CrossRef] [PubMed]
93. Schorr, M.T.; Tietbohl-Santos, B.; de Oliveira, L.M.; Terra, L.; de Borba Telles, L.E.; Hauck, S. Association between different types of childhood trauma and parental bonding with antisocial traits in adulthood: A systematic review. *Child Abuse Negl.* **2020**, *107*, 104621. [CrossRef]
94. Moreno-García, I.; Meneres-Sancho, S.; Camacho-Vara de Rey, C.; Servera, M. A randomized controlled trial to examine the posttreatment efficacy of neurofeedback, behavior therapy, and pharmacology on ADHD measures. *J. Atten. Disord.* **2019**, *23*, 374–383. [CrossRef] [PubMed]
95. van Dongen, J.D. The empathic brain of psychopaths: From social science to neuroscience in empathy. *Front. Psychol.* **2020**, *11*, 695. [CrossRef] [PubMed]

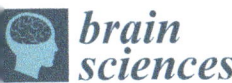

Systematic Review

Biological Bases of Empathy and Social Cognition in Patients with Attention-Deficit/Hyperactivity Disorder: A Focus on Treatment with Psychostimulants

Pamela Fantozzi [1,†], Gianluca Sesso [1,2,†], Pietro Muratori [1], Annarita Milone [1] and Gabriele Masi [1,*]

1. IRCCS Stella Maris Foundation, Scientific Institute of Child Neurology and Psychiatry, Department of Child and Adolescent Psychiatry and Psychopharmacology, 56128 Pisa, Italy; pamela.fantozzi@fsm.unipi.it (P.F.); gianluca.sesso@fsm.unipi.it (G.S.); pietro.muratori@fsm.unipi.it (P.M.); annarita.milone@fsm.unipi.it (A.M.)
2. Department of Clinical and Experimental Medicine, University of Pisa, 56126 Pisa, Italy
* Correspondence: gabriele.masi@fsm.unipi.it; Tel.: +39-050-886293
† Both authors contributed equally to this work.

Abstract: In recent years, there has been growing interest in investigating the effect of specific pharmacological treatments for ADHD not only on its core symptoms, but also on social skills in youths. This stands especially true for ADHD patients displaying impulsive aggressiveness and antisocial behaviors, being the comorbidity with Disruptive Behavior Disorders, one of the most frequently observed in clinical settings. This systematic review aimed to synthesize research findings on this topic following PRISMA guidelines and to identify gaps in current knowledge, future directions, and treatment implications. Search strategies included the following terms: ADHD; methylphenidate and other ADHD drugs; empathy, theory of mind and emotion recognition. Full-text articles were retrieved and data from individual studies were collected. Thirteen studies were finally included in our systematic review. Ten studies assessing changes in empathy and/or theory of mind in patients with ADHD treated after pharmacological interventions were identified. Similarly, seven partially overlapping studies assessing changes in emotion recognition were retrieved. Despite a great heterogeneity in the methodological characteristics of the included studies, most of them reported an improvement in emphatic and theory of mind abilities in youths with ADHD treated with psychostimulants and nonstimulant drugs, as well as positive but less consistent results about emotion recognition performances.

Keywords: empathy; theory of mind; emotion recognition; ADHD; disruptive behavior

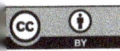

1. Introduction

Attention-Deficit/Hyperactivity Disorder (ADHD) is one of the most common neurodevelopmental disorders, with a pooled worldwide prevalence of 7.2% among children and adolescents [1]. In addition to the core symptoms of inattention, hyperactivity, and impulsivity [2], subjects with ADHD frequently exhibit difficulties in establishing and keeping relationships with peers and are perceived as less socially competent than peers [3]. Particularly, they tend to show a high rate of social and interpersonal problems during their whole life span, since reduced social cognition skills are usually found to be highly associated with the disorder, which may be considered to be an independent risk factor for negative outcome and poor quality of life in ADHD [3].

Interestingly, ADHD core symptoms per se may interfere with adequate social interactions. Indeed, attention deficits interfere with a proper coding and interpretation of social information, i.e., focusing and sustaining attention during conversations or appropriately reading social cues during play [4]. On the other hand, impulsivity involves inappropriately intruding in conversations or play, and disinhibition of motor, verbal, and behavioral responses can lead to fewer opportunities for social interaction due to peer rejection [5].

Moreover, ADHD is commonly associated with the presence of comorbid disruptive behavior disorders such as Oppositional Defiant Disorders (ODD) and/or Conduct Disorders (CD) that may further worsen social impairments and maladjustment [6]. Interestingly, deficits in social cognition skills may be even more challenging when ADHD presents with comorbid ODD/CD [7].

1.1. Empathy and Related Constructs

Social cognition is essential for successful social interaction and, as a whole, refers to the ability to understand other people's behaviors. It involves codification, representation and interpretation of social cues and includes (1) recognizing others' affects from face and prosody perception (i.e., emotion recognition), (2) making inferences regarding others' mental states (i.e., theory of mind (ToM)), (3) sharing and understanding the emotional perspective of others (i.e., empathy) [3]. More complex social cognition abilities include humor processing and further steps of the social information-processing model [8], from which biases may lead individuals to assume the hostile attributions of another's ambiguous behavior and generate aggressive or ineffective solutions to social problems.

Empathy is a complex multidimensional construct including an affective component—affective empathy (AE)—that is, the capacity of sharing emotions and responding to emotional displays of others, and a cognitive one—cognitive empathy (CE)—namely, the ability to understand the perspective of another person [9–13]. AE may involve several related underlying processes, including, among others, emotional contagion, emotion recognition, and shared pain [14]; on the other hand, CE involves making inferences regarding the other's affective and cognitive mental states [15].

These two components may have different neuroanatomical correlates, the former implying the contribution of limbic and paralimbic structures and developing earlier than the latter, which assumes, in turn, a fine-tuned maturation of prefrontal and temporal networks [16]. However, in a study on the anatomical correlates of empathy in patients with focal brain injuries, Shamay-Tsoory and colleagues [17] demonstrated that prefrontal lesions, especially those involving the orbitofrontal and ventromedial regions, were significantly associated with impairments in both cognitive and affective empathic skills, while lesions involving right parietal areas were also associated with deficient empathy. The distinction between the emotional and cognitive empathic subprocesses may also relate to different neurobiological systems. It has been suggested, indeed, that the oxytocinergic system, which has been associated with attachment and pair bonding, may modulate emotional but not cognitive empathy [18], whereas dopaminergic circuitry is associated with cognitive aspects of empathy [19].

Although the two systems work independently, as previously suggested by the Perception–Action Model of empathy [20,21], they interact with each other. The affective component is, indeed, regarded as a bottom-up automatic process, while the cognitive component may be better represented as a top-down modulator. Nonetheless, they also work in synergy with several other distinct but integrated components of social cognition, among which the theory of mind (ToM) stands out first. ToM is defined as the ability to make inferences regarding others' mental states—their knowledge, needs, intentions, and feelings—and is mediated by dissociable though interacting cognitive and affective aspects [22], whereas cognitive ToM, for instance, assessed through the so-called False Belief task, is thought to require cognitive understanding of the difference between the speaker's knowledge and that of the listener. Affective ToM, for example, tested with Faux Pas and Irony tasks, is supposed to require, in addition, an empathic appreciation of the listener's emotional state [23]. ToM functioning critically involves a complex neural network including the medial prefrontal cortex, the superior temporal sulcus region, the temporal pole, and the amygdalae [24–26], and has also been linked to the integrity of the dopaminergic and serotoninergic systems [24].

On the other side, the appropriate recognition of emotional cues represents a fundamental milestone in the early development of social cognition skills. Indeed, the ability to identify emotions from facial expressions and prosody is acquired during childhood and further develops during adolescence. Besides, nonverbal channels of communication seem to play an important role in helping individuals to interact appropriately with each other. Intact emotion recognition is required for the inhibition of aggressive behavior and its deficiencies might lead to aggressive reactions toward others [27]. At the same time, impaired recognition of facial emotions has been suggested to play a central role for social malfunctioning, being a potential cause of low social competence and low popularity in peer groups [28]. In other words, social adaptation is poorer in those who tend to identify emotional expressions less accurately [29].

In healthy individuals, facial expressions usually elicit neural changes over frontotemporal and parieto-occipital cortices, while right-sided peri-sylvian areas are engaged in the processing of emotional prosody [3]. Face emotion recognition has also been linked to temporal, prefrontal (e.g., orbitofrontal), and anterior cingulate regions, as well as the amygdala and the basal ganglia [30]. Finally, a connection between the perception of emotions and the dopaminergic pathway has been demonstrated [31].

1.2. Social Cognition in ADHD

Clinical evidence suggests several psychopathological disorders to be characterized by deficits in social cognition [32,33]. Importantly, empathy/ToM deficits have been implicated, indeed, in neurodevelopmental conditions in childhood and adolescence, among which Autism Spectrum Disorder (ASD) [34–37] and ODD/CD with limited prosocial emotions i.e., callous–unemotional traits [38,39] are the most studied. Empathy and ToM may be also compromised in a proportion of youths with ADHD. Clinical practice usually reveals low levels of social perspective taking and ToM in ADHD children [6,40,41]. Indeed, young people with ADHD may have low CE attitudes, as demonstrated, for instance, by the frequently observed unawareness of other children playing the same game [42]. In this regard, a recent meta-analysis on social cognition findings in ADHD [43] revealed that especially ToM was significantly impaired in ADHD patients. Interestingly, they also reported that social cognition deficits in ADHD lied intermediately between ASD and healthy controls [43].

On the other hand, several studies have also demonstrated that children with ADHD exhibited AE deficits compared to healthy controls [6,41,44], either assessed as trait using parent reports [45] or as a state assessed with affective responses to vignettes [41]. Presumably, a global empathy deficit can be detected in ADHD, involving both components, as shown by Maoz and colleagues [46] through self-report assessments. Interestingly, in another study from the same research group [47], differences in the empathic profile were identified between the Combined (ADHD-C) and the Inattentive (ADHD-I) subtypes of ADHD, with greater impairment in the former.

Children and adolescents with ADHD also exhibit an impaired emotion recognition ability and a nonverbal receptive language deficit [5,48,49], which denotes a difficulty in detecting and interpreting social clues and generates impaired social interactions and interpersonal problems. In particular, individuals with ADHD are significantly poorer in identifying emotional expressions, especially the negative effects of fear, anger and sadness, likely originating from a primary deficiency in encoding social cues and selectively inhibiting irrelevant information in ADHD [43,50].

According to Uekermann and colleagues [3], empathy deficits in ADHD might be explained, at least in part, by the impulsive response modalities typically found in these patients, and thus may be linked to dysfunctions of the fronto-striatal brain networks, functionally related to empathic processing and executive functioning. Interestingly, Barkley [51] argues that deficits in behavioral inhibition might impair social cognition skills, but how much they could affect empathic abilities still remains an unsolved question. In this respect, several studies have demonstrated a significant positive correlation between empathic skills and executive functions in both healthy subjects [52] and clinical samples [7,53,54]. Interestingly, a recent meta-analysis on healthy individuals [52] revealed that executive functioning, i.e., working memory, cognitive flexibility, and sustained attention, was more strongly related to CE; besides, AE was still closely related to inhibitory control. Conversely, Cristofani and colleagues [7] identified an opposite trend in ADHD patients and speculated that these subjects are somewhat constrained by their executive dysfunction in an underdeveloped empathic attitude, which would be limited to the expression of emotional contagion.

1.3. The Systematic Review

Recent literature has suggested that pharmacological interventions in ADHD patients may provide beneficial effects on social cognition deficits. Indeed, psychostimulants, including methylphenidate (MPH), and amphetamines, the gold-standard drug treatment for ADHD [55], have been likely associated with improvements in social judgment and interpersonal relationships [56,57], as well as in empathy and ToM in youths with ADHD [46,47,58–62]. Interestingly, MPH administration has been shown to promote empathy-like behaviors and sociability and reduce aggressiveness in a mouse model of callousness [63]. Moreover, it has been suggested that MPH treatment may possibly provide an improvement in emotion recognition [28,50]. Nonetheless, the evidence on the efficacy of psychostimulants on empathy and ToM, as well as on emotion recognition, is still under debate [64]. Thus, the aim of the present study was to systematically review the available literature on the topic in order to clarify whether the gold-standard drug treatment for ADHD may exert its effects on empathy and related constructs, through and beyond its well-known effects on the core symptoms of the disorder.

2. Materials and Methods

2.1. Search Strategy

The aim of the present study was to perform a systematic review of the literature on the effects of psychostimulants and nonstimulant drugs on empathy and related constructs in patients with ADHD. The review was conducted according to the Preferred Reporting Items for Systematic Reviews and Meta-Analyses (PRISMA) guidelines; the corresponding checklist is available in Supplementary Table S1. The protocol of the present systematic review was preregistered on PROSPERO (CRD42021247024). Three bibliographic databases were searched, namely PubMed, Scopus, and Web of Science, from the inception date to the 10 August 2021. A search strategy was developed including three groups of terms related to the following semantic fields: (1) ADHD; (2) Methylphenidate or other psychostimulants and nonstimulant drugs for ADHD; (3) Social Cognition, Empathy, Theory of Mind and Emotion Recognition. The full search strategy, along with the details of the bibliographic search, is available in Supplementary Table S2. The strategy was thus to include all relevant articles relating to Group 1 and Group 2 and Group 3; terms were consistently adapted for each database. Results of the bibliographic search were then downloaded into Mendeley software, and two authors (GS and PF) reviewed and discussed the scoping search which included both original studies and reviews. If a previous review was already available on the topic, its reference list was carefully searched to retrieve primary studies. Reference lists of the studies included in the final search were also thoroughly inspected to identify relevant citations.

2.2. Screening Procedure

Our search strategy was used to retrieve potentially relevant abstracts; duplicates from different bibliographic databases were initially removed, whereas additional records were identified through reference lists and the inspection of screened articles, as stated above, were also included. Two researchers (GS and PF) screened all titles and abstracts to identify relevant articles. Full texts of selected papers were then retrieved and carefully screened to finally identify the included studies according to eligibility criteria. Any disagreements were resolved by consensus. The PRISMA flowchart (Figure 1) shows the process of identification and selection of papers. Inclusion criteria were defined in order to retrieve clinical studies aimed at assessing the effects of MPH and other psychostimulants and nonstimulant drugs on empathy, theory of mind, and emotion recognition in patients with ADHD, as follows:

(1) Study design: any type of clinical trial;
(2) Comparison: either case versus control, drug versus placebo or pre-to peri-/post-treatment;
(3) Participants: patients non-retrospectively diagnosed with ADHD according to the international classification systems DSM-IV, ICD-9, or later versions; no restriction for participants' age, gender, or IQ;
(4) Intervention: either one-day, single-dose administration or prolonged daily administration of psychostimulants (e.g., Methylphenidate) or nonstimulant drugs (e.g., Atomoxetine);
(5) Measures: any type of measurement (i.e., tasks, rating scales, and parent- or self-rated questionnaires) assessing empathy, theory of mind, and emotion recognition.

Exclusion criteria are detailed in Figure 1 and Supplementary Table S2. Briefly, in order of exclusion, they have been defined as follows: (1) Not clinical trial; (2) Absence of adequate comparison; (3) Subjects not diagnosed with ADHD; (4) Retrospective diagnosis of ADHD; (5) Clinical diagnosis not based on DSM-IV, ICD-9, or later versions; (6) Not intervention with psychostimulant/nonstimulant drugs; (7) Not assessment of empathy, theory of mind, and emotion recognition.

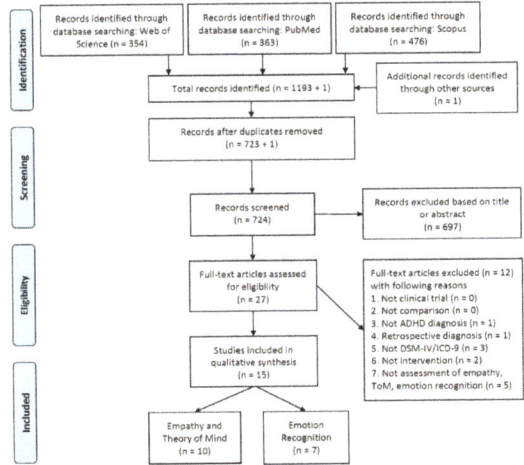

Figure 1. PRISMA flowchart showing the process of identification and selection of studies.

2.3. Data Collection

For each included study, we extracted relevant information, whenever available, including sample size, demographic data (age and gender), ADHD diagnosis and subtypes, intellectual functioning and psychiatric comorbidities, previous and current medication (including dosage and administration), follow-up duration, as well as information about the clinical measure used to assess changes in empathic competencies and related constructs and main findings of the study. When datasets were not fully available, authors of the included studies were contacted to attain the relevant data. Extracted information are available in Tables 1 and 2. Included studies were classified according to the examined construct as follows: (1) empathy and theory of mind and (2) emotion recognition. Emotion recognition is an underlying process related to the affective empathy, often investigated separately from the construct of empathy and theory of mind; for this reason, we decided to group studies into two classification types. Articles were also grouped according to the study design, either (1) single-dose administration of the drug with one-day follow-up or (2) daily administration of the medication with prolonged follow-up.

Table 1. Summary findings of the included studies: empathy and theory of mind.

Study	N	Gender	Age	ADHD	Comorbidity	Treatment	Assessment	Outcome
Coelho et al., 2017 [65]	60 ADHD (30 C, 30 I)	48/12	7–14 (unimodal group = 10.13) (multimodal group = 10.2)	no other medications when recruited	ID excluded	unimodal-medication only vs. multimodal medication + CBT for 20 weeks (prolonged release-MPH 20 mg)	Children's Social Skills Multimedia System	Multimodal treatment showed more improvement in frequency indicators on empathy.
Demirci and Erdogan, 2016 [58]	60 ADHD (21 C, 17 H/I, 22 I) 60 HCs	35/25 ADHD 35/25 HCs	8–15 (ADHD = 10.8) (HCs = 10.8)	drug-naive	ID, ASD, CD excluded	pharmacological treatment for 12 weeks: –38 OROS-MPH (final dose 1.2 mg/kg/day) –32 ATX (final dose 1.2 mg/kg/day)	RMET	The ADHD sample had significantly lower scores in RMET than HCs. ADHD-H/I had a lower number of correct answers in the RMET than ADHD-I. After OROS-MPH/ATX treatment, the ADHD sample showed a significant improvement in RMET.
Fantozzi et al., 2021 [62]	61 ADHD (50 C, 11 I)	51/10	6–17 (10.3)	drug-naive	ID, ASD excluded 14 SLD; 9 ODD; 4 MD; 2 LD; 1 AD; 1 tics; 1 dyspraxia	MPH treatment for 6 months (final dosage 31.6 ± 15.1 mg/day)	BES	Significant improvement in AE and CE. Changes in attention symptoms predicted changes in AE but not in CE.
Golubchik and Weizman, 2017 [59]	52 ADHD		8–18	psychostimulant-medication naive	ID, ASD, schizophrenia, bipolar disorder, suicidal ideation excluded 26 ODD	MPH treatment for 12 weeks (0.5–1 mg/kg/day)	EQ-C	Significant improvement in EQ scores in both groups (ADHD and ADHD/ODD). Only in the ADHD group, a significant correlation between changes in ADHD-RS and in EQ-C was found.
Golubchik and Weizman, 2019 [66]	25 ADHD	21/4	7–17 (10.8)		ID, ASD, psychosis, bipolar disorder excluded	single dose of MPH (1 mg/kg)	RMET	No improvement of RMET.
Gumustas et al., 2017 [60]	65 ADHD 61 HCs	53/12 ADHD 46/15 HCs	8–14 (ADHD = 10.86) (HCs = 11.21)	drug-naive	ID, ASD, psychosis, mood disorders, anxiety disorders, ODD excluded	OROS-MPH treatment for 12 weeks (0.83 ± 0.21 mg/kg/day)	BEI (trait empathy) GEM-PR (trait empathy) ERT (state empathy)	No significant statistical differences in trait and in state empathy skills in the two groups. Following the MPH treatment, the ADHD group showed a significant increase in the ERT (state empathy) interpretation sub-score.
Levi-Shachar et al., 2019 [61]	50 ADHD 40 HCs	28/22 ADHD 22/18 HCs	6–12 (ADHD = 9.42) (HCs = 8.95)	psychotropic medication free	psychosis, affective disorders, CD, substance abuse disorder excluded	single dose of short-acting MPH (0.3–0.5 mg/kg)	ToM test	The ADHD sample displayed significantly poorer ToM performance compared with HCs. Following MPH administration, the ToM performance of the ADHD sample normalized.

Table 1. *Cont.*

Study	N	Gender	Age	ADHD	Comorbidity	Treatment	Assessment	Outcome
Levi-Shachar et al., 2021 [67]	50 ADHD	28/22 ADHD	6–12 (ADHD = 9.42)	psychotropic medication free	psychosis, affective disorders, CD, substance abuse disorder excluded	single dose of short-acting MPH (0.3–0.5 mg/kg)	ToM test FPR	Negative association between severity of behavioral ADHD domains and impairment in ToM. Administration of MPH improved ToM performance, with the greatest improvement in children with more severe behavioral symptoms.
Maoz et al., 2013 [47]	24 ADHD (11 C, 13 I)	16/8	6–12 (10.2)		ID, psychosis, bipolar disorder, major depression, DBD, substance abuse disorder excluded	single-dose of long-acting MPH	IRI FRP TCT	Significant improvement in ToM performance.
Maoz et al., 2019 [46]	24 ADHD 36 HCs	6/8 ADHD 19/17 HCs	6–12 (ADHD = 10.29) (HCs = 9.37)	psychotropic medication free	ID, psychosis, bipolar disorder, major depression, CD, substance abuse disorder excluded	single dose of long-acting MPH	IRI FRP	The ADHD sample showed lower levels of self-reported empathy and FRP scores compared with HCs. In ADHD sample, MPH administration improved FRP scores to a level equal to that in HCs.

Abbreviations: AE, Affective Empathy; ADHD, Attention Deficit/Hyperactivity Disorder; ADHD-RS, Attention Deficit/Hyperactivity Disorder-Rating Scale; ASD, Autism Spectrum Disorder; ATX, Atomoxetine; BEI, Bryant Bryant Index of Empathy; BES, Basic Empathy Scale; C, Attention Deficit/Hyperactivity Disorder-Combined subtype; CD, Conduct Disorder; EQ-C, Empathizing Quotient-Children's version; ERT, Empathy Response Task; FPR, Faux-Pas Recognition task; GEM-PR, Griffith Empathy Measurement-Parent Rating; H/I, Attention Deficit/Hyperactivity Disorder-Hyperactive/Impulsive subtype; HCs, Healthy Controls; I, Attention Deficit/Hyperactivity Disorder-Inattentive subtype; ID, Intellectual Disability; IRI, Interpersonal Reactivity Index; RMET, Reading the Mind in the Eyes Test; MPH, Methylphenidate; ODD, Oppositional Defiant Disorder; OROS-MPH, long acting-Methylphenidate; SLD, Specific Learning Disability; TCT, ToM Computerized Task; ToM, Theory of Mind.

Table 2. Summary details of the included studies: Emotion Recognition.

Study	N	Gender	Age	ADHD	Comorbidity	Treatment	Assessment	Outcome
Demirci and Erdogan, 2016 [58]	60 ADHD (21 C, 17 H/I, 22 I) 60 HCs	35/25 ADHD 35/25 HCs	8–15 years (ADHD = 10.8) (HCs = 10.8)	drug-naive	ID, ASD, CD excluded	pharmacological treatment for 12 weeks: –38 OROS-MPH (final dose 1.2 mg/kg/day) –32 ATX (final dose 1.2 mg/kg/day)	BFRT	ADHD sample had significantly lower scores in BFRT than HCs. ADHD-H/I had a lower number of correct answers in BFRT than ADHD-C and I. After OROS-MPH/ATX treatment, the ADHD sample showed a significant improvement in BFRT.
Gumustas et al., 2017a [60]	65 ADHD 61 HCs	53/12 ADHD 46/15 HCs	8–14 years (ADHD = 10.86)(HCs = 11.21)	drug-naive	ID, ASD, psychosis, mood disorders, anxiety disorders, ODD excluded	OROS-MPH treatment for 12 weeks (0.83 ± 0.21 mg/kg/day)	DANVA-2	No significant statistical differences in facial expression recognition skills in the two groups. Following the MPH treatment, the ADHD group showed a significant decrease in the recognition error of anger and sadness expressions.

Table 2. Cont.

Study	N	Gender	Age	ADHD	Comorbidity	Treatment	Assessment	Outcome
Hall et al., 1999 [68]	15 ADHD (13 C, 2 H/I) 15 ADHD/LD (14 C, 1 H/I) 15 no ADHD or LD	36/9	7–10 years	the ADHD sample was taken MPH (Ritalin) for at least a month at the time of the study	ID excluded	the DANVA was administered twice to each child in the ADHD and ADHD/LD groups: once while the ADHD and ADHD/LD participants were on medication and once off medication	DANVA SPBRS	The ADHD/LD group demonstrated significant difficulty in comparison to their peers in perceiving paralanguage cues effectively. The ADHD/LD group showed significant improvement on the Postures and Paralanguage subtests during on-medication conditions.
Schulz et al., 2018 [69]	25 ADHD (17C, 8I)	14/9	19–52 years (34.8 ± 9.8)	2 participants were on medication at intake, 9 had a history of previous stimulant treatment (2 of whom had also previously been treated with nonstimulant medication)	psychosis, BD, PTSD, substance use disorcierexcluded	3 to 4 weeks of LDX (mean maintenance dose = 64 mg/day–SD = 13 mg) treatment and 3 weeks of medication in a randomized, counterbalanced, hybrid crossover design	participants were scanned twice with event-related fMRI while performing an emotional go/no-go task	No significant differences between the two treatment arms. LDX was associated with an increase in fMRI activation in the right amygdala and reduced interactions with the orbital aspect of the left inferior frontal gyrus specifically for responses to sad faces.
Schwenck et al., 2013 [70]	56 ADHD (10C,2H/I,44I) 28 ADHD-MD− 28 ADHD-MD+ 28 CG	19/9	8.2–17.3 years (MD− = 12.36) (MD+ = 12.31) (CG = 12.49)	47 children in the ADHD group were taken MPH at the time of the study (one child was additionally taken ATX), 6 drug-naive	ID, ASD, ODD, CD excluded	cross-sectional design study	MT	No differences found between ADHD-MD−, ADHD-MD+ and CG on emotion recognition.

Abbreviations: ADHD, Attention Deficit/Hyperactivity Disorder; ADHD-MED−, Attention Deficit/Hyperactivity Disorder no medication; ADHD-MED+, Attention Deficit/Hyperactivity Disorder with medication; ASD, Autism Spectrum Disorder; ATX, Atomoxetine; BD, Bipolar Disorder; BRFT, Breton Face Recognition Test; C, Attention Deficit/Hyperactivity Disorder-Combined subtype; CD, Conduct Disorder; CG, control group; DANVA, Diagnostic Analysis of Nonverbal Accuracy; ERP, event related potential; FEFA, Frankfurt Test and Training of Facial Affect; fMRI, functional magnetic resonance imaging; H/I, Attention Deficit/Hyperactivity Disorder-Hyperactive/Impulsive subtype; HCs, Healthy Controls; I, Attention Deficit/Hyperactivity Disorder-Inattentive subtype; ID, Intellectual Disability; LD, Learning Disability; LDX, lisdexamfetamine; MPH, Methylphenidate; MT, Morphing Task; ODD, Oppositional Defiant Disorder; OROS-MPH, long acting-Methylphenidate; PTSD, Post Traumatic Stress Disorder; SD, standard deviation; SPBRS, Social Perception Behavior Rating Scale.

3. Results

Details of the screening process and the identification and selection of papers are available in Figure 1, along with the main reasons for exclusion. In summary, 1193 abstracts were initially retrieved using our search strategy, plus one additional record identified in the reference lists of the studies included in the final search. After duplicates removal, 724 records were screened by two authors (G.S. and P.F.) and any disagreement was resolved by consensus. Twenty-seven full-text articles were carefully assessed for eligibility, of which 12 were excluded. Fifteen articles were finally included in our systematic review and were non-mutually subdivided into two partially overlapping groups as follows: (1) empathy and theory of mind (n = 10 studies); (2) emotion recognition (n = 7 studies).

3.1. Empathy and Theory of Mind

Ten studies [46,47,58–62,65–67] assessing the effects of MPH (either immediate-release or long-acting formulations) on empathy and ToM in young patients with ADHD were finally identified. One study [58] also assessed the effects of atomoxetine (ATX) treatment, while another one [65] compared unimodal (medication only) versus multimodal (medication plus cognitive behavioral therapy).

All studies were conducted on children and adolescents aged 6 to 18 years old. Diagnoses were based on DSM-IV or DSM-5 systems [2] and included different proportions of ADHD subtypes. Intelligence was on average, while other psychiatric comorbidities were excluded based on standardized criteria, except for the study by Fantozzi and colleagues [62], which also included patients with ADHD and comorbid with language disorders, verbal dyspraxia, Specific Learning Disabilities, tics, affective disorders, and behavioral disruptive disorders, and for the study by Golubchik and Weizman [59], which also included youths with ADHD and comorbid with ODD. Further details of the studies are reported in Table 1.

Five studies [46,47,61,66,67] examined the effect of a single-dose administration of MPH on children and adolescents with ADHD who were already regularly taking the medication at the time of the study. Particularly, one study [47] revealed an improvement in cognitive and affective ToM, as measured with two ToM tests, the Faux Pas Recognition task and the ToM Computerized task, in a group of young patients with ADHD after a single MPH dose administration. The same research group [46] later replicated their findings through a self-report measure, the Interpersonal Reactivity Index, and the Faux Pas test demonstrating that ADHD patients, who initially displayed significant deficits in empathy/ToM skills, improved their performances after a single dose of MPH until they matched their healthy peers.

A recent study [61] corroborated these findings by examining the effect of a single dose of MPH versus placebo on different ToM task performances in a group of children with ADHD versus healthy controls in a double-blind controlled trial. ToM abilities in ADHD children, while initially poorer, normalized only after MPH administration and differences between the two groups were no longer found. The same research group, analyzing later the same ADHD sample [67], found a correlation between the severity of the ADHD behavioral symptoms and deficits in ToM. The authors also found that the administration of a single dose of MPH improved ToM performance, especially in children with more severe behavioral symptoms. Conversely, another research group [66] revealed no significant single-dose MPH effects in children with ADHD on ToM performances, as measured through the commonly used Reading the Mind in the Eyes test.

Five additional studies [58–60,62,65] evaluated the effects of mid-term treatment with daily drug administrations in ADHD patients. Notably, all five studies agreed in demonstrating a significant improvement in empathy/ToM performance after drug treatment. Particularly, a significant increase in empathic abilities, as measured by the Empathizing Quotient, was shown after 12 weeks of daily treatment with MPH [59]; it should be noted, however, that half of the included patients were also diagnosed with comorbid ODD, which implied even lower baseline scores than the ADHD-only group. Though they did not confirm such improvement in trait empathy by means of two paper-and-pencil questionnaires, the Bryant Index of Empathy and the Griffith Empathy Measure-Parent Rating, Gumustas and colleagues [60] found a significant increase in state empathic skills, as measured through the Empathy Response Task, after 12 weeks of MPH treatment in drug-naïve children and adolescents with ADHD. Recently, our research group [62] conducted a study on a sample of drug-naïve young patients with ADHD, naturalistically treated with MPH monotherapy and followed up for 6 months, who showed a significant improvement in AE and CE scores measured with the Basic Empathy Scale. The authors also found that changes in attention symptoms predicted changes in AE but not in CE.

Interestingly, a multimodal approach including drug treatment plus cognitive behavior therapy resulted in significantly greater improvements in frequency indicators on skillful reactions of empathy than the medication-only approach in ADHD patients [65]. Finally, ATX demonstrated a similar effectiveness on ToM skills, as measured with the Reading the Mind in the Eyes test, in a group of young drug-naive patients with ADHD, as compared with long-acting MPH administered for 12 weeks [58].

3.2. Emotion Recognition

Seven studies [31,50,58,60,68–70] assessing the effects of psychostimulants and non-stimulant drugs on emotion recognition abilities in individuals with ADHD were finally identified. Most of the studies were conducted on children and adolescents aged 7 to 17 years old, except for one study [69] that included adult patients. Diagnoses were based on DSM-IV and, in one case [31], on the ICD classification system, and included different proportions of ADHD subtypes; intelligence was generally on average, whereas other psychiatric comorbidities were excluded based on standardized criteria except for two studies [50,68] that included learning disabilities and internalizing disorders, respectively. Further details of the studies are reported in Table 2.

Two studies [31,68] examined the effect of a single-dose administration of MPH on children with ADHD who were already taking the medication regularly at the time of the study. Particularly, the former study [68] compared 30 ADHD patients with and without learning disabilities (LD) to 15 matched controls with no ADHD nor LD and found that, while at baseline only ADHD patients with comorbid LD demonstrated greater difficulties in perceiving paralanguage gesture cues than the other groups, as assessed through the Diagnostic Analysis of Nonverbal Accuracy test, the effect of medication was to equalize such differences. On the other hand, the latter study [31] revealed no significant medication effects on 21 children with ADHD on facial affect recognition abilities, neither with pictures of faces nor with eye pairs for any type of emotions, as assessed through the Frankfurt Test and Training of Social Affect.

Four studies [50,58,60,70] evaluated the effect of a mid-term treatment with daily administration of MPH. The oldest study [50] revealed significant improvements in fear and anger recognition in thirty-three patients with ADHD and comorbid anxiety and depression symptoms—either drug-naïve or under MPH treatment suspended at least three days before the testing session—after four weeks of daily treatment with MPH. Nonetheless, despite such improvements, ADHD patients still displayed deficits in emotion recognition abilities compared to healthy controls. Conversely, in a cross-sectional design study [70], the authors found no significant effects of MPH on emotion recognition reaction times and the number of correct answers in twenty-eight treated versus twenty-eight untreated ADHD patients compared to healthy controls, by means of a morphing task implemented from the Karolinska Directed Emotional Faces Set. The only difference approaching statistical significance concerned the number of sad faces mistaken as angry after MPH treatment.

Two more recent studies [58,60] compared a sample of more than 60 drug-naïve patients treated with MPH for 3 months to matched healthy controls and found significant improvements in emotion recognition abilities, as assessed through the Diagnostic Analysis of Nonverbal Accuracy (for sadness and anger only) and the Benton Face Recognition tests, respectively. Interestingly, the former study [58] confirmed a similar trend also for ATX. Finally, only one study [69] assessed the effects of a 4-week treatment with lisdexamfetamine (LDX) versus placebo in 25 adult patients with ADHD on performances of a mixed task evaluating executive functioning and emotion recognition abilities (i.e., Face Emotion Go/No-Go Task). The authors revealed no significant differences between the two treatment arms; it should be noted, however, that some patients were previously treated with MPH suspended at least 2 weeks before the testing session.

4. Discussion

The present systematic review aimed to synthesize research findings on the effect of psychostimulants and nonstimulant drugs on social cognition in patients with ADHD. As far as we know, our study is the first review that systematically and specifically addressed this topic; former narrative but still comprehensive reviews [3,6] were respectively focused on social dysfunctions in ADHD, with the contribution of comorbid disruptive behavior disorders (i.e., ODD/CD) to social impairments, and on the link between social cognition deficits in ADHD and evidence from neuroimaging and lesion studies. Here, we complementarily aimed at looking for the available evidence from scientific literature on the impact of pharmacological interventions on empathy, theory of mind, and emotion recognition in ADHD. The research interest on such a topic is quite recent since the oldest studies retrieved through our search date back to 1999 for emotion recognition [68] and even later for empathy/ToM [47]. Unfortunately, for this reason, the number of studies dedicated to the assessment of social cognition in ADHD is still limited and even less on the effects of pharmacological treatment.

Most of the studies we identified through our search were conducted on children as expected, since ADHD is a neurodevelopmental condition with greater incidence in childhood [71] and social cognition deficits may become attenuated from adolescence on [53], while only one study was performed on adults [69]. Nonetheless, longitudinal studies are missing to investigate the developmental trajectories of social cognition skills from early childhood to adulthood, thus highlighting a still underexplored field of research on this topic. Study samples included, when clinical details were available, both Combined and Inattentive presentations of ADHD, whereas the Hyperactive/Impulsive type was typically underrepresented; in one study [68], a group of patients with ADHD and comorbid learning disabilities was compared to a pure ADHD group, while DBD and other comorbidities were generally excluded with some notable exceptions [31,50,59,62]. Most studies also included a comparison group variably consisting of healthy or clinical controls without ADHD.

As for the assessment of empathy and ToM, both paper-and-pencil questionnaires, including self (e.g., Basic Empathy Scale) and parent reports (e.g., Griffith Empathy Measurement), and standardized tests (e.g., Reading the Mind in the Eyes Test) were used. On the other hand, only standardized tasks were used instead to assess the emotion recognition abilities of participants (e.g., Diagnostic Analysis of Nonverbal Accuracy). Among the available treatment options for ADHD, most studies assessed the effect of psychostimulants, and first of all MPH, which represents the gold-standard pharmacological intervention for the disorder [55]. Schulz and colleagues [69], instead, evaluated the impact of LDX—an amphetamine derivative—while the study conducted by Demirci and Erdogan [58] was the only one that applied a selective noradrenaline reuptake inhibitor, namely ATX. Finally, Coelho and colleagues [65] assessed the efficacy of a multimodal treatment (medication plus cognitive-behavioral therapy) to investigate a possible additive effect of both types of intervention on social skills.

Study designs significantly varied across the included papers, most of which were based on longitudinal trials. Indeed, several studies assessed the effect of a mid-term treatment with MPH and/or other pharmacological and non-pharmacological interventions administered on a regular daily basis for 3–12 weeks to 4–6 months, typically in drug-naïve ADHD patients, except for a few samples including individuals previously exposed to psychostimulants that were washed-out from 3 days to 1 month prior to testing. Some additional studies assessed the effects of a single-dose administration of MPH, either alone or versus placebo in drug-naïve ADHD patients or subjects that were already regularly taking drugs, whereas only one study [70] applied a cross-sectional design on drug-naïve ADHD patients versus MPH-treated ones.

Eight studies demonstrated significant improvements in empathy and/or ToM skills after a single-dose administration or prolonged treatment [46,47,58–62]. Interestingly, Coelho and colleagues [65] observed a significant effect of a multimodal treatment including medication combined with CBT on measures of social skills. Notably, the only study in which the authors did not find any significant improvement of ToM skills after a single-dose administration of MPH was the one by Golubchik and Weizman [66]. When compared to healthy controls, patients with ADHD displayed significantly lower baseline performances on empathy/ToM measures that greatly improved after pharmacological intervention until they reached those obtained by the comparison group [46,58,61]; interestingly, the greater baseline impairments were identified in Hyperactive/Impulsive and Combined types than in the Inattentive one.

As for emotion recognition abilities, most studies showed a significant improvement after the implementation of pharmacological treatment [50,58,60,68], while one study [31] found a non-significant improvement. Only two studies did not reveal a beneficial effect, though neither was it detrimental, of drugs on the emotion recognition skills in ADHD patients [69,70]; however, the former assessed the effects of LDX, which is not considered the first-line treatment option for the disorder, while the latter was based on a cross-sectional design. Interestingly, Gumustas and colleagues [60] revealed that, following the treatment with MPH, the ADHD group showed a significant improvement in the recognition of anger and sadness expressions. When compared to controls, patients with ADHD exhibited significantly lower baseline performances on emotion recognition that improved after pharmacological implementation until they reached those obtained by the comparison group.

Based on our review, we could speculate that, in patients with ADHD, drug treatment improves social cognition skills, namely emotion recognition, empathy and ToM abilities. Psychostimulant treatment has been also likely associated with a long-term improvement in prosocial behavior and other outcomes of social functioning [72], including social judgment and interpersonal relationships [56]. Empathy is a critical facilitator of prosocial behavior and is disrupted in ADHD patients, as previously reported in Section 1; however, the beneficial impact of pharmacological interventions on social cognition and functioning is likely to result from their effects on brain circuitries known to be involved in ADHD, possibly, but speculatively, not exhaustively mediated by the effects on the core symptoms of the disorder. In the subsequent paragraphs, we try to illustrate a theoretical framework linking psychostimulants mechanisms of action to social cognition outcomes in ADHD that could be hypothesized based on literature findings, which is depicted in Figure 2.

Structural and functional neuroimaging studies have documented abnormalities in brain anatomy and function in individuals with ADHD [73–75]. Meta-analyses of magnetic resonance imaging (MRI) studies show smaller volumes in the ADHD brain, most consistently in the basal ganglia [74,76]. Functional abnormalities are reported by a meta-analysis of 55 task-based functional MRI (fMRI) studies [73], reporting that children with ADHD show a hypoactivation in the fronto-parietal and ventral attentional networks, involved in attention and goal-directed behaviors, and a hyperactivation in the sensorimotor network and default-mode network, involved in lower-level cognitive processes [77]. In high-functioning, drug-naive young adults with ADHD, resting-state fMRI revealed altered connectivity in the orbitofrontal-temporal-occipital and frontal-amygdala-occipital networks, relating to inattentive and hyperactive/impulsive symptoms, respectively, compared with matched controls [78]. Structural MRI studies on children and adolescents with ADHD demonstrated that chronic naturalistic stimulant treatment was associated with attenuation of ADHD-related brain structural abnormalities, the more consistent findings in frontal, striatal, cerebellar and corpus callosum regions [79]. In the review by Spencer et al. [79], analyzed fMRI studies revealed most consistent findings for striatum and anterior cingulate cortex. In the review by Faraone [78], the author reported that MPH treatment was associated with an increased activation of the parietal and prefrontal cortices and with an increased deactivation of the insula and posterior cingulate cortex during visual attention and working memory tasks. The same author indicated that MPH exposure altered connectivity strength across various cortical and subcortical networks.

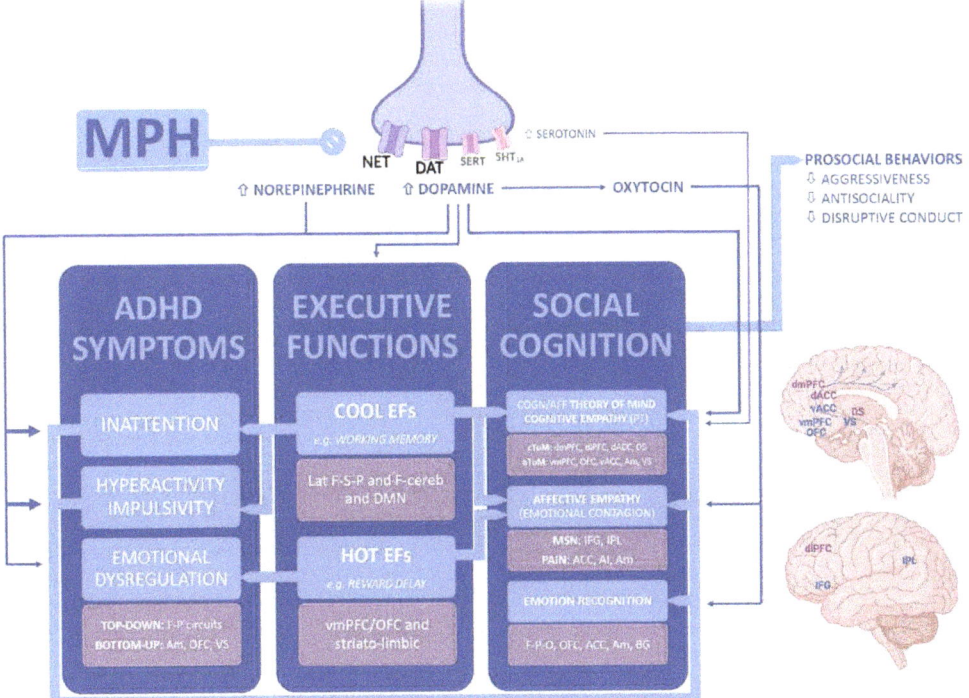

Figure 2. Proposed neurobiological pathways linking methylphenidate pharmacodynamic effects and changes in social cognition in patients with ADHD.

Interestingly, it has been suggested that the efficacy of psychostimulants on the core symptoms of the disorder—i.e., inattention, hyperactivity, and impulsivity—is due to the increased central dopaminergic and noradrenergic activity in the brain regions that include the cortex and the striatum, regions involved in the regulation of attentional and behavioral outcomes [80]. ADHD patients have, indeed, deficits in higher-level cognitive functions necessary for mature adult goal-directed behaviors, that is executive functioning (EF), which are known to be mediated by later developing fronto-striato-parietal and fronto-cerebellar networks [81]. The most consistent deficits are in the so-called "cool" EF, such as motor response inhibition, working memory, sustained attention, response variability, and cognitive switching [81–84], as well as in temporal processing (i.e., motor timing, time estimation, and temporal foresight), with the most consistent deficits in time discrimination and estimation tasks [85,86]. However, impairment has also been found in so-called "hot" EF of motivation control and reward-related decision making, as measured in temporal discounting and gambling tasks, albeit with more inconsistent findings [82,86–88].

Among these, emotion regulation (ER) is also known to be affected in ADHD patients. According to what Posner and colleagues [89] termed the "dyscontrol hypothesis", ER deficits—or simply emotional dysregulation (ED)—in ADHD arise from impairments in hot EF. ED is an altered ability to modulate emotional states in an adaptive and goal-oriented way, with excitability, ease anger, and mood lability [90], which should be considered as pivotal components of ADHD [91]. More specifically, deficits in top-down inhibitory processes, which are found in a sizeable portion of individuals with ADHD, would lead to abnormal emotional reactions, whilst emotional processing per se would be largely normal. The concept proposed by Barkley of "deficient emotional self-regulation" should be considered within this model [92]. Alternatively, the affectivity hypothesis posits that emotional processing per se is abnormal, due to dysfunctions in bottom-up circuits, encompassing the amygdala, the orbitofrontal cortex, and the ventral striatum that processes emotional stimuli.

Interestingly, previous studies demonstrated a positive correlation between EF/ER and empathy/ToM competences in healthy subjects (for a recent review on the topic, please refer to [52]); inhibitory control, working memory, and cognitive flexibility were more strongly related to cognitive empathy, while only inhibitory control was closely related to the affective component. Conversely, a recent paper by our research group [7], which assessed the reciprocal relationship between empathic attitudes and executive functioning in ADHD patients with comorbid conditions, indicated that this latter was more strongly related to the affective empathy. Moreover, a recent meta-analysis [93] that examined the effects of MPH on executive functions in children, youths, and adults with ADHD found that the effects on response inhibition, working memory, and sustained attention were small to moderate. Thus, one may speculate that MPH has a positive effect on EF that, in turn, constitutes a possible mediator for the improvement of empathy and social abilities in youths with ADHD.

From a neuroanatomical point of view, strong evidence supports a model of two separate, yet interacting, systems for empathy, as previously mentioned in Section 1. AE would rely on a large brain network that includes the anterior cingulate cortex, anterior insula, inferior parietal lobule, and inferior frontal gyrus, with its mirror neuron system involved in motor imitation and emotional contagion [14,94]. On the other hand, CE/ToM is subserved by prefrontal and temporal networks: the cognitive ToM network engages the dorsomedial prefrontal cortex, dorsal anterior cingulate cortex, and dorsal striatum; the affective ToM network engages the ventromedial prefrontal cortex, orbitofrontal cortices, ventral anterior cingulate cortex, amygdala, and ventral striatum [94]. A functionally interactive dorsal and ventral attention/selection system at the temporoparietal junction and anterior cingulate cortex modulates the ability to distinguish between self and other mental states [24]. From a neurochemical point of view, AE is modulated in part by oxytocinergic projections [33], while, on the other hand, CE/ToM functioning is dependent on the integrity of the dopaminergic and serotoninergic systems [24].

Pharmacological treatments, especially with MPH, through a direct modulation of central dopaminergic and noradrenergic transmission in cortex and striatum, an indirect action on other neuropeptides such as oxytocin, and by regulating neural activity in these systems acting on top-down and only partly on bottom-up circuits [90], can concurrently improve empathy, theory of mind, executive and emotional regulation in youths with ADHD (see Figure 2). On the other hand, we may speculate that a possible mechanism explaining the social effect of psychostimulants in ADHD youths may be a positive effect of improved attention and EF on empathic abilities.

Little literature evidence is available to discern whether the impacts of stimulants on social cognition could be mediated by the complementary effects on the different core symptoms of ADHD, namely inattention and hyperactivity/impulsivity. Indeed, the studies conducted so far have not specifically addressed the effects of MPH on different ADHD subtypes, but it may be argued that different subtypes could present different empathy profiles. Children with a predominant Inattentive subtype are typically less aggressive and less likely to have comorbid ODD/CD than children with the combined or the Hyperactive/Impulsive subtype that seem to be less empathic than youths with the inattentive one [46,58]. We could speculate that the Inattentive and Hyperactive/Impulsive profile lies intermediate between two extremes, the latter being substantially overlapping with that of ODD/CD. The very few fMRI studies that compared non-comorbid ADHD and ODD/CD children showed that ADHD is associated with dorsolateral prefrontal and inferior frontal under-activation, while ODD/CD was associated with paralimbic under-activation in orbitofrontal, limbic, and superior temporal regions [83,85,88].

Empathy deficits have been implicated in several neurodevelopmental disorders, among which ASD is the most studied [9,95]. Some authors have speculated that performances of individuals with ADHD on social cognition tasks lies intermediate between ASD and healthy controls [43]. Socioemotional problems in ADHD are associated with a more negative prognosis, notably interpersonal and educational problems and an increased risk of developing other psychiatric disorders, while on the other hand, attentional problems at a very early age have been supposed to precede the onset of clinical manifestations of ASD, ADHD, or both disorders [96]. In this perspective, the association between ASD and ADHD traits may be featured by shared attention-related problems (inattention and attentional switching capacity) and biological pathways involving attentional control may be a key factor in the overlapping conditions [97,98]. Future studies are welcome to explore the effects of MPH on empathy/ToM and emotion recognition also in patients with co-occurring ASD.

The current review indicates several limitations of the studies on this topic. First, the limited number of eligible studies. Second, the heterogeneity of the recruited samples and the study protocols (single dose of MPH versus mid-term treatment). Third, the use of self- and parent-rated measures of empathy, which should be integrated with experimental paradigms. In future investigations, empathy/ToM abilities and emotion recognition skills should be assessed in separate samples of ADHD patients including the Inattentive, Hyperactive/Impulsive, and Combined subtype carefully matched on age, gender and medication status. In addition, it would be interesting to investigate possible different responses on the bases of the comorbidity such as other neurodevelopmental disorders, specially ASD, or psychiatric comorbidity.

5. Conclusions

This review provides a contribution for a better understanding of the possible effects of the MPH. Some evidence support the notion that the timely and affective treatment of ADHD symptoms may have beneficial effects not only on core symptoms of ADHD, but also on the social difficulties of youths with ADHD. Future studies on the association of several measures of empathy with comorbid disorders, such as ASD and disruptive behavioral problems, are warranted. At the same time, future studies concerning gender effects are desirable. One important issue for future studies would be the question of whether empathy/Tom/emotion recognition impairments can be observed in all subtypes and, in this case, whether the underlying mechanisms are the same for ADHD subtypes.

Supplementary Materials: The following are available online at https://www.mdpi.com/article/10.3390/brainsci11111399/s1, Table S1: PRISMA checklist, Table S2: search strategy.

Author Contributions: Conceptualization, P.F. and G.S.; methodology, G.S.; validation, G.S.; writing-original draft preparation, P.F. and G.S.; writing-review and editing, P.M., A.M. and G.M.; supervision, A.M.; project administration, G.M. All authors have read and agreed to the published version of the manuscript.

Funding: This research received no external funding.

Institutional Review Board Statement: The study was conducted according to the guidelines of the Declaration of Helsinki and approved by the Institutional Review Board of IRCCS Stella Maris (16 January 2018).

Informed Consent Statement: Not applicable.

Data Availability Statement: The data presented in this study are available on request from the corresponding author.

Acknowledgments: P.F., A.M., P.M. and G.M. are supported by a grant from the IRCCS Fondazione Stella Maris (Ricerca Corrente and the '5 * 1000' voluntary contributions, Italian Ministry of Health).

Conflicts of Interest: G.M. was in advisory boards for Angelini, received institutional research support from Lundbeck and Humana, and was speaker for Angelini, FB Health, Janssen, Lundbeck, and Otsuka. Other authors report no biomedical financial interests or potential conflict of interest.

References

1. Thomas, R.; Sanders, S.; Doust, J.; Beller, E.; Glasziou, P. Prevalence of attention-deficit/hyperactivity disorder: A systematic review and meta-analysis. *Pediatrics* **2015**, *135*, e994–e1001. [CrossRef]
2. American Psychiatric Association. *Diagnostic and Statistical Manual of Mental Disorders, DSM-5*, 5th ed.; American Psychiatric Association: Washington, DC, USA, 2013; ISBN 0-89042-555-8.
3. Uekermann, J.; Kraemer, M.; Abdel-Hamid, M.; Schimmelmann, B.G.; Hebebrand, J.; Daum, I.; Wiltfang, J.; Kis, B. Social cognition in attention-deficit hyperactivity disorder (ADHD). *Neurosci. Biobehav. Rev.* **2010**, *34*, 734–743. [CrossRef] [PubMed]
4. Andrade, B.F.; Waschbusch, D.A.; Doucet, A.; King, S.; MacKinnon, M.; McGrath, P.J.; Stewart, S.H.; Corkum, P. Social Information Processing of Positive and Negative Hypothetical Events in Children with ADHD and Conduct Problems and Controls. *J. Atten. Disord.* **2012**, *16*, 491–504. [CrossRef] [PubMed]
5. Sinzig, J.; Morsch, D.; Lehmkuhl, G. Do hyperactivity, impulsivity and inattention have an impact on the ability of facial affect recognition in children with autism and ADHD? *Eur. Child Adolesc. Psychiatry* **2008**, *17*, 63–72. [CrossRef] [PubMed]
6. Nijmeijer, J.S.; Minderaa, R.B.; Buitelaar, J.K.; Mulligan, A.; Hartman, C.A.; Hoekstra, P.J. Attention-deficit/hyperactivity disorder and social dysfunctioning. *Clin. Psychol. Rev.* **2008**, *28*, 692–708. [CrossRef] [PubMed]
7. Cristofani, C.; Sesso, G.; Cristofani, P.; Fantozzi, P.; Inguaggiato, E.; Muratori, P.; Narzisi, A.; Pfanner, C.; Pisano, S.; Polidori, L.; et al. The role of executive functions in the development of empathy and its association with externalizing behaviors in children with neurodevelopmental disorders and other psychiatric comorbidities. *Brain Sci.* **2020**, *10*, 489. [CrossRef] [PubMed]
8. Crick, N.R.; Dodge, K.A. Social Information-Processing Mechanisms in Reactive and Proactive Aggression. *Child Dev.* **1996**, *67*, 993–1002. [CrossRef]
9. Blair, R.J.R. Fine Cuts of Empathy and the Amygdala: Dissociable Deficits in Psychopathy and Autism. *Q. J. Exp. Psychol.* **2008**, *61*, 157–170. [CrossRef] [PubMed]
10. de Waal, F.B.M. Putting the Altruism Back into Altruism: The Evolution of Empathy. *Annu. Rev. Psychol.* **2008**, *59*, 279–300. [CrossRef] [PubMed]
11. Davis, M.H. A multidimensional approach to individual difference in empathy. *JSAS Cat. Sel. Doc. Psychol.* **1980**, *10*, 85–94.
12. Decety, J.; Moriguchi, Y. The empathic brain and its dysfunction in psychiatric populations: Implications for intervention across different clinical conditions. *Biopsychosoc. Med.* **2007**, *1*, 22. [CrossRef] [PubMed]
13. Decety, J.; Jackson, P.L. The Functional Architecture of Human Empathy. *Behav. Cogn. Neurosci. Rev.* **2004**, *3*, 71–100. [CrossRef]
14. Shamay-Tsoory The neural bases for empathy. *Neuroscientist* **2011**, *17*, 18–24. [CrossRef]
15. Shamay-Tsoory, S.; Harari, H.; Szepsenwol, O.; Levkovitz, Y. Neuropsychological evidence of impaired cognitive empathy in euthymic bipolar disorder. *J. Neuropsychiatry Clin. Neurosci.* **2009**, *21*, 59–67. [CrossRef] [PubMed]
16. Singer, T.; Seymour, B.; O'Doherty, J.P.; Stephan, K.E.; Dolan, R.J.; Frith, C.D. Empathic neural responses are modulated by the perceived fairness of others. *Nature* **2006**, *439*, 466–469. [CrossRef]
17. Shamay-Tsoory, S.; Tomer, R.; Goldsher, D.; Berger, B.D.; Aharon-Peretz, J. Impairment in cognitive and affective empathy in patients with brain lesions: Anatomical and cognitive correlates. *J. Clin. Exp. Neuropsychol.* **2004**, *26*, 1113–1127. [CrossRef] [PubMed]
18. Hurlemann, R.; Patin, A.; Onur, O.A.; Cohen, M.X.; Baumgartner, T.; Metzler, S.; Dziobek, I.; Gallinat, J.; Wagner, M.; Maier, W.; et al. Oxytocin enhances amygdala-dependent, socially reinforced learning and emotional empathy in humans. *J. Neurosci.* **2010**, *30*, 4999–5007. [CrossRef]
19. Lackner, C.L.; Bowman, L.C.; Sabbagh, M.A. Dopaminergic functioning and preschoolers' theory of mind. *Neuropsychologia* **2010**, *48*, 1767–1774. [CrossRef] [PubMed]
20. Preston, S.D.; de Waal, F.B.M. Empathy: Its ultimate and proximate bases. *Behav. Brain Sci.* **2002**, *25*, 1–20; discussion 20–71.
21. Decety, J.; Skelly, L.R.; Kiehl, K.A. Brain response to empathy-eliciting scenarios involving pain in incarcerated individuals with psychopathy. *JAMA Psychiatry* **2013**, *70*, 638–645. [CrossRef]
22. Frith, U. *Autism and "Theory of Mind."* In *Diagnosis and Treatment of Autism*; Springer US: Boston, MA, USA, 1989; pp. 33–52.
23. Shamay-Tsoory, S.; Aharon-Peretz, J.; Perry, D. Two systems for empathy: A double dissociation between emotional and cognitive empathy in inferior frontal gyrus versus ventromedial prefrontal lesions. *Brain* **2009**, *132*, 617–627. [CrossRef] [PubMed]
24. Abu-Akel, A.; Shamay-Tsoory, S. Neuroanatomical and neurochemical bases of theory of mind. *Neuropsychologia* **2011**, *49*, 2971–2984.
25. Frith, U.; Frith, C.D. Development and neurophysiology of mentalizing. *Philos. Trans. R. Soc. B Biol. Sci.* **2003**, *358*, 459–473. [CrossRef]

26. Siegal, M.; Varley, R. Neural systems involved in "theory of mind". *Nat. Rev. Neurosci.* **2002**, *3*, 463–471. [CrossRef]
27. Blair, R.J.R. Neurocognitive models of aggression, the antisocial personality disorders, and psychopathy. *J. Neurol. Neurosurg. Psychiatry* **2001**, *71*, 727–731. [CrossRef]
28. Hermens, D.F.; Rowe, D.L.; Gordon, E.; Williams, L.M. Integrative neuroscience approach to predict ADHD stimulant response. *Expert Rev. Neurother.* **2006**, *6*, 753–763.
29. Nelson, A.L.; Combs, D.R.; Penn, D.L.; Basso, M.R. Subtypes of social perception deficits in schizophrenia. *Schizophr. Res.* **2007**, *94*, 139–147. [CrossRef] [PubMed]
30. Pera-Guardiola, V.; Contreras-Rodriguez, O.; Batalla, I.; Kosson, D.; Menchon, J.M.; Pifarre, J.; Bosque, J.; Cardoner, N.; Soriano-Mas, C. Brain Structural Correlates of Emotion Recognition in Psychopaths. *PLoS ONE* **2016**, *11*, e0149807. [CrossRef]
31. Beyer Von Morgenstern, S.; Becker, I.; Sinzig, J. Improvement of facial affect recognition in children and adolescents with attention-deficit/hyperactivity disorder under methylphenidate. *Acta Neuropsychiatry* **2014**, *26*, 202–208. [CrossRef]
32. Muratori, P.; Lochman, J.E.; Lai, E.; Milone, A.; Nocentini, A.; Pisano, S.; Righini, E.; Masi, G. Which dimension of parenting predicts the change of callous unemotional traits in children with disruptive behavior disorder? *Compr. Psychiatry* **2016**, *69*, 202–210. [CrossRef]
33. Gonzalez-Liencres, C.; Shamay-Tsoory, S.G.; Brüne, M. Towards a neuroscience of empathy: Ontogeny, phylogeny, brain mechanisms, context and psychopathology. *Neurosci. Biobehav. Rev.* **2013**, *37*, 1537–1548. [CrossRef]
34. Blair, R.J.R. Responding to the emotions of others: Dissociating forms of empathy through the study of typical and psychiatric populations. *Conscious. Cogn.* **2005**, *14*, 698–718. [CrossRef]
35. Gillberg, C.L. The Emanuel Miller Memorial Lecture 1991: Autism and Autistic-like Conditions: Subclasses among Disorders of Empathy. *J. Child Psychol. Psychiatry* **1992**, *33*, 813–842. [CrossRef] [PubMed]
36. Preti, A.; Vellante, M.; Baron-Cohen, S.; Zucca, G.; Petretto, D.R.; Masala, C. The Empathy Quotient: A cross-cultural comparison of the Italian version. *Cogn. Neuropsychiatry* **2011**, *16*, 50–70. [CrossRef] [PubMed]
37. Vellante, M.; Baron-Cohen, S.; Melis, M.; Marrone, M.; Petretto, D.R.; Masala, C.; Preti, A. The "reading the Mind in the Eyes" test: Systematic review of psychometric properties and a validation study in Italy. *Cogn. Neuropsychiatry* **2013**, *18*, 326–354. [CrossRef] [PubMed]
38. Jolliffe, D.; Farrington, D.P. Development and validation of the Basic Empathy Scale. *J. Adolesc.* **2006**, *29*, 589–611. [CrossRef] [PubMed]
39. Milone, A.; Cerniglia, L.; Cristofani, C.; Inguaggiato, E.; Levantini, V.; Masi, G.; Paciello, M.; Simone, F.; Muratori, P. Empathy in youths with conduct disorder and callous-unemotional traits. *Neural Plast.* **2019**, *2019*, 9638973. [CrossRef] [PubMed]
40. Abikoff, H.; Hechtman, L.; Klein, R.G.; Gallagher, R.; Fleiss, K.; Etcovitch, J.; Cousins, L.; Greenfield, B.; Martin, D.; Pollack, S. Social functioning in children with ADHD treated with long-term methylphenidate and multimodal psychosocial treatment. *J. Am. Acad. Child Adolesc. Psychiatry* **2004**, *43*, 820–829. [CrossRef] [PubMed]
41. Braaten, E.B.; Rosén, L.A. Self-regulation of affect in attention deficit-hyperactivity disorder (ADHD) and non-ADHD boys: Differences in empathic responding. *J. Consult. Clin. Psychol.* **2000**, *68*, 313–321. [CrossRef] [PubMed]
42. Cordier, R.; Bundy, A.; Hocking, C.; Einfeld, S. Empathy in the play of children with attention deficit hyperactivity disorder. *OTJR Occup. Particip. Heal.* **2010**, *30*, 122–132. [CrossRef]
43. Bora, E.; Pantelis, C. Meta-analysis of social cognition in attention-deficit/hyperactivity disorder (ADHD): Comparison with healthy controls and autistic spectrum disorder. *Psychol. Med.* **2016**, *46*, 699–716.
44. Parke, E.M.; Becker, M.L.; Graves, S.J.; Baily, A.R.; Paul, M.G.; Freeman, A.J.; Allen, D.N. Social Cognition in Children with ADHD. *J. Atten. Disord.* **2018**, *25*, 519–529. [CrossRef] [PubMed]
45. Marton, I.; Wiener, J.; Rogers, M.; Moore, C.; Tannock, R. Empathy and social perspective taking in children with attention-deficit/hyperactivity disorder. *J. Abnorm. Child Psychol.* **2009**, *37*, 107–118. [CrossRef] [PubMed]
46. Maoz, H.; Gvirts, H.Z.; Sheffer, M.; Bloch, Y. Theory of Mind and Empathy in Children with ADHD. *J. Atten. Disord.* **2019**, *23*, 1331–1338. [CrossRef]
47. Maoz, H.; Tsviban, L.; Gvirts, H.Z.; Shamay-Tsoory, S.G.; Levkovitz, Y.; Watemberg, N.; Bloch, Y. Stimulants improve theory of mind in children with attention deficit hyperactivity disorder. *J. Psychopharmacol.* **2014**, *28*, 212–219. [CrossRef] [PubMed]
48. Staff, A.I.; Luman, M.; van der Oord, S.; Bergwerff, C.E.; van den Hoofdakker, B.J.; Oosterlaan, J. Facial emotion recognition impairment predicts social and emotional problems in children with (subthreshold) ADHD. *Eur. Child Adolesc. Psychiatry* **2021**. [CrossRef]
49. Pelc, K.; Kornreich, C.; Foisy, M.L.; Dan, B. Recognition of Emotional Facial Expressions in Attention-Deficit Hyperactivity Disorder. *Pediatr. Neurol.* **2006**, *35*, 93–97. [CrossRef]
50. Williams, L.M.; Hermens, D.F.; Palmer, D.; Kohn, M.; Clarke, S.; Keage, H.; Clark, C.R.; Gordon, E. Misinterpreting Emotional Expressions in Attention-Deficit/Hyperactivity Disorder: Evidence for a Neural Marker and Stimulant Effects. *Biol. Psychiatry* **2008**, *63*, 917–926. [CrossRef]
51. Barkley, R.A. The relevance of the Still lectures to attention-deficit/hyperactivity disorder: A commentary. *J. Atten. Disord.* **2006**, *10*, 137–140. [CrossRef]
52. Yan, Z.; Hong, S.; Liu, F.; Su, Y. A meta-analysis of the relationship between empathy and executive function. *PsyCh J.* **2020**, *9*, 34–43. [CrossRef]
53. Abdel-Hamid, M.; Niklewski, F.; Heßmann, P.; Guberina, N.; Kownatka, M.; Kraemer, M.; Scherbaum, N.; Dziobek, I.; Bartels, C.; Wiltfang, J.; et al. Impaired empathy but no theory of mind deficits in adult attention deficit hyperactivity disorder. *Brain Behav.* **2019**, *9*, e01401. [CrossRef] [PubMed]

54. Pineda-Alhucema, W.; Aristizabal, E.; Escudero-Cabarcas, J.; Acosta-López, J.E.; Vélez, J.I. Executive Function and Theory of Mind in Children with ADHD: A Systematic Review. *Neuropsychol. Rev.* **2018**, *28*, 341–358. [CrossRef] [PubMed]
55. Cortese, S.; Adamo, N.; Del Giovane, C.; Mohr-Jensen, C.; Hayes, A.J.; Carucci, S.; Atkinson, L.Z.; Tessari, L.; Banaschewski, T.; Coghill, D.; et al. Comparative efficacy and tolerability of medications for attention-deficit hyperactivity disorder in children, adolescents, and adults: A systematic review and network meta-analysis. *Lancet Psychiatry* **2018**, *5*, 727–738. [CrossRef] [PubMed]
56. Whalen, C.K.; Henker, B.; Granger, D.A. Social judgment processes in hyperactive boys: Effects of methylphenidate and comparisons with normal peers. *J. Abnorm. Child Psychol.* **1990**, *18*, 297–316. [CrossRef] [PubMed]
57. Whalen, C.K.; Henker, B. Social impact of stimulant treatment for hyperactive children. *J. Learn. Disabil.* **1991**, *24*, 231–241. [CrossRef] [PubMed]
58. Demirci, E.; Erdogan, A. Is emotion recognition the only problem in ADHD? Effects of pharmacotherapy on face and emotion recognition in children with ADHD. *ADHD-Atten. Deficit Hyperact. Disord.* **2016**, *8*, 197–204. [CrossRef]
59. Golubchik, P.; Weizman, A. The Possible Effect of Methylphenidate Treatment on Empathy in Children Diagnosed with Attention-Deficit/Hyperactivity Disorder, Both with and Without Comorbid Oppositional Defiant Disorder. *J. Child Adolesc. Psychopharmacol.* **2017**, *27*, 429–432. [CrossRef]
60. Gumustas, F.; Yilmaz, I.; Yulaf, Y.; Gokce, S.; Sabuncuoglu, O. Empathy and facial expression recognition in children with and without attention-deficit/hyperactivity disorder: Effects of stimulant medication on empathic skills in children with attention-deficit/hyperactivity disorder. *J. Child Adolesc. Psychopharmacol.* **2017**, *27*, 433–439. [CrossRef]
61. Levi-Shachar, O.; Gvirts, H.Z.; Goldwin, Y.; Bloch, Y.; Shamay-Tsoory, S.; Zagoory-Sharon, O.; Feldman, R.; Maoz, H. The effect of methylphenidate on social cognition and oxytocin in children with attention deficit hyperactivity disorder. *Neuropsychopharmacol. Off. Publ. Am. Coll. Neuropsychopharmacol.* **2020**, *45*, 367–373. [CrossRef]
62. Fantozzi, P.; Muratori, P.; Caponi, M.C.; Levantini, V.; Nardoni, C.; Pfanner, C.; Ricci, F.; Sesso, G.; Tacchi, A.; Milone, A.; et al. Treatment with Methylphenidate Improves Affective but Not Cognitive Empathy in Youths with Attention-Deficit/Hyperactivity Disorder. *Children* **2021**, *8*, 596. [CrossRef]
63. Zoratto, F.; Franchi, F.; Macri, S.; Laviola, G. Methylphenidate administration promotes sociability and reduces aggression in a mouse model of callousness. *Psychopharmacology* **2019**, *236*, 2593–2611. [CrossRef] [PubMed]
64. Uekermann, J.; Kraemer, M.; Krankenhaus, A.K.; Abdel-Hamid, M.; Hebebrand, J.; Uekermann, J.; Kraemer, M.; Abdel-Hamid, M.; Schimmelmann, B.G.; Hebebrand, J.; et al. *Social Cognition in Attention-Deficit Hyperactivity Disorder (ADHD) Essener Interview zur Schulzeitbezogenen Biographie bei ADHS im Erwachsenenalter View Project COMPAS Study View Project Social Cognition in Attention-Deficit Hyperactivity Disorder (ADHD)*; Elsevier: Amsterdam, The Netherlands, 2009. [CrossRef]
65. Coelho, L.F.; Barbosa, D.L.F.; Rizzutti, S.; Bueno, O.F.A.; Miranda, M.C. Group cognitive behavioral therapy for children and adolescents with ADHD. *Psicol. Reflex. Crit. Rev. Semest. Dep. Psicol. UFRGS* **2017**, *30*, 11. [CrossRef]
66. Golubchik, P.; Weizman, A. Poor performance of the "child Reading the Mind in the Eyes Test" correlates with poorer social-emotional functioning in children with attention-deficit/hyperactivity disorder. *Int. Clin. Psychopharmacol.* **2020**, *35*, 105–108. [CrossRef] [PubMed]
67. Levi-Shachar, O.; Gvirts, H.Z.; Goldwin, Y.; Bloch, Y.; Shamay-Tsoory, S.; Boyle, D.; Maoz, H. The association between symptom severity and theory of mind impairment in children with attention deficit/hyperactivity disorder. *Psychiatry Res.* **2021**, *303*, 114092. [CrossRef] [PubMed]
68. Hall, C.W.; Peterson, A.D.; Webster, R.E.; Bolen, L.M.; Brown, M.B. Perception of nonverbal social cues by regular education, adhd, and adhd/ld students cathy w. hall, andrea d. peterson, raymond e. webster, larry m. bolen, and michael b. brown. *Psychology* **1999**, *36*, 505–514.
69. Schulz, K.P.; Krone, B.; Adler, L.A.; Bédard, A.C.V.; Duhoux, S.; Pedraza, J.; Mahagabin, S.; Newcorn, J.H. Lisdexamfetamine Targets Amygdala Mechanisms That Bias Cognitive Control in Attention-Deficit/Hyperactivity Disorder. *Biol. Psychiatry Cogn. Neurosci. Neuroimaging* **2018**, *3*, 686–693. [CrossRef]
70. Schwenck, C.; Schneider, T.; Schreckenbach, J.; Zenglein, Y.; Gensthaler, A.; Taurines, R.; Freitag, C.M.; Schneider, W.; Romanos, M. Emotion recognition in children and adolescents with attention-deficit/hyperactivity disorder (ADHD). *ADHD Atten. Deficit Hyperact. Disord.* **2013**, *5*, 295–302. [CrossRef]
71. Meier, S.M.; Pavlova, B.; Dalsgaard, S.; Nordentoft, M.; Mors, O.; Mortensen, P.B.; Uher, R. Attention-deficit hyperactivity disorder and anxiety disorders as precursors of bipolar disorder onset in adulthood. *Br. J. Psychiatry* **2018**, *213*, 555–560. [CrossRef]
72. Shaw, M.; Hodgkins, P.; Caci, H.; Young, S.; Kahle, J.; Woods, A.G.; Arnold, L.E. A systematic review and analysis of long-term outcomes in attention deficit hyperactivity disorder: Effects of treatment and non-treatment. *BMC Med.* **2012**, *10*, 99. [CrossRef]
73. Cortese, S.; Castellanos, F.X. Neuroimaging of attention-deficit/hyperactivity disorder: Current neuroscience-informed perspectives for clinicians. *Curr. Psychiatry Rep.* **2012**, *14*, 568–578. [CrossRef]
74. Frodl, T.; Skokauskas, N. Meta-analysis of structural MRI studies in children and adults with attention deficit hyperactivity disorder indicates treatment effects. *Acta Psychiatr. Scand.* **2012**, *125*, 114–126. [CrossRef] [PubMed]
75. Greven, C.U.; Bralten, J.; Mennes, M.; O'Dwyer, L.; Van Hulzen, K.J.E.; Rommelse, N.; Schweren, L.J.S.; Hoekstra, P.J.; Hartman, C.A.; Heslenfeld, D.; et al. Developmentally stable whole-brain volume reductions and developmentally sensitive caudate and putamen volume alterations in those with attention-deficit/hyperactivity disorder and their unaffected siblings. *JAMA Psychiatry* **2015**, *72*, 490–499. [CrossRef]

76. Hoogman, M.; Bralten, J.; Hibar, D.P.; Mennes, M.; Zwiers, M.P.; Schweren, L.S.J.; van Hulzen, K.J.E.; Medland, S.E.; Shumskaya, E.; Jahanshad, N.; et al. Subcortical brain volume differences in participants with attention deficit hyperactivity disorder in children and adults: A cross-sectional mega-analysis. *Lancet Psychiatry* **2017**, *4*, 310–319. [CrossRef] [PubMed]
77. Franke, B.; Michelini, G.; Asherson, P.; Banaschewski, T.; Bilbow, A.; Buitelaar, J.K.; Cormand, B.; Faraone, S.V.; Ginsberg, Y.; Haavik, J.; et al. Live fast, die young? A review on the developmental trajectories of ADHD across the lifespan. *Eur. Neuropsychopharmacol.* **2018**, *28*, 1059–1088. [CrossRef]
78. Faraone, S.V. The pharmacology of amphetamine and methylphenidate: Relevance to the neurobiology of attention-deficit/hyperactivity disorder and other psychiatric comorbidities. *Neurosci. Biobehav. Rev.* **2018**, *87*, 255–270. [PubMed]
79. Spencer, T.J.; Brown, A.; Seidman, L.J.; Valera, E.M.; Makris, N.; Lomedico, A.; Faraone, S.V.; Biederman, J. Effect of psychostimulants on brain structure and function in ADHD: A qualitative literature review of magnetic resonance imaging-based neuroimaging studies. *J. Clin. Psychiatry* **2013**, *74*, 902–917. [CrossRef] [PubMed]
80. Faraone, S.V.; Asherson, P.; Banaschewski, T.; Biederman, J.; Buitelaar, J.K.; Ramos-Quiroga, J.A.; Rohde, L.A.; Sonuga-Barke, E.J.S.; Tannock, R.; Franke, B. Attention-deficit/hyperactivity disorder. *Nat. Rev. Dis. Prim.* **2015**, *1*, 15020. [CrossRef]
81. Rubia, K. Functional brain imaging across development. *Eur. Child Adolesc. Psychiatry* **2013**, *22*, 719–731. [CrossRef]
82. Sonuga-Barke, E.J.S.; Sergeant, J.A.; Nigg, J.; Willcutt, E. Executive Dysfunction and Delay Aversion in Attention Deficit Hyperactivity Disorder: Nosologic and Diagnostic Implications. *Child Adolesc. Psychiatr. Clin. N. Am.* **2008**, *17*, 367–384.
83. Rubia, K. "Cool" inferior frontostriatal dysfunction in attention-deficit/hyperactivity disorder versus "hot" ventromedial orbitofrontal-limbic dysfunction in conduct disorder: A review. *Biol. Psychiatry* **2011**, *69*, e69–e87. [CrossRef]
84. Pievsky, M.A.; McGrath, R.E. The Neurocognitive Profile of Attention-Deficit/Hyperactivity Disorder: A Review of Meta-Analyses. *Arch. Clin. Neuropsychol.* **2018**, *33*, 143–157.
85. Rubia, K.; Halari, R.; Christakou, A.; Taylor, E. Impulsiveness as a tinning disturbance: Neurocognitive abnormalities in attention-deficit hyperactivity disorder during temporal processes and normalization with methylphenidate. *Philos. Trans. R. Soc. B Biol. Sci.* **2009**, *364*, 1919–1931. [CrossRef] [PubMed]
86. Noreika, V.; Falter, C.M.; Rubia, K. Timing deficits in attention-deficit/hyperactivity disorder (ADHD): Evidence from neurocognitive and neuroimaging studies. *Neuropsychologia* **2013**, *51*, 235–266. [CrossRef]
87. Plichta, M.M.; Scheres, A. Ventral-striatal responsiveness during reward anticipation in ADHD and its relation to trait impulsivity in the healthy population: A meta-analytic review of the fMRI literature. *Neurosci. Biobehav. Rev.* **2014**, *38*, 125–134. [CrossRef] [PubMed]
88. Rubia, K.; Criaud, M.; Wulff, M.; Alegria, A.; Brinson, H.; Barker, G.; Stahl, D.; Giampietro, V. Functional connectivity changes associated with fMRI neurofeedback of right inferior frontal cortex in adolescents with ADHD. *Neuroimage* **2019**, *188*, 43–58. [CrossRef] [PubMed]
89. Posner, J.; Kass, E.; Hulvershorn, L. Using Stimulants to Treat ADHD-Related Emotional Lability. *Curr. Psychiatry Rep.* **2014**, *16*, 478. [CrossRef] [PubMed]
90. Lenzi, F.; Cortese, S.; Harris, J.; Masi, G. Neuroscience and Biobehavioral Reviews Pharmacotherapy of emotional dysregulation in adults with ADHD: A systematic review and meta-analysis. *Neurosci. Biobehav. Rev.* **2018**, *84*, 359–367. [CrossRef] [PubMed]
91. Retz, W.; Stieglitz, R.D.; Corbisiero, S.; Retz-Junginger, P.; Rösler, M. Emotional dysregulation in adult ADHD: What is the empirical evidence? *Expert Rev. Neurother.* **2012**, *12*, 1241–1251. [PubMed]
92. Barkley, R.A.; Murphy, K.R. Impairment in occupational functioning and adult ADHD: The predictive utility of executive function (EF) ratings versus EF tests. *Arch. Clin. Neuropsychol.* **2010**, *25*, 157–173. [CrossRef]
93. Tamminga, H.G.H.; Reneman, L.; Huizenga, H.M.; Geurts, H.M. Effects of methylphenidate on executive functioning in attention-deficit/hyperactivity disorder across the lifespan: A meta-regression analysis. *Psychol. Med.* **2016**, *46*, 1791–1807.
94. Arioli, M.; Cattaneo, Z.; Ricciardi, E.; Canessa, N. Overlapping and specific neural correlates for empathizing, affective mentalizing, and cognitive mentalizing: A coordinate-based meta-analytic study. *Hum. Brain Mapp.* **2021**, *42*, 4777–4804. [CrossRef]
95. Jones, A.P.; Happé, F.G.E.; Gilbert, F.; Burnett, S.; Viding, E. Feeling, caring, knowing: Different types of empathy deficit in boys with psychopathic tendencies and autism spectrum disorder. *J. Child Psychol. Psychiatry* **2010**, *51*, 1188–1197. [CrossRef] [PubMed]
96. Visser, J.C.; Rommelse, N.N.J.; Greven, C.U.; Buitelaar, J.K. Autism spectrum disorder and attention-deficit/hyperactivity disorder in early childhood: A review of unique and shared characteristics and developmental antecedents. *Neurosci. Biobehav. Rev.* **2016**, *65*, 229–263. [CrossRef]
97. Polderman, T.J.C.; Hoekstra, R.A.; Vinkhuyzen, A.A.E.; Sullivan, P.F.; Van Der Sluis, S.; Posthuma, D. Attentional switching forms a genetic link between attention problems and autistic traits in adults. *Psychol. Med.* **2013**, *43*, 1985–1996. [CrossRef] [PubMed]
98. Sokolova, E.; Oerlemans, A.M.; Rommelse, N.N.; Groot, P.; Hartman, C.A.; Glennon, J.C.; Claassen, T.; Heskes, T.; Buitelaar, J.K. A causal and mediation analysis of the comorbidity between attention deficit hyperactivity disorder (ADHD) and autism spectrum disorder (ASD). *J. Autism Dev. Disord.* **2017**, *47*, 1595–1604. [CrossRef] [PubMed]

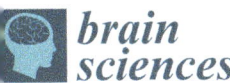

Study Protocol

Neuropsychological Characterization of Aggressive Behavior in Children and Adolescents with CD/ODD and Effects of Single Doses of Medications: The Protocol of the Matrics_WP6-1 Study

Carla Balia [1,2,*,†], Sara Carucci [1,2,*,†], Annarita Milone [3], Roberta Romaniello [1], Elena Valente [3], Federica Donno [1,2], Annarita Montesanto [3], Paola Brovedani [3], Gabriele Masi [3], Jeffrey C. Glennon [4,5,‡], David Coghill [6,7,8,‡], Alessandro Zuddas [1,2,‡] and the MATRICS Consortium [§]

[1] Department of Biomedical Science, Section of Neuroscience & Clinical Pharmacology, University of Cagliari, 09042 Cagliari, Italy; roberta.romaniello@gmail.com (R.R.); federica.donno87@gmail.com (F.D.); azuddas.unica@gmail.com (A.Z.)
[2] Child & Adolescent Neuropsychiatric Unit, "A. Cao" Paediatric Hospital-ARNAS "G. Brotzu" Hospital Trust, Department of Paediatrics, 09121 Cagliari, Italy
[3] IRCCS Stella Maris Foundation, 56128 Pisa, Italy; annarita.milone@fsm.unipi.it (A.M.); elenavalente86@gmail.com (E.V.); ar.montesanto@gmail.com (A.M.); paola.brovedani@fsm.unipi.it (P.B.); gabriele.masi@fsm.unipi.it (G.M.)
[4] Conway Institute of Biomolecular and Biomedical Research, School of Medicine, University College Dublin, D04 V1W8 Dublin, Ireland; jeffrey.glennon@ucd.ie
[5] Radboud University Medical Centre, Department of Cognitive Neuroscience, Radboud University, 6525 EN Nijmegen, The Netherlands
[6] Division of Neuroscience, School of Medicine, University of Dundee, Dundee DD1 4HN, UK; david.coghill@unimelb.edu.au
[7] Murdoch Children's Research Institute, Melbourne 3052, Australia
[8] Departments of Paediatrics and Psychiatry, Faculty of Medicine, Dentistry and Health Sciences, University of Melbourne, Melbourne 3052, Australia
* Correspondence: balia.carla@gmail.com (C.B.); sara.carucci@gmail.com (S.C.)
† Equal contributing authors.
‡ Equal senior authors.
§ Membership of the MATRICS Consortium is provided in the Acknowledgments.

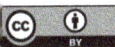

Abstract: Aggressive behaviors and disruptive/conduct disorders are some of the commonest reasons for referral to youth mental health services; nevertheless, the efficacy of therapeutic interventions in real-world clinical practice remains unclear. In order to define more appropriate targets for innovative pharmacological therapies for disruptive/conduct disorders, the European Commission within the Seventh Framework Programme (FP7) funded the MATRICS project (Multidisciplinary Approaches to Translational Research in Conduct Syndromes) to identify neural, genetic, and molecular factors underpinning the pathogenesis of aggression/antisocial behavior in preclinical models and clinical samples. Within the program, a multicentre case-control study, followed by a single-blind, placebo-controlled, cross-over, randomized acute single-dose medication challenge, was conducted at two Italian sites. Aggressive children and adolescents with conduct disorder (CD) or oppositional defiant disorder (ODD) were compared to the same age (10–17 y) typically developing controls (TDC) on a neuropsychological tasks battery that included both "cold" (e.g., inhibitory control, decision making) and "hot" executive functions (e.g., moral judgment, emotion processing, risk assessment). Selected autonomic measures (heart rate variability, skin conductance, salivary cortisol) were recorded before/during/after neuropsychological testing sessions. The acute response to different drugs (methylphenidate/atomoxetine, risperidone/aripiprazole, or placebo) was also examined in the ODD/CD cohort in order to identify potential neuropsychological/physiological mechanisms underlying aggression. The paper describes the protocol of the clinical MATRICS WP6-1 study, its rationale, the specific outcome measures, and their implications for a precision medicine approach.

Keywords: aggression; conduct disorder; oppositional defiant disorder; medications for aggression; callous-unemotional traits; D2 receptor modulators; ADHD medications; neuropsychological functioning; autonomic functioning; control design; acute placebo-controlled single-blind challenge clinical trial

1. Introduction

Aggression toward others is a behavior developed as part of our defense and protection [1,2]. As such, it can be considered a normal dimension of the repertoire conferring adaptive advantages contributing to survival [3]. In humans, aggressive behavior is frequent during early years: growing older, most children learn to socialize and tend to inhibit or suppress aggressive behaviors [4]; following normal morphological and functional development of the human cerebral cortex, infants learn to suppress aggressive behaviors increases while in parallel impulsive behaviors tend to diminish with increasing age, evolving into the "age of reason" [1].

Failure in suppressing aggressive behaviors and in learning effective age-appropriate self-regulation abilities may lead to pathological aggression, which can arise as an excessive response to the stimulus, causing harm to the other or toward self. Pathological aggressive behaviors often occur in individuals falling in the diagnostic category of disruptive, impulse-control and conduct disorders (DICCDs), including both conduct disorder (CD) and oppositional defiant disorder (ODD) (American Psychiatric Association, Diagnostic and Statistical Manual of Mental Disorders Fifth Edition—DSM-5, 2013) [5].

DICCDs are characterized by repetitive and persistent patterns of antisocial, aggressive, and/or defiant behavior that amounts to significant and persistent global impairment. Problems of aggression, oppositionality, and impulsivity, with or without attention deficit or hyperactivity, constitute frequent psychopathology in children and adolescents and are associated with a significant global burden [6]: they imply a worrisome impact on functioning and quality of life with strong long-term negative effects on the individual, on families and on society in general.

Aggressive behaviors are sometimes associated with callous-unemotional traits (CU). Individuals with CD showing CU traits are defined in the DSM-5 by the additional specifier "with limited prosocial emotions" (APA 2013) [5]. To qualify for this specifier, a child must have displayed in multiple relationships and settings at least two out of the following four characteristics, for at least 12 months: lack of remorse or guilt; callousness-lack of empathy; unconcern about performance (for example, at school); shallow or deficient effect (a lack of or insincere expression of feelings to others). These characteristics must reflect the individual's typical (persistent) pattern of interpersonal and emotional functioning and not an occasional behavior [5].

Considering the poor pharmacological response of those with CU traits and the scarce availability of specific treatments [7], in the last decade, many efforts have been made to obtain a better neuropsychological characterization of subtypes of CD.

In CD, the literature suggests a strong correlation between aggressive symptoms and specific neuropsychological deficits: individuals with CD have been found to have important deficits in verbal skills and executive functions, including selective attention, cognitive flexibility, concept formation, and planning abilities [8–11]. Cognitive experimental data suggest that children with CD may also be characterized by impairments in punishment and reward processing and, more generally, in cognitive control [12–14] and in emotional processing [15,16]. Heart rate, skin conductance, and cortisol levels also appear to be altered in this population, in particular in children and adolescents with aggressive CD [17–27].

Although subjects with CD may exhibit different levels of deficits in both *cold* (i.e., working memory, response inhibition, attentional control, planning..) and *hot* (i.e., motivation, delay aversion, sensitivity to reward and punishment, emotional processing), executive functions and may show abnormal physiological parameters (such as heart rate, electrodermal activity, and cortisol levels), data on the prevalence of these characteristics are still conflicting, and the relationships between the different types of deficits have not been completely clarified. Results of the recent largest psychophysiological study to date in this field revealed no evidence for emotional under-responsiveness in CD and a very small effect for respiratory sinus arrhythmia response to sadness [28]. No difference has been found between CD subjects and controls in both sexes also on baseline heart rate, heart rate variability, and pre-ejection period, while only respiratory rate resulted higher in CD female participants [29].

Disruptive/conduct disorders are, in fact, a heterogeneous group of disorders both in terms of pathophysiology and clinical expression, and their neurobiological bases have yet to be completely clarified. Different mechanisms can lead to either CD with callous-unemotional (CU) traits with predominant instrumental aggression (low emotional reactivity, dysfunction in emotional/cognitive empathy, and deficit in decision making), or, on the other hand, to a CD characterized by reactive aggression (impulsive aggression, exaggerated effective response, deficit in processing of social-affective stimuli and in cognitive control). Blair has proposed a model delineating CD physiopathology that defines the aetiological (genetic and environmental), neural, cognitive factors associated with the behavioral aspects of CD [30]. Blair and colleagues describe the interplay of various aetiological factors and the resulting cognitive and behavioral phenotypes and define two main phenotypes: "CD with psychopathic traits" (mainly associated with decreased amygdala, striatal and ventromedial prefrontal cortex (vmPFC) reactivity, and including CU traits, antisocial behavior and instrumental behavior, and frustration-based reactive aggression) and "CD associated with anxiety and emotional lability" (mainly associated with increased amygdala reactivity, and including threat-based reactive aggression and anxiety). Both forms are likely to show under-regulated responses to social provocation. More recently, another large EU-funded study evidenced that amygdala activity in response to negative faces was not significantly influenced by aggression-related subtypes while it was decreased in the high CU traits group [31].

A crucial issue in these models is how specific neurotransmitters (noradrenaline, serotonin, and dopamine) may be involved in the modulation of the major brain areas implicated in the control of aggressive behavior (anterior cingulate cortex, prefrontal cortex, insula, amygdala, striatum, and hypothalamus) and in the underlying neuropsychological functioning. Animal models show that even a single dose of medication can induce a significant change of brain monoamine levels modifying specific neuropsychological functioning during selected tasks [32–36]. The available studies on humans confirm that acute doses of different medications (all able to modulate monoaminergic systems) can have specific effects on specific neuropsychological functions by modulating the neurotransmitters that regulate those processes, independently of their actual observable clinical impact [37–42]. This indicates that the acute administration of monoaminergic drugs may modulate specific regional activities, suggesting their potentially specific role in regulating the neuropsychological functioning in aggressive subjects.

In fact, some clinical evidence suggests that the use of different medications may reduce aggressive symptoms in CD. Evidence confirms that stimulant medications can improve aggression when ADHD co-occurs with disruptive behavior disorders [43,44] and in subjects with a primary diagnosis of CD [45]. Antipsychotics are the most used medication for managing aggressive behaviors in clinical practice, with risperidone being the most studied and effective within this category [46–50]. In addition, mood stabilizers [51–54] and other agents have been proved to exert a certain control on aggression. However, data are limited and often contradictory: no clear indications on the effectiveness of treatments depending on the specific subtype of aggression and their underlying neuropsychological mechanisms have yet been formulated [7].

On the basis of the current literature, further research is required to understand how aggressive CD/ODD patients differ from neuro-typical subjects, and exploring the putative correlations between aggressive behaviors, specific neuropsychological functions, and the physiological measures of the autonomic nervous system activity is required and may provide important information on the biological mechanisms underlying the different subtypes of aggression.

In order to enhance current knowledge on the mechanisms of pathological aggression/antisocial behaviors and their treatment, the European Commission, through the FP7-HEALTH-2013-INNOVATION-1 program, funded the European MATRICS project (Multidisciplinary Approaches to Translational Research In Conduct Syndromes), including different studies finalized to identify neural, genetic and molecular factors involved in the pathogenesis of aggression/antisocial behavior in preclinical (animal) models and clinical samples (stratified for the presence of CU traits), and proof-of-concept clinical studies aimed to define the effects of medication on specific neuropsychological domains.

Considering the limited evidence on the efficacy of medication on the treatment of aggression in the ODD/CD population, the WP6-1 study "The neuropsychological characterization of aggressive behaviour in children and adolescents with CD/ODD" was designed to highlight the neuropsychological differences between aggressive youths with CD/ODD and healthy subjects and to investigate the acute effects of a single dose of different medications on multiple neuropsychological domains, as well as their effects on the autonomic functions that are known to be impaired in these patients [19]. This may allow the identification of cognitive and physiological pathways underlying the disorders and improve the strategies for the management of aggression in clinical practice.

1.1. Aims of the MATRICS WP-6-1 Study

1.1.1. Primary Objectives

The primary objective of the study is to compare the neuropsychological and autonomic functioning in children and adolescents with a diagnosis of ODD or CD who have clinically relevant levels of aggression with that of typically developing (TD) controls.

We primarily aim to explore if conduct problems and aggression symptoms are related to specific neuropsychological profiles (attention, working memory, decision making and risk taking, social cognition, delay aversion, emotional processing, motivation, cooperation, reward-punishment sensitivity), and autonomic functioning (heart rate, skin conductance, salivary cortisol).

1.1.2. Secondary Objectives

As a secondary objective, we aim to investigate the acute effects of medications (known to impact positively on aggression in the context of CD/ODD) on specific neuropsychological and physiological features. For this purpose, we specifically explore the responses to an acute medication challenge by the administration of a single dose of a stimulant with action on monoamine reuptake (methylphenidate), a nonstimulant Serotonin and norepinephrine reuptake inhibitor (SNRI) (atomoxetine) and two antipsychotic medications with partially different mechanisms (risperidone, a full D2, and 5-HT2A antagonist; aripiprazole, a partial D2 agonist).

A further secondary objective is to evaluate the moderating or modulating role on both the neuropsychological/autonomic profile and the corresponding medication effect of socio-demographic and clinical variables such as comorbidities, SES, age and sex, previous medication, source of information (patient, parents, teacher, clinician evaluation), family structure, presence of CU traits.

Details of the protocol of the clinical MATRICS WP6-1 study are described below, including the specific outcome measures and their implications for future precision medicine approaches.

2. Materials and Methods

2.1. Study Design

This is a multicentre, phase II, control design, and acute, placebo-controlled, single-blind, challenge clinical study, employing the following 3 study periods (Table 1, see Section 2.4 study procedures for details):

Phase I: a screening and clinical assessment visit;
Phase II: a case-control design;
Phase III: a randomized, single-blind, placebo-controlled, single-dose, cross-over, acute medication challenge.

This study (EudraCT registration number: 2015-001916-37) was conducted at two Italian sites (Università degli Studi di Cagliari and IRCCS Stella Maris, Pisa) in accordance with the Declaration of Helsinki and the good clinical practice (GCP) parameters. The study protocol, informed consents, and any other appropriate documents were submitted to the competent authority AIFA (Agenzia Italiana del Farmaco) and to the local ethical review boards (Comitato Etico Indipendente of the Cagliari University Hospital, Comitato Etico per la Sperimentazione Clinica of the Tuscany Region). AIFA approval was obtained on 4 July 2017. The ethical review board(s) reviewed the protocol as required. Before the first subject was enrolled in the trial, all ethical and legal requirements were met, and the study was approved on 29 December 2017 for the Cagliari site and on 22 January 2018 for the Pisa site.

Table 1. Single-blind, placebo-controlled, acute dose, cross-over, randomized medication challenge.

Baseline Assessment [1] and Randomization [2] Group A/B	Randomization Drug/Placebo Sequence	Acute Challenge		
Week 0	Week 1	Week 1	Week 2	Week 3
Aggressive ODD/CD Group A (N = 60)	Group A1	Placebo	Drug A	Drug B
	Group A2	Drug B	Placebo	Drug A
	Group A3	Drug A	Drug B	Placebo
Aggressive ODD/CD Group B (N = 60)	Group B1	Placebo	Drug C	Drug D
	Group B2	Drug D	Placebo	Drug C
	Group B3	Drug C	Drug D	Placebo
Controls (N = 40)	No further follow up			

[1] ODD/CD patients and TD controls. [2] Only ODD/CD patients. Group A: received a single dose of a stimulant (Drug A), a single dose of antipsychotic (Drug B), and placebo, each one in a different week, according to their allocation to group A1, A2, or A3. Group B: received a single dose of nonstimulant (Drug C), a single dose of antipsychotic (Drug D), and placebo, each one in a different week, according to their allocation to group B1, B2, or B3. Drug A = MPH; Drug B = Aripiprazole; Drug C = ATX; Drug D = Risperidone.

2.2. Study Population

2.2.1. Population

The target population was 120 ODD/CD children (age 10–17 years and 10 months at screening visit; e.g., 50% 10–14 and 50% 15–17) and 40 TD controls. ODD/CD participants were inpatient or outpatient or referred by other centers. Our aim was to obtain a representative sample including both male and female subjects, considering that CD occurs in approximately 2.5% of boys and 1.5% of girls (Rowe et al., 2010). The TD group was matched to the ODD/CD group based on age, sex, and IQ.

The planned number of participants was supposed to be split equally between two Italian sites: Università degli Studi di Cagliari and IRCCS Stella Maris, Calambrone, Pisa.

2.2.2. Inclusion Criteria

In order to be eligible to participate in this study within the **ODD/CD group**, patients should have an IQ ≥ 80 and comply with DSM-5 criteria for a diagnosis of ODD or CD, documented by the semi-structured K-SADS-PL interview; also, they must show significant levels of aggression, measured by a T score of ≥ 70 at the aggression or delinquency subscale of the Teacher Report Form (TRF), Youth Self Report (YSR), or Child Behavior Checklist (CBCL); or a score of ≥ 27 on the Nisonger-CBRF D-Total (a total composite score for disruptive behavior (D-Total) derived from the Oppositional and the Conduct Problems subscales). Subjects with a primary diagnosis of schizophrenia-related disorders, bipolar disorder, autistic spectrum disorder, depression or anxiety, and subjects having any psychotropic medications within the last six months before screening visit were excluded.

Subjects could be enrolled in the **TDC group** if they were the same age range, intelligent (IQ ≥ 80), drug-naïve for psychotropic medications, and with aggression below the clinical range. Subjects were excluded if they presented any psychiatric condition.

The rest of the specific inclusion criteria and the exclusion ones are listed in Tables 2 and 3.

Table 2. Inclusion and exclusion criteria for ODD/CD group.

Inclusion Criteria
IQ ≥ 80 (Wechsler intelligence scale, within the last two years before enrollment);
Aged between 10 and 17 years and 10 months at the screening visit;
Diagnosis of ODD or CD, based on the DSM-5 criteria, documented by the semi-structured K-SADS-PL interview; patients meeting criteria for comorbid ADHD, depression, anxiety, or PTSD (as to the clinical judgment of the investigator) will not be excluded from study participation;
Significant levels of aggression, measured by a T score of ≥ 70 at the aggression or delinquency subscale of the Teacher Report Form (TRF), Youth Self Report (YSR), or Child Behavior Checklist (CBCL); or a score of ≥ 27 on the Nisonger-CBRF D-Total (a total composite score for disruptive behavior (D-Total) derived from the Oppositional and the Conduct Problems subscales);
Eligibility to be treated with a pharmacological therapy based on previous medical and instrumental cardiological assessments and based on previous blood chemistry (performed within the last six months), current physical and neurological examination;
Drug-naïve for psychotropic medications (psychostimulants, antipsychotics, SNRI, antidepressants, mood stabilizers) or off any psychotropic medication within the last six months;
Sexually active and of childbearing-potential subjects (WOCBP: women of childbearing potential) must have a negative urine pregnancy test at the screening visit and at the baseline visit, and at each week, during the acute challenge phase of the study;
Subjects' parents/legal guardians must provide and sign informed consent documents; patients must provide informed consent and sign consent or assent documents.
Exclusion Criteria
Primary DSM-5 diagnosis of schizophrenia-related disorders, schizophrenia, bipolar disorder, autistic spectrum disorder, depression or anxiety;
Any psychotropic medications (psychostimulants, antipsychotics, SNRI, antidepressants, mood stabilizers) within the last six months before screening visit;
The subject is pregnant or nursing;
Body weight < 30 Kg;
Any acute or unstable medical condition that, in the opinion of the investigator, would compromise participation in the study;
History of severe allergies to medications, in particular hypersensitivity to neuroleptics, or of multiple adverse drug reactions, or the patient has any contraindications to the use of methylphenidate, atomoxetine, risperidone, or aripiprazole.

Table 3. Inclusion and exclusion criteria for the TDC group.

Inclusion Criteria
IQ $\geq$ 80 (Wechsler intelligence scale, within the last two years before enrollment);
Age between 10 and 17 years and 10 months at the screening visit;
Aggression below the clinical range, T < 70 on the aggression or delinquency subscale of the Teacher Report Form (TRF), Youth Self Report (YSR), Child Behavior Checklist (CBCL), and score of <27 on the Nisonger-CBRF D-Total (composite of Disruptive Behavior Disorder subscales);
Drug-naïve for psychotropic medications;
Subjects' parents/legal guardians must provide and sign informed consent documents; TD control must provide informed consent and sign consent or assent documents;
If the patient is a girl who is sexually active and WOCBP, she must have a negative urine pregnancy test at the screening visit and at the baseline visit.
Exclusion Criteria
A primary DSM-5 diagnosis of ADHD, ODD, CD, or any other psychiatric condition;
Any psychotropic medications (psychostimulants, antipsychotics, SNRI, antidepressants, mood stabilizers) within the last six months before screening visit;
The subject is pregnant or nursing.

2.2.3. Sample Size Calculation

Our approach to calculating sample size for this study is two-fold.

As per protocol, in order to analyse the case-control contrast on the dependent variables, setting alpha at 0.05 (two-tailed), we calculated that a sample size of 120 ODD/CD cases and 40 TD has 80.5% statistical power to detect a group difference with an effect size 0.30, allowing to include the covariates (sex, site, children vs. adolescents, IQ, comorbidity with ADHD). However, hypothesizing an effect size at 0.35 with a variance of 0.32, the 80.5% statistical power to detect group differences with a sample size of 88 ODD/CD subjects and 40 TD would be preserved.

For the acute medication challenge phase of the study, setting alpha at 0.05 (two-tailed), a sample size of 52 participants in each of the two studies has 80% power to detect a difference between the different conditions with an effect size of 0.4.

2.3. Recruitment

CD/ODD group participants were inpatient or outpatient or clinical referrals from community centers; TD controls were enrolled on a voluntary basis referred from schools or other clinical departments. TD controls were also recruited within the families of the ODD/CD group, with investigators asking the parents if they would agree to nominate a cousin or other family members or a classmate of their children who may be willing to join the study. The nominated person's parent was asked to contact the study team, who provided information leaflets and proposed participation.

The planned number of participants was split between two Italian sites: Università degli Studi di Cagliari and IRCCS Stella Maris, Pisa.

2.4. Study Procedures

Study procedures and their timing are summarized in the study schedule of events (Supplementary Table S1).

Phase I = Screening and clinical assessment visit.

All subjects (CD/ODD and TD controls) visited the study site for a screening evaluation (Visit -1). During this visit, before starting any procedures, the study was explained to the patient and his or her parent or legal guardian, who then personally signed and dated the informed consent and assent documents. Patients underwent psychiatric screening assessments, and all criteria for enrollment were verified.

Phase II = Case-control design.

CD/ODD children/adolescents and TD controls underwent a baseline assessment (Table 4) at the study site with their parent/guardian for two subsequent days (Visit 0a and 0b) in order to complete the clinical and neuropsychological testing battery. Neuropsychological testing was split up into 3 sessions. The first session included 5 tasks and lasted about sixty minutes; it was administered during the first of the two days planned for baseline assessment. The second session, composed of 4 tasks and lasting about 50 min, was administered during the second of the two days planned for baseline assessment. The third session, composed of 4 tasks and lasting about 50 min, was administered 45 min after the end of the second session to allow for resting time.

Table 4. Neuropsychological assessment.

Task	Battery
First Day (Visit 0a): Testing Session (aprx 60 min)	
Intra-Extra Dimensional Set Shift (IED)	CANTAB
Face and Eyes Emotional Recognition Task (FEERT)	EMOTICOM
Delay Discounting (DD)	EMOTICOM
Moral Judgment (MJ)	EMOTICOM
Prisoners Dilemma (PD)	EMOTICOM
Second Day (Visit 0b, 1, 2, 3): First Session (aprx 50 min.)	
Rapid Visual Information Processing (RVP)	CANTAB
Delayed Matching to Sample (DMS)	CANTAB
Progressive Ratio Task (PRT)	EMOTICOM
New Cambridge Gambling Task (NCGT)	EMOTICOM
Second Day (Visit 0b, 1, 2, 3): Second Session (aprx 50 min)	
Face Affective Go/NoGo (FAGNG)	EMOTICOM
Reinforcement Learning Task (RLT)	EMOTICOM
Theory of Mind (ToM)	EMOTICOM
Ultimatum Game (UG)	EMOTICOM

During these baseline visits, participants were also assessed on selected autonomic measures (heart rate, skin conductance, salivary cortisol) at rest and during the testing session.

Phase III = Randomized, single-blind, placebo-controlled, single-dose, cross-over, acute medication challenge.

CD/ODD children/adolescents were enrolled in one of the two randomized, single-blind, placebo-controlled, single-dose, cross-over, acute challenge arms (Table 1). The control cohort did not take part in this phase. Each subject was randomly exposed to a single dose of the drug each week for three consecutive weeks according to the condition of their randomization group (A or B). Patients randomized to group A received a single dose of a stimulant, a single dose of antipsychotic medication, and a single dose of placebo, each one in a different week (Visit 1, 2, and 3), according to the order of their allocation to group A1, A2 or A3. Following the same procedure, patients randomized to group B received a single dose of a nonstimulant, a single dose of antipsychotic medication, and a single dose of placebo, each one in a different week, according to their allocation to group B1, B2, or B3.

After the administration of a single dose of one of the four selected medication (methylphenidate, atomoxetine, risperidone, aripiprazole) or placebo, patients underwent a subset of the tasks performed during the baseline assessment (only the second and the third session tasks, for a total task time of about one hour and forty minutes; Table 4).

During this phase, participants were also reassessed on selected autonomic measures (heart rate, skin conductance, salivary cortisol) at rest and during the testing session as in the baseline assessment.

We controlled for practice effects by using a modified Latin square design, using parallel versions of tasks where available, and having a one-week medication-free break between testing sessions.

2.4.1. Method of Assignment to Treatment

At the baseline visit, CD/ODD patients were randomly assigned to Group A or Group B: each subject was given a precise sequence of drug administration within the group (e.g., A1/A2/A3) as shown in Table 1. Assignment to medication groups was determined by a computerized randomization list generator, set by the pharmacist from the Cagliari University hospital, not directly involved in patient screening and assessment.

To ensure groups were balanced among sites, the randomization had been stratified by age and sex.

2.4.2. Blinding

During the acute single-dose medication challenge study, at each testing session, the patient was unaware of the specific nature of medication or placebo tablet (single-blind phase; Study Period III). Investigators were unblinded to the patient's treatment.

The single-blind design and the unblinding of the investigator will not affect the outcome of the study as the task administration is automated with set scripts, and outcome measures are objectively determined by the computer.

2.4.3. Concomitant Therapy

No concomitant psychotropic medication (i.e., psychostimulants, antipsychotics, SNRI, mood stabilizers, and antidepressant medication) was allowed during baseline visit or study period III, nor permitted during the previous six months. If the patient was on any other medication for any chronic condition, the investigator, according to his clinical judgment and upon consent by the patient and patient's parent, could allow the co-administration of the two drugs or suggest tapering off, stopping, or completely washing out the concomitant medication six months before the baseline visit.

2.4.4. Screening and Clinical Assessment

The screening and clinical assessment session (I) included the following evaluations:

- *K-SADS-PL* [55]: a semi-structured diagnostic interview assessing psychopathology based on DSM-IV categories. This interview was used to assess the primary diagnosis and the possible comorbid conditions, including substance (ab)use. The presence/absence of an abuse of tobacco, alcohol, and/or illegal psychotropic drugs was investigated, and the frequency of use during the last 12 months was recorded separately within the CRF.
- *Wechsler Intelligence Scales*: To obtain an estimate of IQ, WISC-IV (Wechsler Intelligence Scale for Children—Fourth Edition) [56] or WAIS-IV (Wechsler Adult Intelligence Scale) [57] was administered, depending on age, for an estimate of global intelligence functioning.
- *Questionnaires:*
    - Child Behavior Checklist (CBCL), Teacher Report Form (TRF) Youth Self Report (YSR) [58]: these questionnaires are part of the Achenbach System of Empirically Based Assessment (ASEBA) and provide a measure of general functioning as well as internalizing and externalizing problems.
    - Conners' Parent Rating Scale-Revised Short Form (CPRS-RS) [59]: an abbreviated version of the factor-derived subscales that assess a cross-section of ADHD-related symptoms and problem behaviors. The parent or caregiver typically responds on the basis of the subject's behavior over the past month.
    - Behavior Rating Inventory of Executive Function (BRIEF) [60]: an 86-item questionnaire fulfilled by parents on executive function behaviors at home and at school for children and adolescents ages 5–18.

- Inventory of Callous-Unemotional Traits (ICU) [61]: a 24-item questionnaire administered to parents designed to provide a comprehensive assessment of CU traits and including three subscales (Callousness, Uncaring, and Unemotional).
- Rating scales:
  - Modified Overt Aggression Scale (MOAS) [62]: a short, widely used rating instrument for assessment of verbal aggression, aggression against property, auto-aggression, and physical aggression. It needs to be administered by the clinician to the parent/caregiver
  - The Nisonger Child Behavior Rating Form (NCBRF-TIQ) parent version: a 66-item measure used to assess child and adolescent behavior in children with disruptive behavior disorder; it needs to be administered by the clinician to the parents/caregiver [63].
- Other:
  - The Clinical Global Impressions-Severity (CGI-S) [64]: a single-item rating of the clinician's assessment of the severity of symptoms in relation to the clinician's total experience (Guy, 1976; NIMH, 1985). Severity is rated on a 7-point scale (1 = normal, not at all ill; 7 = among the most extremely ill subjects).
  - The Children's Global Assessment (C-GAS) [65]: a global, one-dimensional clinician rating of social, family, academic and psychiatric functioning. Scores on the measure range from 1 (most impaired, persistent risk to hurt) to 100 (healthiest; no symptoms).

2.4.5. Risk Assessment for Pharmacological Treatments (Patients Only)

The screening session (I) included the following evaluations to assess the risk of cardiological contraindications and the risk of cardiac adverse events:

- Assessment of the history of exercise syncope, undue breathlessness, and other cardiovascular symptoms;
- Heart rate and blood pressure;
- Family history of cardiac disease and examination of the cardiovascular system;
- An ECG, performed within the last six months;
- A cardiological consultation if considered necessary by the investigator.

A check of previous blood chemistry (within the last six months), exhaustive medical history, and a physical and neurological examination were performed in order to exclude any contraindication to the use of psychotropic medications.

2.4.6. The Neuropsychological Task Battery

Three of the tasks used in this study, which mainly assess "cold" executive functions (set-shifting ability, sustained attention, and working memory), are from the Cambridge Neuropsychological Test Automated Battery (CANTAB RESEARCH SUITE https://www.cambridgecognition.com/cantab/ (accessed on 1 December 2021) [66]), a well-known and validated cognitive software. CANTAB includes highly sensitive, precise, and objective measures of cognitive function correlated to neural networks and is widely used in the clinical research field.

The other ten tasks, mainly assessing "hot" executive functions, are instead derived from EMOTICOM [67], an innovative and not yet commercialized neuropsychological battery developed by the same research group that developed the CANTAB. These tasks assess 4 core domains of affective cognition (emotion processing, motivation, impulsiveness, and social cognition).

All computerized tests were administered using a touchscreen tablet (10.1-inch screen). Apart from the first one (motor screening (MOT) from Cantab), the other tasks were administered on a random sequence for each subject in order to minimize any impact of fatigue across the study. During Phase III, each subject belonging to the CD/ODD group was re-tested by using the same sequence he/her was administered during the baseline assessment.

Baseline assessment (First session) neuropsychological tasks:

- Motor screening (MOT)
  A simple reaction time screening test from the CANTAB battery, the first one to be administered. It aims to familiarize the subject with the test material and to assess the presence of any limitations in the use of the device (vision problems, hearing problems, motors, etc.).
- Intra-Extra Dimensional Set Shift (IED):
  IED (Cantab) is a test that assesses visual discrimination and attentional set formation, maintenance, shifting, and flexibility of attention.
  Outcome measures: This test has many outcome measures; the main ones include accuracy (total errors) and shift ability (numbers of stages completed).
- Face and Eyes Emotional Recognition Task (FEERT)
  The FEERT (Emoticom) measures the ability to identify emotions in facial/eyes expressions. Target emotions are presented using ten different images for each of the four basic emotions (happiness, sadness, anger, and fear), each showing different levels of intensity. Choice accuracy and latency are recorded.
  Outcome Measures: The outcome measures are accuracy across emotions and intensities, overall response latencies (mean reaction times), and effective bias.
- Delay Discounting (DD)
  DD (Emoticom) is a measure of inhibition/impulsivity and delay aversion that assesses the rate of discounting across delays and probabilities.
  Outcome Measures: Area under the curve (AUC) and k calculated from indifference points.
- Moral Judgment (MJ)
  MJ (Emoticom) uses cartoon figures to depict moral scenarios; it assesses normative emotional reactions to being a victimizer (agent) or a victim in the moral situation.
  Outcome Measures: The outcome measures of the task are ratings for the four emotions (guilt, shame, annoyance, and good/bad), which can be looked at across all conditions: agent/victim condition (situations in which the subject is asked to identify himself with the victimizer or with the victim, respectively) combined with intentional/unintentional condition (situations in which an intentional or accidental harm is acted) in order to explore the effect of intention upon moral emotions in moral scenarios.
- Prisoner Dilemma (PD)
  PD (Emoticom) assesses cooperation.
  Outcome Measures: Split and steal behavior across three different opponents (each with a different strategy: aggressive (tit for tat but starts with steal), tit for two tats (starts with split, then changes behavior after the player stolen two times consecutively) and a cooperative player who always splits) and for each type of contribution (win, lose, draw). Response latency is also an outcome variable.

Baseline (second session) and each medication trial visit assessment neuropsychological tasks:

- Rapid Visual Information Processing (RVP)
  RVP (Cantab) is a measure of visual sustained attention.
  Outcome measures: The nine RVP outcome measures cover latency (mean reaction times), response accuracy, and target sensitivity.
- Delayed Matching to Sample (DMtS)
  DMtS (Cantab) assesses forced-choice recognition memory for non-verbalizable patterns, testing both simultaneous matching and short-term visual memory.
  Outcome measures: This test has several outcome measures, the main ones assessing latency (the participant's speed of response) and the proportion of correct patterns

selected when the patterns are presented simultaneously or after brief delays from the stimulus.
- Progressive Ratio Task (PRT)
PR Task (Emoticom) assesses participants' motivational 'breakpoint'.
Outcome measures: main measures are trials completed, post-reinforcement pause (average time taken to initiate the next trial following a reward), and running rate (time taken to complete the block of trials).
- Face Affective Go/NoGo Task (FAGNG)
FAGNG (Emoticom) assesses information processing biases for positive and negative facial expressions (biased emotional attention).
Outcome Measures: The task records proportions of hits, misses, correct rejections, and false alarms. This is used to calculate accuracy, reaction times, and effective bias across conditions.
- New Cambridge Gambling Task (New CGT)
NCGT (Emoticom) assesses decision-making and risk-taking behavior and investigates reward-seeking and punishment avoidance separately.
Outcome Measures: The six outcome measures cover risk taking, quality of decision making, deliberation time, and overall proportion bet, split in loss condition, and win condition.
- Reinforcement Learning Task (RLT)
RLT Task (Emoticom) assesses reward and punishment sensitivity.
Outcome Measures: Outcome measures include learning rate and response times.
- Theory of Mind (TOM)
TOM (Emoticom) assesses information sampling in socially ambiguous situations.
Outcome Measures: Information sampling, preference for feelings, thoughts, and facts (proportion of faces/thoughts/facts selected by the subjects to help resolve ambiguity), outcome choice (negative, positive, or neutral), and outcome choice confidence.
- Ultimatum Game (UG)
UG (Emoticom battery) assesses fairness sensitivity and punishment tendency.
Outcome Measures: Outcome measures include "accept" percentage for each level of opponent offers (90%, 80%, 75%, 70%, 65%, 60%, or 50%) used to assess risk adjustment.

2.4.7. Physiological Measures

- *Saliva cortisol samples collection*: Participants were asked to collect saliva using a "passive drool" method in order to measure salivary cortisol. The saliva cortisol samples were collected during V0a and V0b visits and, for the CD/ODD sample only, during each subsequent visit (V1, V2, V3). Each visit was scheduled in the morning. One baseline sample and one stress sample were collected before and after the testing session, respectively. The baseline sample was collected before the testing session in a time window between 8:00 and 9:30 a.m. while the stress sample was collected at the end of the testing session (exact time was supposed to vary based on the time needed for the execution of the whole neuropsychological battery for each subject). The sampling time was recorded in the patient's CRF. If the participant had trouble spitting, sugar- and flavor-free chewing gum were provided to assist salivation. They were asked to rinse their mouths with water and then waited approximately 1 min before producing each sample. All samples were centrifuged after collection and then frozen and stored at $-20\ °C$ until assay. Cortisol levels were assessed by an external lab (Ospedale San Raffaele, Milano);
- *Autonomic measures by using Empatica E4*: During the performance of all abovementioned tasks, subjects underwent an autonomic profile measurement by a wristband able to record heart rate (HR) and heart rate variability by a photoplethysmography technique. HR was recorded for five minutes while the participant was at rest to yield baseline and continuously during the performance of the whole neuropsycholog-

ical battery. The same wristband allowed to record the electrodermal activity in terms of skin conductance (referred to as galvanic skin response), arousal, and excitement.

2.4.8. Vital Signs, Body Temperature, Height, and Weight

Fifteen minutes before the beginning and 15 min after the conclusion of the neuropsychological testing sessions, vital signs (blood pressure, heart rate) were recorded. Body temperature, height, and weight were recorded, and physical examination was also performed.

2.4.9. Single Acute Medication Administration

Within the single-blind, randomized, placebo-controlled, single-dose, cross-over medication challenge, the ODD/CD subjects were randomly assigned to have a single dose of placebo or two of the following medications once a week for three consecutive weeks: methylphenidate, atomoxetine, risperidone, aripiprazole.

The investigator or his/her designee was responsible for explaining the characteristics of the investigational agent(s) and possible adverse effects to the patients and his/her parents/legal guardian, maintaining accurate records of study drug dispensing at each visit.

Patients received a single dose of medication at the investigator study site one hour and a half before the beginning of the first testing session (e.g., 8.00 a.m. if the testing session is supposed to start at 9:30 a.m.). The time of administration had been estimated as the best time in order to evaluate the change of the performance on the various tasks during the pharmacodynamics window for these medications.

Dosages of each medication had been chosen according to the available literature considering the safety and tolerability of each drug on a single administration. Single doses were assigned to the participants according to their weight range (Table 5).

Table 5. IMP dosages for specific weight ranges.

Weight (kg)	MPH (Medikinet)	ATX (Strattera)	RISPERIDONE (Risperdal)	ARIPIPRAZOLE (Abilify)
≥50	20 mg	40 mg	1 mg	5 mg
≥35–<50	15 mg	25 mg	0.5 mg	2.5 mg

2.5. Outcome Measures: Study Parameters/Endpoints

2.5.1. Main Outcome Measures

Main outcome measures include the following:

- Quantitative and qualitative measures from the neuropsychological tasks: reaction times (response latency), accuracy (number/percentage of errors), test completion, learning rate, motivation, cooperation, reward-punishment sensitivity on the neuropsychological tasks from CANTAB and EMOTICOM batteries;
- Physiological measures: heart rate, skin conductance, and salivary cortisol levels at rest and during test performance.

2.5.2. Secondary Study Parameters/Endpoints

Secondary endpoints include measures to investigate the association between severity, type of aggression, and performance on the neuropsychological tasks:

- Screening questionnaires: TRF, YSR, CBCL, CPRS, BRIEF, ICU;
- Screening rating scales: MOAS and Nisonger interview;
- CGI-S, C-GAS.

2.6. Handling and Storage of Data and Documents

Data were handled confidentially and anonymously. A subject identification code list was used to link the data to the subject. The code was not based on the patient's initials and birth date. The key to the code was safeguarded by the investigators. Demographic data (name, address, etc.) and identification numbers were coupled in a file, which was saved on a pc protected by a password, only accessible to the investigators. The handling of personal data complies with Personal Data Protection Acts.

Salivary samples were received by the laboratory, which performed the analyses. Samples were given a unique code, consisting of the type of sample, the visit and the date of collection, and a unique, consecutive number.

2.7. Statistical Analysis

2.7.1. Primary Study Parameter(s)

Cognitive-behavioral measures

For each task, mean reaction time, accuracy rate, and other quantitative parameters for every participant will be calculated.

Chi-square or one-way analysis of variance (ANOVA) tests will be used to assess group differences in case of data meeting assumptions of normality and homogeneity of variance, while covariates will be explored by using analysis of covariance (ANCOVA) and, thereafter, by determination of simple effects or interactions. All other data will be compared using appropriate non-parametric tests (e.g., Mann–Whitney U test) or by using a bootstrap-based non-parametric ANOVA. Simple and multiple regression models will be applied on the whole sample and on the CD/ODD group with the descriptive measures of CU traits and aggression as dependent variables and all outcome measures as the main predictors. Subjects with an ICU score ≥ 32 will be considered as having high CU traits based on previous studies where a cut-off score of 32 on the ICU was used to split groups of subjects with psychopathic tendencies [68], CD [69], or non-CD diagnosis [70].

Covariates will include age, sex, IQ. The primary diagnosis of ODD or CD separately for a between-group comparison as well as a binary covariate will be explored within the total sample; comorbidities as ADHD, anxiety, and depression, etc., will also be analyzed as covariates.

To explore the potential effects of medication, data from the medication acute challenge will be entered into a bootstrap repeated-measures ANOVA for analysis.

Neuropsychopharmacological response to medication is defined as the score change on the primary measures from each task.

Correlations, simple and multiple regressions, and ANCOVAs will be used to investigate demographic, clinical, neuropsychological, and neurophysiological predictors of acute pharmacological response to establish their role as moderating or modulating variables and to define the correlation between severity, CU traits, and neuropsychological/autonomic profiles.

Autonomic measures

If, as expected, the raw cortisol values are positively skewed, they will be normalized using a log transformation. To assess group differences in cortisol, HR, and skin conductance during task performance, repeated-measures ANOVAs will be performed with the group as a between-subjects factor and session as a within-subjects factor. To quantify cortisol, HR, and skin conductance responsiveness to the stress related to the performance during tasks, change relative to baseline will be calculated. With regard to cortisol levels, the collection time of the samples will be used as a covariate. A one-way ANOVA will be used for group comparisons.

2.7.2. Secondary Study Parameters

Chi-square or one-way ANOVA tests will be used to assess group differences in demographic variables, as appropriate.

We will use (I) ANOVA to compare the ODD/CD group and TD group on all outcome measures and (II) multiple regression models on the whole sample (N = 160) with the descriptive measures of CU traits, aggression, and conduct problems as dependent variables, and all outcome measures as the main predictors. Covariates will include age, sex, SES, IQ, previous medication, ADHD symptoms, source of information, family structure.

3. Discussion and Clinical Implications

ODD and CD have significant long-term implications for affected patients and their families and represent a significant public health problem. While there is some evidence to support the use of medications in reducing conduct problems, such evidence across adolescent development is limited and contradictory [71]. Clear indications on the effectiveness of treatments for specific subtypes of aggression have not yet been formulated, with many clinicians prescribing medications off-label. Currently, in randomized controlled trials, a relatively large pharmacological effect on aggression has been reported for risperidone [72] and methylphenidate [43]. There is some limited evidence for clinical efficacy in CD for other D-2 modulators, including aripiprazole, and there is some low-quality evidence, mainly derived from open-label trials, to support a small effect of mood stabilizers. Only a few studies investigated patients with CD as the primary diagnosis, and very few discriminated between different types of aggression or reported measures of CU traits, thus providing inconclusive results on the modulating role of CU traits on the efficacy of medications [7].

Considering the poor knowledge in the field, the high heterogeneity of the two disorders, and the fact that the neurobiological bases of disruptive/conduct disorders have not been completely clarified, the present study was designed to develop a better understanding of the neuropsychological and autonomic characteristics underpinning conduct and oppositional defiant disorder and to identify specific pharmacological responses for the development of novel targeted pharmacological treatments.

Previous single-dose cross-over studies in children and adolescents on stimulant medications have been performed in patients with ADHD, showing important effects of MPH on various aspects of cognition beyond clinical symptoms [39]. These data suggested that the administration of single doses of medication can have immediate effects on neurobiological correlates and that clinical and neuropsychological effects may not necessarily coincide, with consequent important implications for treatment planning.

In the present study, we include subjects with a primary diagnosis of CD or ODD and aggression, thus trying to trace specific phenotypes for ADHD and for disruptive/conduct disorders, despite the frequent overlap between the two disorders in the clinical population. The high comorbidity with ADHD and the impact of inattention and impulsiveness on the global impairment of CD/ODD subjects can, in fact, explain the severity of the disease and the predisposition to the persistence of antisocial behaviors [73,74]. Based on this understanding, several clinical variables (including ADHD comorbidity, family history of psychiatric disorders, or previous treatments) will be explored to investigate their effects on predictive models for conduct problems and aggression. In particular, the role of inattention in mediating some of the executive function deficits known to be present in CD/ODD subjects [75,76] will be investigated.

Apart from ADHD core symptoms, another complicating factor in the management and treatment of CD is related to the presence of CU traits. Although many youths with CD and CU traits seem to respond to treatment, most studies have found that CU traits predict relatively poor treatment outcomes, independently of conduct problem severity before treatment [77,78]. An advantage of the present protocol is the possibility of investigating if and how CU traits may modulate the effects of medications, considering that a poorer response for patients with high CU traits may be expected [77].

Considering the absence of drugs registered for this specific indication (aggression) in this particular population (pediatric ODD and CD with normal IQ), the enrollment into the present study represents an important opportunity to strictly monitor these patients and stimulate their awareness and compliance to therapeutic interventions. Moreover, besides the effects of the single doses of the medications on the outcome measures (positive and negative effects, such as cognitive impairment), the data collected on adverse events may also be of particular interest, considering the impact that the appearance of side effects usually has on patient compliance with chronic treatments.

3.1. Strengths and Limitations of the Present Study

Considering the current lack of evidence on pharmacological effects on cognitive functioning in the ODD and CD population with and without CU traits, the main strength of the present protocol is to investigate the acute effects of different medications on different neuropsychological functions within the same study, as well as the medication effects on the autonomic functions that are known to be impaired in these patients. This may allow us to verify the putative role of cognitive and physiological pathways underlying the disorder in order to improve the knowledge on aggression management. The information derived from the modulation of different monoaminergic systems (noradrenergic, serotoninergic, and dopaminergic) by different medications could be crucial for personalized medicine strategies and the development of more effective treatments.

The main limitations of this study protocol include that the Emoticom tasks are not yet standardized in a pediatric population and that the battery administered in this study is an "experimental" version. Furthermore, some of the Emoticom tasks include reading words (especially Theory of Mind and Moral Judgment), which could be less suitable for younger patients or those with specific reading disabilities, therefore requiring additional effort, which might interfere with their performances. Another important limitation is that while the study protocol includes a measure of CU traits (the ICU questionnaire), no specific measures for impulsive vs. proactive aggression assessment have been included: we are aware that their inclusion would have clarified the association between subtypes of aggression and CU traits, possibly adding useful information on drug effects profiles.

3.2. Benefits and Risks for Participants

The present study aims at collecting scientific information rather than assessing immediate therapeutic benefits for patients: no efficacy on clinical symptoms was foreseen from the administration of single doses of the study drugs, and patients were not provided chronic pharmacotherapy within the study.

Medications used in the present protocol are indicated for comorbid disorders: and, with the exception of risperidone (registered for behavioral problems in children and adolescents with autism or intellectual disability), are not currently specifically indicated for the treatment of aggression for either conduct disorder or oppositional defiant disorder: the benefits for the enrolled patients could be related to the possibility of identifying their potentially most effective treatment on the basis of their pharmacological response to the neuropsychological tasks and of their autonomic profile.

4. Conclusions

Validating the hypothesis that specific neuropsychological and autonomic features found in CD/ODD aggressive children and adolescents are responsive to an acute dose of medication may lead to a specific targeted precision medicine approach for CD with and without CU traits.

Based on the results of this study, the more promising medications may be studied in future prolonged, controlled trials to test their efficacy in modifying cognitive and behavioral symptoms as well as the clinical progress of the psychiatric disorder. Taken together, the results of the present study may contribute to the development of specific guidelines for selecting appropriate medications according to patients' aggressive profiles.

Finally, the results of this study could lead to the definition of a neuropsychopharmacological toolkit, which would include the tests found as more useful and sensitive for predicting efficacious responses to medications to be used in clinical practice.

Supplementary Materials: The following are available online at https://www.mdpi.com/article/10.3390/brainsci11121639/s1. Table S1: Matrics WP6-1 study schedule of events.

Author Contributions: D.C. and A.Z. designed the study protocol, C.B. and S.C. wrote the manuscript, P.B., G.M., J.C.G. and D.C. worked on the editing and added minor corrections, J.C.G., D.C. and A.Z. supervised the writing, J.C.G. contributed to the project administration. C.B., S.C., A.M. (Annarita Milone), R.R., E.V., F.D., A.M. (Annarita Montesanto), P.B., G.M., J.C.G., D.C. and A.Z. contributed to the revision of the manuscript. All authors have read and agreed to the published version of the manuscript.

Funding: This research was funded by the European Community's Seventh Framework Programme (FP7/2007–2013) under grant agreement number 603016.

Institutional Review Board Statement: The study was conducted according to the guidelines of the Declaration of Helsinki and approved by the national competent authority AIFA (Agenzia Italiana del Farmaco) on 4 July 2017. Approval from the local ethical review boards (Comitato Etico Indipendente of the Cagliari University Hospital and Comitato Etico per la Sperimentazione Clinica of the Tuscany Region) was obtained on 29 December 2017 for the Cagliari site and on 22 January 2018 for Pisa (Tuscany) site. EudraCT registration number: 2015-001916-37.

Informed Consent Statement: Informed consent was obtained from all subjects' parents/legal guardians before starting any study procedure; patients and control subjects were also provided informed consent and signed assent documents according to the national law.

Data Availability Statement: Data are not publicly available at the moment. They could be available on request from the corresponding authors.

Acknowledgments: MATRICS Consortium members not included in the author list: Jan Buitelaar, Tom Heskes, Carmen Sandi, Giovanni Laviola, Angélique Heckmann, Steven Williams, Declan Murphy, Jack Price, Gunter Schumann, Paramala J Santosh, Tobias Banaschewski, Ralf W. Dittmann, Pieter Hoekstra, Jonathan Mill, Klaus Schellhorn, Joerg Fegert, Diane Purper-Ouakil, York Winter, Nina Donner, Josefina Castro-Fornieles, Celso Arango, Greg Prescott, Geert Poelmans. Authors want also to thank Trevor W. Robbins, Barbara J. Sahakian, Rebecca Elliott, and Amy Blend for developing and sharing the EMOTICOM neuropsychological test battery. The authors are also grateful to Christiana Krammer and Caterina Medda involved in the project management, and Francesca Placini and all the MDs who contributed to the recruitment phase and organization processes of the study.

Conflicts of Interest: C.B. had collaborations within projects from the European Union (7th Framework Program) and as a sub-investigator in sponsored clinical trials by Lundbeck, Otsuka, Janssen Cilag, and Angelini. S.C. had collaborations within projects from the European Union (7th Framework Program) and as sub-investigator in sponsored clinical trials by Shire Pharmaceutical Company, Lundbeck, Otuka, Janssen Cilag, and Angelini. R.R. had a collaboration as sub-investigator in a sponsored clinical trial by Lundbeck. F.D. had collaborations as sub-investigator in clinical trials sponsored by Lundbeck and as an independent rater in clinical trials sponsored by Servier. G.M. was on advisory boards for Angelini, received institutional grants from Lundbeck and Humana, and was a speaker for Angelini, FB Health, Janssen, Lundbeck, and Otsuka. J.C.G. has been a consultant to Boehringer Ingelheim GmbH. D.C. has received consultancy, research support, or speaker fees from Takeda/Shire, Novartis, Bial, Servier, Medice, and royalties from Oxford University Press and Cambridge University. A.Z. served in an advisory or consultancy role for Angelini, EduPharma, Servier, Taked. He received conference support or speaker's fee from Angelini and Janssen. He has been involved in clinical trials conducted by Angelini, Janssen, Lundbeck, Otsuka, Roche, Sevier, and Shire. He received royalties from Giunti OS, Oxford University Press. All other authors declare no conflict of interest.

References

1. Blake, P.; Grafman, J. The neurobiology of aggression. *Lancet* **2004**, *364* (Suppl. S1), S12–S13. [CrossRef]
2. Vaeroy, H.; Schneider, F.; Fetissov, S.O. Neurobiology of aggressive behaviour—role of autoantibodies reactive with stress-related peptide hormones. *Front. Psychiatry* **2019**, *10*, 872. [CrossRef] [PubMed]
3. Berkowitz, L. *Aggression: Its Causes, Consequences, and Control*; McGraw-Hill: New York, NY, USA, 1993.
4. Tremblay, R.E. Developmental origins of disruptive behaviour problems: The 'original sin' hypothesis, epigenetics and their consequences for prevention. *J. Child Psychol. Psychiatry* **2010**, *51*, 341–367. [CrossRef] [PubMed]
5. American Psychiatric Association. *Diagnostic and Statistical Manual of Mental Disorders*, 5th ed.; American Psychiatric Association: Washington, DC, USA, 2013.

6. Erskine, H.E.; Ferrari, A.J.; Polanczyk, G.V.; Moffitt, T.E.; Murray, C.J.; Vos, T.; Whiteford, H.A.; Scott, J.G. The global burden of conduct disorder and attention-deficit/hyperactivity disorder in 2010. *J. Child Psychol. Psychiatry* **2014**, *55*, 328–336. [CrossRef]
7. Balia, C.; Carucci, S.; Coghill, D.; Zuddas, A. The pharmacological treatment of aggression in children and adolescents with conduct disorder. Do callous—unemotional traits modulate the efficacy of medication? *Neurosci. Biobehav. Rev.* **2018**, *91*, 218–238. [CrossRef]
8. Lynam, D.R.; Henry, B. The role of neuropsychological deficits in conduct disorders. In *Conduct Disorders in Childhood and Adolescence*; Hill, J., Maughan, B., Eds.; Cambridge University Press: Cambridge, MA, USA, 2000; pp. 235–263.
9. Teichner, G.; Golden, C.J. Neuropsychological impairment in conduct-disordered adolescents: A conceptual review. *Aggress. Viol. Behav.* **2000**, *5*, 509–528. [CrossRef]
10. Johnson, V.A.; Kemp, A.H.; Heard, R.; Lennings, C.J.; Hickie, I.B. Childhood-versus adolescent- onset antisocial youth with conduct disorder: Psychiatric illness, neuropsychological and psychosocial function. *PLoS ONE* **2015**, *10*, e0121627. [CrossRef]
11. Blair, R.J.; Leibenluft, E.; Pine, D.S. Conduct disorder and callous- unemotional traits in youth. *N. Engl. J. Med.* **2014**, *371*, 2207–2216. [CrossRef]
12. Matthys, W.; Vanderschuren, L.J.; Schutter, D.J.; Lochman, J.E. Impaired neurocognitive functions affect social learning processes in oppositional defiant disorder and conduct disorder: Implications for interventions. *Clin. Child Fam. Psychol. Rev.* **2012**, *15*, 234–246. [CrossRef]
13. Matthys, W.; Vanderschuren, L.J.M.J.; Schutter, D.J.L.G. The neurobiology of oppositional defiant disorder and conduct disorder: Altered functioning in three mental domains. *Dev. Psychopathol.* **2013**, *25*, 193–207. [CrossRef]
14. Blair, R.J. The neurobiology of impulsive aggression. *J. Child Adolesc. Psychopharmacol.* **2016**, *26*, 4–9. [CrossRef]
15. Sharp, C.; Petersen, N.; Goodyer, I. Emotional reactivity and the emergence of conduct problems and emotional symptoms in 7- to 11-year-olds: A 1-year follow-up study. *J. Am. Acad. Child Adolesc. Psychiatry* **2008**, *47*, 565–573. [CrossRef]
16. Herpers, P.C.M.; Bakker-Huvenaars, M.J.; Greven, C.U.; Wiegers, E.C.; Nijhof, K.S.; Baaneders, A.N.; Buitelaar, J.K.; Rommelse, N.N.J. Emotional valence detection in adolescents with oppositional defiant disorder/conduct disorder or autism spectrum disorder. *Eur. Child Adolesc. Psychiatry* **2019**, *28*, 1011–1022. [CrossRef]
17. Raine, A.; Venables, P.H.; Mednick, S. Low resting heart rate at age 3 predisposes to aggression at age 11 years: Evidence from the Mauritius child health project. *J. Am. Acad. Child Adolesc. Psychiatry* **1997**, *36*, 1457–1464. [CrossRef]
18. Ortiz, J.; Raine, A. Heart rate level and antisocial behaviour in children and adolescents: A meta-analysis. *J. Am. Acad. Child Adolesc. Psychiatry* **2004**, *43*, 154–162. [CrossRef]
19. Lorber, M.F. Psychophysiology of aggression, psychopathy, and conduct problems: A meta-analysis. *Psychol. Bull.* **2004**, *130*, 531–552. [CrossRef]
20. Portnoy, J.; Farrington, D.P. Resting heart rate and antisocial behavior: An updated systematic review and meta-analysis. *Aggress. Violent Behav.* **2015**, *22*, 33–45. [CrossRef]
21. Van Goozen, S.H.M.; Matthys, W.; Cohen-Kettenis, P.T.; Buitelaar, J.K.; van Engeland, H. Hypothalamic–pituitary–adrenal axis and autonomic nervous system activity in disruptive children and matched controls. *J. Am. Acad. Child Adolesc. Psychiatry* **2000**, *39*, 1438–1445. [CrossRef]
22. Van de Weil, N.M.H.; Van Goozen, S.H.M.; Matthys, W.; Snoek, H.; van Engeland, H. Cortisol and treatment effect in children with disruptive behaviour disorders: A preliminary study. *J. Am. Acad. Child Adolesc. Psychiatry* **2004**, *43*, 1011–1018. [CrossRef]
23. Van Bokhoven, I.; van Goozen, S.H.M.; van Engeland, H.; Schaal, B.; Arseneault, L.; Seguin, J.R.; Nagin, D.S.; Vitaro, F.; Tremblay, R.E. Salivary cortisol and aggression in a population-based longitudinal study of adolescent males. *J. Neural Transm.* **2005**, *112*, 1083–1096. [CrossRef]
24. Herpertz, S.C.; Vloet, T.; Mueller, B.; Domes, G.; Willmes, K.; Herpertz- Dahlmann, B. Similar autonomic responsivity in boys with conduct disorder and their fathers. *J. Am. Acad. Child Adolesc. Psychiatry* **2007**, *46*, 535–544. [CrossRef]
25. Vanyukov, M.M.; Moss, H.B.; Plail, J.A.; Blackson, T.; Mezzich, A.C.; Tarter, R.E. Antisocial symptoms in preadolescent boys and in their parents: Associations with cortisol. *Psychiatry Res.* **1993**, *46*, 9–17. [CrossRef]
26. Shoal, G.D.; Giancola, P.R.; Kirillova, G.P. Salivary cortisol, personality, and aggressive behaviour in adolescent boys: A 5-year longitudinal study. *J. Am. Acad. Child Adolesc. Psychiatry* **2003**, *42*, 1101–1107. [CrossRef]
27. Oosterlaan, J.; Geurts, H.M.; Knol, D.L.; Sergeant, J.A. Low basal salivary cortisol is associated with teacher-reported symptoms of conduct disorder. *Psychiatry Res.* **2005**, *134*, 1–10. [CrossRef]
28. Oldenhof, H.; Jansen, L.; Ackermann, K.; Baker, R.; Batchelor, M.; Baumann, S.; Bernhard, A.; Clanton, R.; Dochnal, R.; Fehlbaum, L.V.; et al. Psychophysiological responses to sadness in girls and boys with conduct disorder. *J. Abnorm. Psychol.* **2020**. ahead of print. [CrossRef]
29. Oldenhof, H.; Prätzlich, M.; Ackermann, K.; Baker, R.; Batchelor, M.; Baumann, S.; Bernhard, A.; Clanton, R.; Dikeos, D.; Dochnal, R.; et al. Baseline autonomic nervous system activity in female children and adolescents with conduct disorder: Psychophysiological findings from the FemNAT-CD study. *J. Crim. Justice* **2019**, *65*, 101564. [CrossRef]
30. Blair, R.J.R. The neurobiology of psychopathic traits in youths. *Nat. Rev. Neurosci.* **2013**, *14*, 786–799. [CrossRef]
31. Aggensteiner, P.M.; Holz, N.E.; Böttinger, B.W.; Baumeister, S.; Hohmann, S. The effects of callous-unemotional traits and aggression subtypes on amygdala activity in response to negative faces. *Psychol. Med.* **2020**, *6*, 1–9.
32. Winstanley, C.A. The utility of rat models of impulsivity in developing pharmacotherapies for impulse control disorders. *Br. J. Pharmacol.* **2011**, *164*, 1301–1321. [CrossRef]

33. Bari, A.; Mar, A.C.; Theobald, D.E.; Elands, S.A.; Kelechi Oganya, C.N.A.; Eagle, D.M.; Robbins, T.W. Prefrontal and monoaminergic contributions to stop-signal task performance in rats. *J. Neurosci.* **2011**, *31*, 9254–9263. [CrossRef]
34. Bari, A.; Theobald, D.E.; Caprioli, D.; Mar, A.C.; Aidoo-Micah, A.; Dalley, J.W.; Robbins, T.W. Serotonin modulates sensitivity to reward and negative feedback in a probabilistic reversal learning task in rats. *Neuropsychopharmacology* **2010**, *35*, 1290–1301. [CrossRef] [PubMed]
35. Seu, E.; Jentsch, J.D. Effect of acute and repeated treatment with desipramine or methylphenidate on serial reversal learning in rats. *Neuropharmacology* **2009**, *57*, 665–672. [CrossRef] [PubMed]
36. Jager, A.; Kanters, D.; Geers, F.; Buitelaar, J.K.; Kozicz, T.; Glennon, J.C. Methylphenidate dose-dependently affects aggression and improves fear extinction and anxiety in BALB/cJ mice. *Front. Psychiatry* **2019**, *10*, 768. [CrossRef] [PubMed]
37. Chamberlain, S.R.; Muller, U.; Blackwell Clark, L.; Robbins, T.; Sahakian, B. Neurochemical modulation of response inhibition and probabilistic learning in humans. *Science* **2006**, *311*, 861–863. [CrossRef]
38. Chamberlain, S.R.; Del Campo, N.; Dowson, J.; Müller, U.; Clark, L.; Robbins, T.W.; Sahakian, B.J. Atomoxetine improved response inhibition in adults with attention deficit/hyperactivity disorder. *Biol. Psychiatry* **2007**, *62*, 977–984. [CrossRef]
39. Coghill, D.R.; Seth, S.; Pedroso, S.; Usala, T.; Currie, J.; Gagliano, A. Effects of methylphenidate on cognitive functions in children and adolescents with attention-deficit/hyperactivity disorder: Evidence from a systematic review and a meta-analysis. *Biol. Psychiatry* **2014**, *76*, 603–615. [CrossRef]
40. Fosco, W.D.; White, C.N.; Hawk, L.W., Jr. Acute stimulant treatment and reinforcement increase the speed of information accumulation in children with ADHD. *J. Abnorm. Child Psychol.* **2017**, *45*, 911–920. [CrossRef]
41. Alcorn, J.L., 3rd; Rathnayaka, N.; Swann, A.C.; Moeller, F.G.; Lane, S.D. Effects of intranasal oxytocin on aggressive responding in antisocial personality disorder. *Psychol. Rec.* **2015**, *65*, 691–703. [CrossRef]
42. Cherek, D.R.; Lane, S.D. Effects of d,l-fenfluramine on aggressive and impulsive responding in adult males with a history of conduct disorder. *Psychopharmacology* **1999**, *146*, 473–481. [CrossRef]
43. Pappadopulos, E.; Woolston, S.; Chait, A.; Perkins, M.; Connor, D.F.; Jensen, P.S. Pharmacotherapy of aggression in children and adolescents: Efficacy and effect size. *J. Can. Acad. Child Adolesc. Psychiatry* **2006**, *15*, 27–39.
44. Ipser, J.; Stein, D.J. Systematic review of pharmacotherapy of disruptive behavior disorders in children and adolescents. *Psychopharmacology* **2007**, *191*, 127–140. [CrossRef]
45. Klein, R.G.; Abikoff, H.; Klass, E.; Ganeles, D.; Seese, L.M.; Pollack, S. Clinical efficacy of methylphenidate in conduct disorder with and without attention deficit hyperactivity disorder. *Arch. Gen. Psychiatr.* **1997**, *54*, 1073–1080. [CrossRef]
46. Findling, R.L.; McNamara, N.K.; Branicky, L.A.; Schluchter, M.D.; Lemon, E.; Blumer, J.L. A double-blind pilot study of risperidone in the treatment of conduct disorder. *J. Am. Acad. Child Adolesc. Psychiatry* **2000**, *39*, 509–516. [CrossRef]
47. Snyder, R.; Turgay, A.; Aman, M.; Binder, C.; Fisman, S.; Carroll, A.; Risperidone Conduct Study Group. Effects of risperidone on conduct and disruptive behaviour disorders in children with subaverage IQs. *J. Am. Acad. Child Adolesc. Psychiatry* **2002**, *41*, 1026–1036. [CrossRef]
48. Connor, D.F.; McLaughlin, T.J.; Jeffers-Terry, M. Randomized controlled pilot study of quetiapine in the treatment of adolescent conduct disorder. *J. Child Adolesc. Psychopharmacol.* **2008**, *18*, 140–156. [CrossRef]
49. Gadow, K.D.; Arnold, L.E.; Molina, B.S.; Findling, R.L.; Bukstein, O.G.; Brown, N.V.; McNamara, N.K.; Rundberg-Rivera, E.V.; Li, X.; Kipp, H.L.; et al. Risperidone added to parent training and stimulant medication: Effects on attention-deficit/hyperactivity disorder, oppositional defiant disorder, conduct disorder, and peer aggression. *J. Am. Acad. Child Adolesc. Psychiatry* **2014**, *53*, 948–959. [CrossRef]
50. Juárez-Treviño, M.; Esquivel, A.C.; Isida, L.; Delgado, D.; de la Ocavazos, M.E.; Ocañas, L.G.; Sepúlveda, R.S. Clozapine in the treatment of aggression in conduct disorder in children and adolescents: A randomized, double-blind, controlled trial. *Clin. Psychopharmacol. Neurosci. Off. Sci. J. Korean Coll. Neuropsychopharmacol.* **2019**, *17*, 43–53. [CrossRef]
51. Campbell, M.; Adams, P.B.; Small, A.M.; Kafantaris, V.; Silva, R.R.; Shell, J.; Perry, R.; Overall, J.E. Lithium in hospitalized aggressive children with conduct disorder: A double-blind and placebo-controlled study. *J. Am. Acad. Child Adolesc. Psychiatry* **1995**, *34*, 445–453. [CrossRef]
52. Carlson, G.A.; Rapport, M.D.; Pataki, C.S.; Kelly, K.L. Lithium in hospitalized children at 4 and 8 weeks: Mood, behaviour and cognitive effects. *J. Child Psychol. Psychiatry* **1992**, *33*, 411–425. [CrossRef]
53. Malone, R.P.; Delaney, M.A.; Luebbert, J.F.; Cater, J.; Campbell, M. A double-blind placebo-controlled study of lithium in hospitalized aggressive children and adolescents with conduct disorder. *Arch. Gen. Psychiatry* **2000**, *57*, 649–654. [CrossRef]
54. Rifkin, A.; Karajgi, B.; Dicker, R.; Perl, E.; Boppana, V.; Nasan, N.; Pollack, S. Lithium treatment of conduct disorders in adolescents. *Am. J. Psychiatry* **1997**, *154*, 554–555.
55. Kaufman, J.; Birmaher, B.; Brent, D.; Rao, U.; Flynn, C.; Moreci, P.; Williamson, D.; Ryan, N. Schedule for affective disorders and schizophrenia for school-age children-present and lifetime version (K-SADS-PL): Initial reliability and validity data. *J. Am. Acad. Child Adolesc. Psychiatry* **1997**, *36*, 980–988. [CrossRef]
56. Wechsler, D. *Wechsler Intelligence Scale for Children-Fourth Edition*; Pearson Education, Inc.: San Antonio, TX, USA, 2003.
57. Wechsler, D. *Wechsler Adult Intelligence Scale-Fourth Edition: Technical and Interpretive Manual*; Pearson Education, Inc.: San Antonio, TX, USA, 2008.
58. Achenbach, T.M. *Integrative Guide for the 1991 CBCL/4-18, YSR, and TRF Profiles*; Department of Psychiatry, University of Vermont: Burlington, VT, USA, 1991.

59. Conners, K.C.; Nobile, M. *CRS-R Conners' Rating Scales-Revised: Manuale*; Giunti O.S. Organizzazioni Speciali: Firenze, Italy, 2007.
60. Gioia, G.; Isquith, P.; Guy, S.; Kenworthy, L. *BRIEF–Behavior Rating Inventory of Executive Function. Professional Manual*; Psychological Assessment Resources: Odessa, FL, USA, 2000.
61. Essau, C.A.; Sasagawa, S.; Frick, P.J. Callous- unemotional traits in a community sample of adolescents. *Assessment* **2006**, *13*, 454–469. [CrossRef]
62. Kay, S.R.; Wolkenfeld, F.; Murrill, L.M. Profiles of aggression among psychiatric patients. *J. Nerv. Ment. Dis.* **1998**, *176*, 539–546. [CrossRef]
63. Aman, M.; Leone, S.; Lecavalier, L.; Park, L.; Buican, B.; Coury, D. The Nisonger child behavior rating form: Typical IQ version. *Int. Clin. Psychopharmacol.* **2008**, *23*, 232–242. [CrossRef]
64. Guy, W. (Ed.) *ECDEU Assessment Manual for Psychopharmacology, Rev. Ed.*; U.S. Department of Health, Education and Welfare: Washington, DC, USA, 1976. (Reprinted 1991).
65. Shaffer, D.; Gould, M.S.; Brasic, J.; Ambrosini, P.; Fisher, P.; Bird, H.; Aluwahlia, S. A Children's Global Assessment Scale (CGAS). *Arch. Gen. Psychiatry* **1983**, *40*, 1228–1231. [CrossRef]
66. Morris, R.G.; Evenden, J.L.; Sahakian, B.J.; Robbins, T.W. Computer-aided assessment of dementia: Comparative studies of neuropsychological deficits in Alzheimer-type dementia and Parkinson's disease. In *Cognitive Neurochemistry*; Stahl, S.M., Iversen, S.D., Goodman, E.C., Eds.; Oxford University Press: Oxford, UK, 1987; pp. 21–36.
67. Bland, A.R.; Roiser, J.P.; Mehta, M.A.; Schei, T.; Boland, H.; Campbell-Meiklejohn, D.K.; Emsley, R.A.; Munafo, M.R.; Penton-Voak, I.S.; Seara-Cardoso, A.; et al. EMOTICOM: A neuropsychological test battery to evaluate emotion, motivation, impulsivity, and social cognition. *Front. Behav. Neurosci.* **2016**, *10*, 25. [CrossRef]
68. Jones, A.P.; Happé, F.G.; Gilbert, F.; Burnett, S.; Viding, E. Feeling, caring, knowing: Different types of empathy deficit in boys with psychopathic tendencies and autism spectrum disorder. *J. Child Psychol. Psychiatry* **2010**, *51*, 1188–1197. [CrossRef]
69. Schwenck, C.; Mergenthaler, J.; Keller, K.; Zech, J.; Salehi, S.; Taurines, R.; Romanos, M.; Schecklmann, M.; Schneider, W.; Warnke, A.; et al. Empathy in children with autism and conduct disorder: Group-specific profiles and developmental aspects. *J. Child Psychol. Psychiatry* **2012**, *53*, 651–659. [CrossRef]
70. Herpers, P.C.M.; Klip, H.; Rommelse, N.N.J.; Greven, C.U.; Buitelaar, J.K. Associations between high callous–unemotional traits and quality of life across youths with non-conduct disorder diagnoses. *Eur. Child Adolesc. Psychiatry.* **2016**, *25*, 547–555. [CrossRef]
71. Schur, S.B.; Sikich, L.; Findling, R.L.; Malone, R.P.; Crismon, M.L.; Derivan, A.; Macintyre, J.C.; Pappadopulos, E.; Greenhill, L.; Schooler, N.; et al. Treatment recommendations for the use of antipsychotics for aggressive youth (TRAAY). Part I: A review. *J. Am. Acad. Child Adolesc. Psychiatry* **2003**, *42*, 132–144. [CrossRef] [PubMed]
72. Loy, J.H.; Merry, S.N.; Hetrick, S.E.; Stasiak, K. Atypical antipsychotics for disruptive behaviour disorders in children and youths. *Cochr. Database Syst. Rev.* **2017**, *8*, CD008559. [CrossRef] [PubMed]
73. Noordermeer, S.D.; Luman, M.; Oosterlaan, J.A. Systematic review and meta-analysis of neuroimaging in Oppositional Defiant Disorder (ODD) and Conduct Disorder (CD) taking Attention-Deficit Hyperactivity Disorder (ADHD) into account. *Neuropsychol. Rev.* **2016**, *26*, 44–72. [CrossRef] [PubMed]
74. Dolan, M.; Lennox, C. Cool and hot executive function in conduct-disordered adolescents with and without co-morbid attention deficit hyperactivity disorder: Relationships with externalizing behaviours. *Psychol. Med.* **2013**, *43*, 2427–2436. [CrossRef] [PubMed]
75. Blair, R.J.; Mitchell, D.G. Psychopathy, attention and emotion. *Psychol. Med.* **2009**, *39*, 543–555. [CrossRef] [PubMed]
76. Newman, J.P.; Baskin-Sommers, A.R. Early Selective Attention Abnormalities in Psychopathy: Implications for Self-Regulation. In *Cognitive Neuroscience of Attention*; Posner, M.I., Ed.; Guilford Press: New York, NY, USA, 2012; pp. 421–440.
77. Frick, P.J.; Ray, J.V.; Thornton, L.C.; Kahn, R.E. Can callous-unemotional traits enhance the understanding, diagnosis, and treatment of serious conduct problems in children and adolescents? A comprehensive review. *Psychol. Bull.* **2014**, *140*, 1–57. [CrossRef] [PubMed]
78. Hawes, D.J.; Price, M.J.; Dadds, M.R. Callous-unemotional traits and the treatment of conduct problems in childhood and adolescence: A comprehensive review. *Clin. Child Fam. Psychol. Rev.* **2014**, *17*, 248–267. [CrossRef]

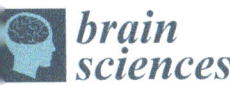

Article

Substance Use Outcomes from Two Formats of a Cognitive-Behavioral Intervention for Aggressive Children: Moderating Roles of Inhibitory Control and Intervention Engagement

John E. Lochman [1,2,3,*], Caroline L. Boxmeyer [4], Chuong Bui [3], Estephan Hakim [1], Shannon Jones [2], Francesca Kassing [1], Kristina McDonald [1], Nicole Powell [2], Lixin Qu [2] and Thomas Dishion [5,†]

1 Department of Psychology, University of Alabama, Tuscaloosa, AL 35487, USA; eahakim@crimson.ua.edu (E.H.); fkassing@crimson.ua.edu (F.K.); klmcdonald2@ua.edu (K.M.)
2 Center for Youth Development and Intervention, University of Alabama, Tuscaloosa, AL 35487, USA; jones178@ua.edu (S.J.); npowell@ua.edu (N.P.); lxqu@ua.edu (L.Q.)
3 Alabama Life Research Institute, University of Alabama, Tuscaloosa, AL 35487, USA; cnbui@ua.edu
4 Department of Psychiatry and Behavioral Medicine, University of Alabama, Tuscaloosa, AL 35487, USA; boxmeyer@ua.edu
5 REACH Institute, Department of Psychology, Arizona State University, Tempe, AZ 85281, USA; tomd@darkwing.uoregon.edu
* Correspondence: jlochman@ua.edu
† Deceased on 2018.

Abstract: Although cognitive-behavioral interventions have reduced the risk of substance use, little is known about moderating factors in children with disruptive behaviors. This study examined whether aggressive preadolescents' inhibitory control and intervention engagement moderates the effect of group versus individual delivery on their substance use. Following screening for aggression in 4th grade, 360 children were randomly assigned to receive the Coping Power intervention in either group or individual formats. The sample was primarily African American (78%) and male (65%). Assessments were made of children's self-reported substance use from preintervention through a six-year follow-up after intervention, parent-reported inhibitory control at preintervention, and observed behavioral engagement in the group intervention. Multilevel growth modeling found lower increases in substance use slopes for children with low inhibitory control receiving individual intervention, and for children with higher inhibitory control receiving group intervention. Children with low inhibitory control but who displayed more positive behavioral engagement in the group sessions had slower increases in their substance use than did similar children without positive engagement. Aggressive children's level of inhibitory control can lead to tailoring of group versus individual delivery of intervention. Children's positive behavioral engagement in group sessions is a protective factor for children with low inhibitory control.

Keywords: substance use; aggression; cognitive-behavioral; group intervention

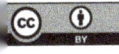

1. Introduction

Youth with behavioral symptoms of the disruptive behavior disorders of conduct disorder (CD) or oppositional defiant disorder (ODD) use substances earlier than peers and are more likely than their peers to develop substance use problems [1,2], and, once established, these substance use problems can remain stable through middle adulthood [3]. In a meta-analysis examining how childhood psychiatric disorders were a risk factor for later substance abuse, Groenman and colleagues [4] found that children with CD or ODD were at increased risk of developing a drug-related disorder compared to children without these diagnoses. One common factor underlying both CD and substance use was behavioral undercontrol or dysregulation [4]. Furthermore, both child externalizing behavior and behavioral undercontrol have been found to independently predict problematic substance use in adolescence [5]. Thus, it may be particularly important to consider how interventions designed to prevent CD conduct disorder are useful in preventing or prolonging onset to substance use initiation in adolescence, and how behavioral control processes may work in conjunction with interventions.

1.1. Prevention and Treatment of Substance Use in Aggressive Youth

Preventive and treatment interventions with aggressive and conduct problem youth can affect their substance use behaviors. When the effects of outpatient treatment on youth who have already established substance abuse have been examined through meta-analysis, group counseling has been found to be effective in reducing marijuana and mixed substance use [6]. Multidimensional and family systems interventions have also demonstrated a positive impact on substance use in youth with conduct problems and delinquent behavior. In a meta-analysis, Baldwin, Christian, Berkeljon, and Shadish [7] found that family therapy interventions for adolescents with behavioral and substance use problems were more effective than no-treatment control and were modestly more effective than care-as-usual and other forms of treatment. As an example of one such comprehensive family- and community-based treatment for youth with serious conduct problems, multisystemic therapy (MST) has been found to reduce substance use in adolescents with conduct problems and delinquent behavior [8–10] and in adolescents who are involved in juvenile drug court services [11].

With regard to preventive interventions, several interventions have been shown to reduce substance abuse in at-risk aggressive youth. Godwin and the Conduct Problems Prevention Research Group [12] found that Fast Track (FT), a comprehensive long-lasting program designed to decrease aggression and delinquency with at-risk kindergartners who were then followed in preventive intervention through 10th grade, decreased the probability of hazardous drinking in adolescence and young adulthood as well as opioid use in young adulthood. FT intervention-driven improvements in children's interpersonal, intrapersonal, and academic skills were found to partially mediate the program's direct effects on adolescent and young adult outcomes, with a strong indirect pathway through children's earlier acquisition of interpersonal skills. Reviews of research on briefer, school-based prevention programs addressing youth's social, coping, and social resistance skills have also found that prevention programs led to reduced risk for drug and alcohol problems in either universal classroom programs or in groups with other at-risk youth [13,14]. Key transition points, such as transition to middle school, can be especially important opportunities for focal prevention programs to produce beneficial effects among high-risk children and families [15,16], in part because the acquired problem-solving skills can help the children to better manage frequent conflicts in middle school settings that have high rates of peer antisocial behavior and less intense teacher management [17]. One such cognitive-behavioral prevention program at the middle school transition that has demonstrated preventive effects on youth substance abuse for at-risk aggressive youth is Coping Power [18].

1.1.1. Coping Power

Coping Power evolved from the Anger Coping program, a cognitive behavioral skills-training program for children that can be delivered in schools [19]. Fourth through 6th grade boys with aggressive and disruptive behavior who participated in the Anger Coping program had lower rates of drug and alcohol involvement compared to untreated peers three years postintervention, as well as higher levels of self-esteem and social problem-solving skills [20]. Coping Power (CP) is a multicomponent child [21] and parent [22] program that builds upon the Anger Coping program. In a study of 183 preadolescent boys with aggressive behavior, Coping Power produced lower rates of substance use and delinquent behavior compared to the control condition at one-year follow-up, with the strongest effects for boys who received the combined child and parent Coping Power program [18]. In an effectiveness study with 245 students with aggressive behavior in the 4th through 6th grades, children who participated in Coping Power or Coping Power plus an enhanced universal prevention component displayed reduced rates of substance use compared to children in a care-as-usual control condition [23]. After one year, children in both Coping Power conditions exhibited reductions in delinquency and substance use compared to children in the care-as-usual condition [24].

Coping Power intervention effects on multiple indices of problem behavior have also been found with youth diagnosed with disruptive behavior disorders [25–29], with students with behavior problems in dissemination and implementation studies in schools and community settings [30–35], and with children in other cultural environments [36–38]. When Coping Power has been implemented as a treatment for children with disruptive behavior disorders, it may also have a subsequent preventive effect for adolescent substance abuse and delinquent behavior. Zonnevylle-Bender, Matthys, Van De Wiel, and Lochman [39] found that Coping Power, when implemented with children with disruptive behavior disorder diagnoses in psychiatric outpatient clinics, reduced cigarette smoking and marijuana use initiation relative to care-as-usual five years after the start of treatment. Furthermore, Coping Power participants' substance use was in the range of the matched healthy control group at long-term follow-up.

1.1.2. Moderators of Coping Power Group Intervention for Aggressive Children

Children's association with peers who are engaged in antisocial behavior in adolescence becomes one of the strongest proximal risk predictors for growth in subsequent delinquency [40] and substance use [41]. These findings have raised questions about the potential ineffectiveness of group interventions that aggregate antisocial youth. In one notable example, a follow-up of the Adolescent Transitions Program found that youth randomized to a cognitive-behavioral group focusing on self-regulation resulted in improvements in observed family interaction, but, unfortunately, also resulted in increases in youth-reported smoking and teacher-reported problem behavior at school at one-year [42] and three-year follow-ups [43]. Analyses of the group conditions revealed that subtle dynamics of deviancy training during unstructured transitions in the groups predicted growth in self-reported smoking and teacher ratings of delinquency [44].

To examine whether and the extent to which aggregating aggressive youth in group treatment might impact treatment effects, Lochman and colleagues [45] randomly assigned aggressive youth to group or individual formats of Coping Power. The existing evidence base for group-administered Coping Power and the program's structured cognitive-behavioral approach provided a unique and unprecedented opportunity to rigorously compare the effects of group versus individual formats. Although there were no overall iatrogenic program effects in the prior Coping Power studies, and in fact there were significant prevention effects, the group format may have minimized the strength of the intervention's potential effects, especially for children with certain characteristics [46]. Research examining this issue, comparing group versus individual delivery formats for Coping Power, has indeed found weaker group effects for children with certain characteristics [47,48], including children's preintervention levels of inhibitory control [45], and their behavioral engagement in group sessions [49]. The following sections focus on these two central intervention moderators: children's inhibitory control, associated with their executive functioning, and behavioral engagement in the intervention.

Child Inhibitory Control

Inhibitory control can be defined as a process of effortful or willful control of behavior, capable of regulating both approach and avoidance [50,51]. It is a central component of executive functioning and involves the active inhibition of a dominant implicit or explicit response or impulse [52]. While conceptually similar to behavioral impulsivity, inhibitory control focuses on the more positive influences of constraint and not the reckless and daring behaviors affiliated with impulsivity [53]. Thus, while the ability to inhibit behavior is necessary to respond adaptively, problems with inhibitory control have been shown to predict adolescents externalizing problems such as aggression [54] and substance use [55–57].

Inhibitory control dysfunction has been noted as a common characteristic of aggressive youth [58,59]. Youth and adolescent studies have also shown that inhibitory control may moderate the relationship between various negative emotions and externalizing problems [60,61], including substance use [62]. Specifically, in discriminating between three separate components of negative emotionality (fear, anger, depressed mood) in a sample of aggressive youth, Pardini and colleagues [62] observed that, at high levels of inhibitory control, alcohol use initiation was significantly predicted by increased levels of depressed mood. However, at moderate/low levels of inhibitory control, alcohol initiation was predicted by increased levels of anger and decreased levels of fear, suggesting the role that greater inhibitory control plays in protecting youth high in anger and low in fear from alcohol use initiation [62].

Inhibitory control has been found to moderate the effects of individual versus group delivery of Coping Power on forms of externalizing behavior [45]. Youth who were lower in inhibitory control and who received Coping Power individually showed steeper declines in teacher-rated externalizing behaviors than children low on inhibitory control in the group condition. Children high in inhibitory control benefited similarly from either group or individual Coping Power. However, this pattern was no longer significant in a four-year follow-up [46].

Child Intervention Engagement

A series of studies have examined the role of children's engagement and therapeutic alliance on Coping Power outcomes. In a study of Coping Power delivered in individual sessions, Mitchell and colleagues [63] examined the role of therapeutic alliance, as rated by independent raters of video-recorded sessions. One aspect of therapeutic alliance, child–therapist bonding (in early Coping Power sessions), predicted better externalizing behavior outcomes.

Similar findings about the positive effects of early child behavioral engagement in Coping Power has also emerged for children receiving group sessions. For example, Ellis, Lindsey, Barker, Boxmeyer, and Lochman [64] found that intervention engagement fluctuated differentially across the group Coping Power intervention for children and parents. Better child engagement early in Coping Power positively influenced parent engagement midway through the intervention. This held even after accounting for contextual risk factors in the family environment, underscoring the importance of maximizing early child intervention engagement. In the same sample, Lindsey and colleagues [65] found that children's engagement during early Coping Power sessions was significantly related to their completion of out-of-session activities (e.g., behavioral goal attainment and Coping Power homework). Early engagement in these out-of-session activities was significantly related to later in-session engagement, which in turn predicted decreased externalizing behavior postintervention. In a study of child and therapist behaviors in group Coping Power sessions that predicted children's slopes of externalizing behavior through a one-year follow-up, children's negative and positive behaviors in sessions were independently coded, and children's negative behaviors, indicating weak engagement with the intervention, predicted escalating externalizing problems by the follow-up [49].

1.2. The Current Study

In the current study, we sought to determine whether inhibitory control moderates the effects of intervention format (group versus individual delivery of Coping Power) on youth substance use through a long-term follow-up, six years after the completion of intervention (i.e., following the youth's 11th grade in high school). Based on our prior findings [45], we hypothesized that children's preintervention inhibitory control would moderate the effects of intervention format (individual versus group) on children's long-term self-reported substance use outcomes. Children with poor inhibitory control in the group Coping Power condition were expected to have greater increases in the growth curves for substance use than children of similar risk status who received individual intervention. It was also hypothesized that, within the group format condition, children with poor inhibitory control would have slower increases in growth curves for substance use if the individual children had displayed fewer negative behaviors and more positive behaviors during the group sessions, indicating greater intervention engagement.

2. Method

2.1. Sample

Children included in the analyses were the full sample from a randomized controlled trial (RCT) examining the relative effectiveness of group and individual formats of Coping Power. The RCT involved 360 children recruited from 20 public elementary schools. Schools were matched based on demographic factors (percent receiving free or reduced-price lunch and percent minority) and within each matched pair, one school was randomly assigned to either Group Coping Power (GCP) or Individual Coping Power (ICP).

Recruitment involved screening by teachers and parents for eligibility; because teacher screenings have been found to be more predictive of later externalizing problems [66,67], they were considered the primary screening and were more stringent, whereas the parent screening was used to exclude children who showed few signs of aggression in the home setting. Fourth grade teachers completed the Reactive and Proactive Aggression Questionnaire (RPQ) [68] on each student in their classrooms. Ratings were compiled across all 20 schools, and a cutoff score corresponding to the 25th percentile was determined, indicating moderate to high levels of aggressive behavior. A randomized list of eligible children was created for each school, and families were contacted according to their placement on the list. Study procedures were described to families over the phone, and face-to-face assessments were scheduled for interested families. The Behavior Assessment System for Children, Second Edition (BASC-II) [69]. Aggression scale (parent-rated) was the second screening. Children whose parents rated them within the average range or above on the BASC Aggression scale were invited to enroll in the study. Families were contacted and assessed until six children were enrolled at each school. Of the 1131 students eligible from the teacher screening, 499 were successfully contacted. Of those, 139 were excluded because they did not schedule or missed the initial appointment (45), did not pass the parent screening (41), declined to participate (32), moved (15), were a sibling of another participant (three), or had cognitive limitations (three).

Three cohorts of 120 youth were recruited over a span of three years, resulting in a total sample of 360 students. At Time 1, the mean age for the sample was 10.17 years (range of 9.17–11.79). The race and ethnicity of the sample was as follows: 78.1% African American, 20.3% Caucasian, 1.4% Hispanic, and 0.3% other. Sixty-five percent of the sample were boys. Family income was below $15,000 for 29.9% of the sample, in the $15,000–$29,999 range for 31.8% of the sample, in the $30,000–$49,999 range for 20.5% of the sample, and above $50,000 for 17.6% of the sample.

2.2. Intervention

The Coping Power child component is an evidence-based manualized intervention developed by Lochman and colleagues [21] to target social-cognitive deficits in youth exhibiting aggressive behavior. Coping Power uses cognitive-behavioral strategies to address social problem solving, goal setting, emotion regulation, and social informational-processing distortions (e.g., hostile attribution bias) and challenges. The intervention consisted of 32 weekly sessions conducted at school from late spring of 4th grade into 5th grade. In the ICP condition, children met individually with a Coping Power leader for 30 min sessions. In the GCP condition, groups included the six children at each school and lasted for 50–60 min. Children in GCP also received monthly individual meetings (15–30 min each) to build rapport, assess comprehension of program materials, and address individual concerns. Both conditions covered the same content; however, specific activities were adapted to condition. For example, children in GCP practiced specific skills through roleplays with their peers and received feedback from their peers at the end of each session, while children in ICP participated in roleplays individually with the Coping Power leader and received feedback from the leader at the end of each session.

Coping Power group leaders were trained in and delivered both conditions and were provided with weekly supervision from two doctoral-level psychologists to ensure high implementation fidelity. Group leaders were also provided with monthly supervisory feedback on video recordings of their sessions to ensure treatment fidelity, quality, and consistency across conditions.

2.3. Procedure

Time 1 (preintervention) measures were completed during the enrollment process. Time 2 (midintervention) assessments were completed during the summer after 4th grade. Time 3 (postintervention) assessments were completed in the summer after 5th grade. Time 4 (one-year follow up), Time 5 (two-year follow up), Time 6 (four-year follow up), Time 7 (five-year follow up), and Time 8 (six-year follow-up) assessments were completed after 6th, 7th, 9th, 10th, and 11th grades, respectively. Children and parents completed interviews separately with research staff who were blind to children's treatment condition. Parents received $50 for each assessment interview and children received $10.

2.4. Measures

2.4.1. Inhibitory Control

Inhibitory control was assessed using the inhibitory control subscale from the parent-rated Early Adolescent Temperament Questionnaire–Parent Report (EATQ) [70] at Time 1 (preintervention). The inhibitory control subscale is an average score of eight items rated on a five-point Likert scale, with higher scores indicating greater inhibitory control. Items include waiting to start an activity when asked, waiting in line, sitting still when told to do so, refraining from smiling/laughing when inappropriate, and easily stopping an activity when asked. Internal consistency for this subscale was good in prior Coping Power samples ($\alpha = 0.78$) [62].

2.4.2. Substance Use

Substance use outcomes were assessed using the Center for Substance Abuse Prevention (CSAP) Study Survey, which was adapted from the California Student Survey [71]. The CSAP Student Survey is a 14-item child-report questionnaire that measures students' attitudes toward and use of alcohol, tobacco, and other drugs. The current study focused on children's reports of daily use of alcohol, tobacco, and other drugs. Children reported how many times they used each substance per day. Number of times used daily was summed and averaged across the three substance types. Internal consistency and test-retest reliability of youth self-reported substance use have been high with youth from 10 years of age through adolescence [72,73]. Substance use measured with the CSAP Student Survey has been found to validly relate to children's proactive and reactive aggressive behaviors in samples of children first assessed at 10 years of age [74,75].

2.4.3. Group Behavior

Behaviors in group were assessed using the Cognitive Behavioral Group Coding System (CBGCS) [76]. Trained coders used the CBGCS to make ratings of children's behaviors from video recordings of GCP sessions. Ratings were made for each child during the first ten minutes, middle ten minutes, and last ten minutes of each session, and the ratings were aggregated for analyses. Items were rated on a five-point Likert scale. Positive child behaviors included showing involvement and interest in group discussion and activities, initiating positive and friendly interactions with other group members, and other children initiating reciprocal positive and friendly interactions toward the child. Negative child behaviors included: deviant talk about antisocial ideas or behaviors; exhibiting off-task, inattentive behavior; engaging in silly or disruptive behavior; demonstrating a negative, hostile attitude; exhibiting verbal or physical aggression; and appearing to trigger these negative behaviors in other group members. Coders were required to rate nine training videos and establish 80% agreement (agreement was defined as ratings falling within one point of the comparison rating) to establish proficiency. To ensure that agreement remained at 80% or higher for the study sessions, 7% of group sessions were double-coded. Furthermore, coders met regularly to prevent coder drift and remediation training videos were required for coders whose ratings fell below 80% agreement. Interrater reliability was adequate during coding (post-training), with agreement rates of 87.1% for child behaviors (across 146 10-min observation segments). There was acceptable internal consistency for the five-item positive behaviors variable (alpha: 0.90) and for the nine-item negative behaviors variable (0.77).

2.5. Analytic Strategy

Three-level growth curve models were used to examine the hypotheses. Repeated measures formed level 1, which were nested in children (level 2), nested in intervention units (i.e., three annual cohorts in each school). As each wave of data collection straddled several months, time was coded as the actual time lapse from baseline. Each adolescent, as a result, had a unique set of values for the time variable. The substance use trajectory was modeled with a quadratic time trend. The fixed intercept represented the mean baseline value. The fixed linear and quadratic time effects represented the overall trajectory. Variations in the growth parameters were partitioned into variation among children within the same intervention unit, and variation among intervention units. Models were estimated using Hierarchical Linear Modeling (HLM) 7.0 with full maximum likelihood (FML) estimation [77]. FML permitted all 360 children to be included in the growth analyses.

Regarding the hypothesized moderation effect of inhibitory control, of interest was the cross-level interaction of *IGCP × inhibitory control* (IGCP = 1 if individual format, and 0 if group format—the reference category) on the growth rate of substance use changes over time. The model was estimated using the full sample of 360 children. Race (1 if African American, 0 otherwise) was included as a control variable. Age and gender were nonsignificant control variables in the initial model and were dropped from the final model. For the second hypothesis regarding children's in-session behaviors, the focus was the cross-level interactions of *inhibitory control × positive behavior* and *inhibitory control × negative behavior* on growth rates of changes in substance use over time. The model was estimated using the subsample of 180 children randomized to the group format of the intervention. Race, gender, and age were included as control variables.

3. Results

Table 1 provides the means and standard deviations for the youth-reported substance use outcome measure by intervention condition at each of the eight time points. To address missing data, the HLM analyses used FML to estimate model parameters, and all 360 participants were included in the analyses. The data collection rates (indicating rate of data completion at each time point, based on the percentage of the full sample at T1) were similar for GCP (99%, 94%, 86%, 78%, 79%, 76%, 78% for T2–T8, respectively), and for ICP (98%, 91%, 83%, 77%, 76%, 76%, 81% for T2–T8, respectively). There were no significant differences in the data collection rates between the two conditions at any of the seven postbaseline time points for the substance use outcome. Data collection bias was tested by examining whether children's characteristics (gender, race, initial level of substance use at baseline) and intervention condition status differentiated those with data at each time point from those without data at that timepoint using logistic regression. There was little evidence of association between data collection rates and children's characteristics or intervention conditions. One exception was race with African American children having higher rates of data collection at time points 4, 6, 7, and 8 than children of other races.

Table 1. Means and standard deviations of substance use across time points.

Time	Group Format (GCP)			Individual Format (ICP)		
	Mean	S.D	n	Mean	S.D	n
1	0.05	0.26	179	0.04	0.20	180
2	0.04	0.21	179	0.03	0.13	176
3	0.02	0.11	170	0.01	0.10	163
4	0.04	0.14	155	0.05	0.26	149
5	0.11	0.34	140	0.12	0.42	139
6	0.18	0.47	142	0.20	0.62	137
7	0.17	0.54	136	0.16	0.43	137
8	0.23	0.61	141	0.29	0.66	146

3.1. Hypothesized Moderation Effect of Inhibitory Control on ICP Versus GCP

Table 2 summarizes the results of the growth curve analysis testing the hypothesized moderation effect of inhibitory control. Race was a significant predictor of the substance use outcome, with African American youth having lower rate of increases in substance use over time than other youth. The analysis found that children's baseline inhibitory control moderated the effect of the intervention delivery formats ($p = 0.053$). As depicted in Figure 1, youth with higher inhibitory control had lower rates of increases in substance use if they had been in the GCP condition. The reverse was true for youth with lower inhibitory control: the ICP condition had lower rates of increases in substance use compared to the GCP condition.

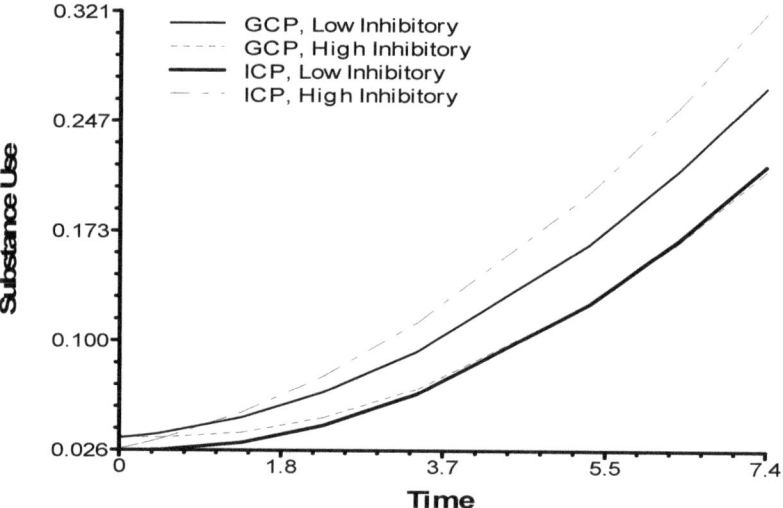

Figure 1. Inhibitory control moderating effects of delivery formats on youth-reported substance use.

Table 2. Growth curve analysis of the inhibitory control moderation effect on substance use.

	Fixed Effect				Random Effect							
						Level-3			Level-2			Level-1
	Coef.	SE	t-Value	df	p-Value	Var	x^2	df	p-Value	Var	x^2	df	p-Value	
Substance use													
Linear growth rate	0.001	0.011	0.06	58	0.951	0.000	50.85	58	>0.500	0.111	425.75	282	0.000	0.069
IGCP (1 = I-CP 0 = G-CP)	0.005	0.009	0.571	58	0.570								
Race (1 = African American, 0 = other)	−0.036	0.015	−2.48	175	0.014								
Inhibitory control	−0.008	0.008	−0.93	175	0.356								
IGCP × nhibitory control	0.022	0.011	1.95	175	0.053								
Quadratic curve growth rate	0.004	0.001	2.544	59	0.014								

3.2. Child In-Session Behaviors Predicting Substance Use within the GCP Condition

Table 3 summarizes the results of the growth curve analysis testing the interaction between inhibitory control and in-session positive and negative behaviors of children in the GCP condition, indicating their engagement with the intervention. The analysis found that children's baseline inhibitory control interacted with children's positive in-session behaviors ($p = 0.028$). As depicted in Figure 2, the combination of lower inhibitory control and lower rates of positive in-session behaviors predicted higher increases in slopes for substance use than lower inhibitory control in combination with higher rates of positive behaviors, as well as for higher inhibitory control.

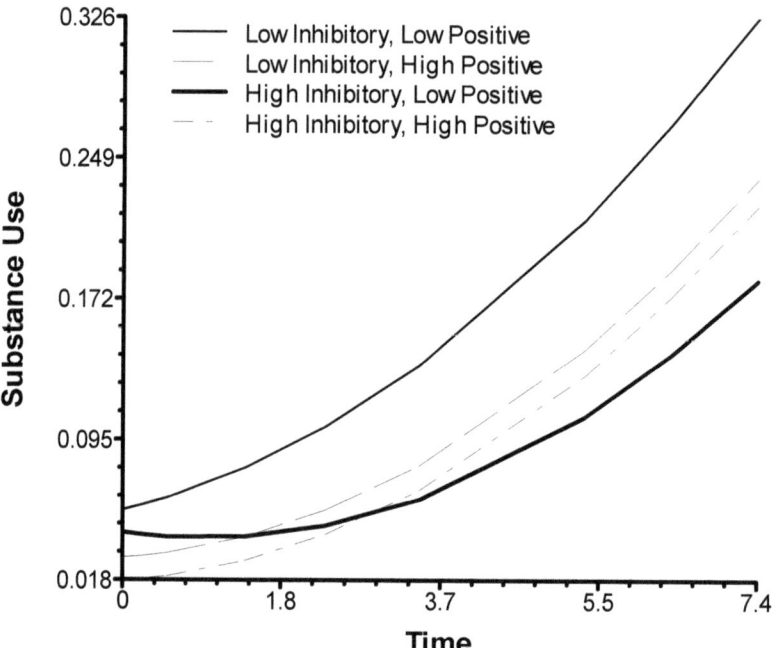

Figure 2. Inhibitory control moderating effects of children's in-session behaviors on youth-reported substance use.

Table 3. Growth curve analysis of interaction between children's inhibitory control and in-session behaviors on rate of substance use within GCP.

	Fixed Effect				Random Effect							
						Level-3			Level-2			Level-1
	Coef.	SE	t-Value	df	p-Value	Var	x^2	df	p-Value	Var	x^2	df	p-Value
Substance use						0.000	26.31	27	>0.500	0.008	170.30	137	0.028	0.071
Linear growth rate	0.003	0.014	0.19	27	0.851								
Positive behavior	0.000	0.005	0.05	27	0.964								
Negative behavior	−0.001	0.001	−0.09	27	0.930								
Race	−0.029	0.022	−1.29	80	0.202								
Age	0.004	0.011	0.34	80	0.735								
Gender	−0.009	0.014	−0.66	80	0.514								
Inhibit control	−0.007	0.009	−0.79	80	0.434								
Positive behav*inhibitory control	0.013	0.006	2.24	80	0.028								
Negative behav × inhibitory control	0.007	0.007	1.11	80	0.272								
Quadratic curve growth rate	0.003	0.002	1.722	29	0.096								

4. Discussion

This study examined whether the format of intervention delivery (group versus individual) could influence youth substance use rates through a six-year follow-up period after a cognitive-behavioral intervention for aggressive youth had been completed and whether two hypothesized child characteristics could affect how the youth responded, in terms of substance use, to the two formats. Overall, as developmentally anticipated, slopes of youth self-reported substance use increased across time, from the intervention baseline when youth were in 4th grade through their adolescent development, ending after 11th grade. In typical adolescents, there are increases in substance use, especially from middle school to high school, similar to the findings with this current sample [78]. Although the group versus individual format of delivery did not have a significant main effect on youth self-reported substance use, children who had lower levels of inhibitory control did have slower rates of increases in their substance use if they received intervention in an individual format. Unexpectedly, the reverse pattern was evident for aggressive children with higher levels of baseline inhibitory control, as they had slower increases in their substance use slopes if they had received intervention in the group format. In addition, for children in the group format, the hypothesis predicting that risk related to low inhibitory control would be moderated by behavioral indicators of children's engagement in intervention sessions was partially supported as children's positive behaviors in group sessions, but not their negative behaviors, predicted a reduced rate of increase in substance use over time. Earlier research has indicated that Coping Power generally delays the onset of substance abuse in middle school [18,24], and the variability in rate of increases in substance use observed in the current study is important, as earlier first-time use of alcohol and marijuana predicts elevated substance use disorders into adulthood [78].

4.1. Effects of Group Versus Individual Format of Cognitive-Behavioral Intervention

Aggressive children with lower levels of inhibitory control prior to the intervention had more rapid increases in substance use through adolescence if they had received intervention in a group format rather than in an individual format. Inhibitory control is believed to be especially important in regulating the expression of negative emotions, in being able to selectively attend to key information in our environment, and in resisting temptations to act impulsively [79], all of which can contribute to children's behavior. Children with lower levels of inhibitory control have less willful control of their behavior and anger [50] and are at risk for early increases in substance use through the adolescent years [62].

The negative association of the group format with lower levels of inhibitory control in children in this sample was evident in their rates of externalizing behavior through a one-year follow-up after intervention [45], and the current findings indicate that the group format can have a more generalized effect for these children on another key outcome, their substance use rates. Children with poor inhibitory control may be less likely to profit from being in a group intervention rather than being seen individually by the therapist for several reasons. Aggressive children with weak inhibitory control may be distracted by their peers in the group and thus be less attentive to and have resultant less recall (and internalization) of discussions and activities about key skills [45]. Children with poor inhibitory control may be more easily aroused by peers' negative behaviors during group sessions. In addition, children with weak inhibitory control may be more easily influenced by deviancy training from antisocial peers in their group sessions [42] and less able to resist the temptation to be affected by peer reinforcement of their poorly controlled and potentially deviant talk and behavior in sessions.

Although the finding that youth with poor inhibitory control had better long-term substance use outcomes when receiving individual rather than group-based intervention was expected, the opposite pattern for children with higher levels of inhibitory control was unexpected. If children had higher levels of inhibitory control (relative to other children in this aggressive sample) they had relatively slower rates of increase in substance use if they received group intervention than if they received individual intervention. Aggressive children with greater inhibitory control may be able to better regulate their emotions and selectively attend to key group activities and tasks. Thus, they could profit more from activities that are unique to the group format, especially activities that involve coping with negative peer pressure and temptations to use substances. The Coping Power group format includes roleplay with peers on emotion regulation and problem-solving tasks and unique opportunities to receive social and tangible rewards. Children can receive rewards for the whole group if group members attain sufficient goal points, and they have potential for receiving spontaneous and structured peer social reinforcement for cooperative and positively engaged behavior in sessions. Individual delivery of Coping Power covers the same content as the group format but lacks these features that could further generalize skills and enhance motivation to try out more competent interpersonal behaviors, inside and outside the group. We had not found that an individual intervention format increased negative outcomes, in comparison to the group format, with high inhibitory control youth on other outcomes, such as externalizing behavior problems, in this sample [45]. However, substance use initiation can be encouraged by peers in important ways [2,80], and thus behavioral practice in refusing peer pressure and in positively engaging peers may be more essential for substance use outcomes.

4.2. Interaction of Children's Inhibitory Control and Their Behavioral Engagement in Groups

If aggressive children have lower inhibitory control and have received cognitive-behavioral intervention in groups, they are at risk for earlier initiation and increase of substance use. However, the current findings indicate these at-risk youth have better outcomes (i.e., lower substance use slopes) if youth display higher observed positive behavior in group sessions. Youth with observed positive behavior were coded as showing involvement and interest in group discussion and activities, initiating positive and friendly interaction with other group members, and receiving reciprocal positive and friendly interactions from their peers in the group.

The protective effects of better engagement in group when a youth has low inhibitory control can occur for several reasons. When children are more actively involved in group activities and discussions, they can receive more social reinforcement from group leaders and their peers and can receive more tangible rewards if the group uses a "prize box" as youth earn participation points in their group, as is the case in Coping Power. Thus, external reinforcement can assist children who have poor inhibitory control, and who by nature may be less engaged in group tasks, to be more actively involved in group tasks involving emotion regulation and problem solving. As a result of their enhanced engagement, they can cope with some of the characteristics of their low level of general inhibitory control and have better potential attention to, and recall of, group activities and discussion. They can more firmly acquire skills that can slow their increase in substance use in the years ahead.

Finally, their positive involvement in group activities can enhance their therapeutic alliance with their group leader, and a strong therapeutic alliance has been found to be predictive of improved behavior following intervention [63]. In a related way, we have found that aggressive children who have group therapists who are engaged in warm, nonirritable ways with them are more likely to display reductions in externalizing behaviors in the years following intervention [49]. Group therapists who handle difficult interpersonal provocations from their child clients by exerting inhibitory control over their expression of their own frustration and by effectively regulating their arousal can be developing stronger therapeutic alliances with the children in the group and are modeling key processes that can be instrumental for children learning to improve their own emotional regulation over time [81]. As children's frustration tolerance and self-regulation abilities develop due to their modeling of the group leader, they may be more likely to positively engage with group activities [49].

4.3. Limitations and Future Directions

There are four limitations to this study that indicate the current results can be regarded with caution and lead to future research opportunities. First, the assessment of youth substance use in the present study was youth self-report. Although youth self-report of substance use has displayed at least moderate reliability and validity during the preadolescent and adolescent age periods [72–75,82], objective measures such as biochemical corroboration using urinalysis [83] and use of parent reports would strengthen the validity of the assessment of substance use and would be useful in future longitudinal research. Second, the youth and parents received stipends to participate in assessments. Although the sizes of the stipends were not deemed to be coercive by the university's Institutional Review Board, the stipends may have influenced parents' and youths' desire to participate in the study and could have skewed the sample toward having more individuals with limited incomes. Third, the current study was unable to determine if the effects were directly affected by mediating factors such as therapeutic alliance and active participation in roleplaying activities, and future research could include a methodological focus on assessment and analysis of mediating factors. Fourth, there was no untreated control or comparison group in this study. The randomized design of this study was specifically focused on differential effects of group versus individual format of intervention; therefore, it cannot confirm if either format performed better than an untreated control or comparison group through the follow-up years. Although prior randomized trial research testing the Coping Power program in comparison to control conditions has found children who had completed the full Coping Power program to have lower substance use at one- and four-year follow-ups after intervention [18,24,39], future research could determine if the Coping Power child component by itself could produce long-term relatively lower rates of increases in substance use through a six-year follow-up in comparison to a control group.

4.4. Clinical Implications

The differential effect for high versus low inhibitory control in group versus individual format suggests that tailoring of intervention format could be important for adolescent substance use for aggressive children who display symptoms of disruptive behavior disorders. When focused on preventing substance abuse, it is important to consider personalizing intervention format (individual versus group) depending on children's level of inhibitory control. In addition, if an aggressive child with poor inhibitory control is receiving group-based cognitive-behavioral intervention, the current results indicate the importance of stimulating and reinforcing children's early positive engagement in group sessions. The essential attention to children's behavioral engagement in group intervention is consistent with prior research that has found that aggressive children's engagement through the middle set of group sessions can predict reductions in externalizing behavior problems [65]. It is important for clinical trainings to emphasize the transformative potential of bonding and therapeutic alliance when working with youth exhibiting aggressive behaviors, even in the context of a manualized intervention [63]. The training of group leaders should not only emphasize skill training in a traditional sense but also focus on how group leaders can promote children's positive behavioral engagement and practice emotional regulation themselves while engaged in group work that can be inherently stressful and frustrating at times [46,84].

5. Conclusions

When considering long-term substance use outcomes, aggressive children's level of inhibitory control can lead to tailoring of group versus individual delivery of intervention, with children having weaker inhibitory benefitting more from individually-delivered intervention, but children with stronger inhibitory control benefitting more from group intervention. Children's positive behavioral engagement in group sessions is a protective factor for children with low inhibitory control.

Author Contributions: Conceptualization, J.E.L. and T.D.; methodology, C.L.B., S.J., J.E.L. and N.P.; software, C.B. and L.Q.; formal analysis, C.B. and L.Q.; investigation, S.J.; resources, C.L.B., T.D., S.J., J.E.L. and N.P.; data curation, L.Q.; writing—original draft preparation, C.L.B., E.H., F.K., J.E.L., K.M. and L.Q.; writing—review and editing, C.L.B., C.B., E.H., F.K., J.E.L., K.M., N.P. and L.Q.; visualization, L.Q.; supervision, J.E.L.; project administration, C.L.B., S.J., J.E.L. and N.P.; funding acquisition, J.E.L. All authors have read and agreed to the published version of the manuscript, except T.D. who is deceased.

Funding: The research in this paper was funded by grants from the National Institute of Drug Abuse (grant number, R01 DA023156) and the National Institute of Child Health & Human Development (grant number, R01 HD079273).

Institutional Review Board Statement: The study was conducted according to the guidelines of the Declaration of Helsinki and approved by the Institutional Review Board (or Ethics Committee) of The University of Alabama (IRB protocol 08-016; original approval on 23 October 2008 and most recent renewal on 28 October 2020).

Informed Consent Statement: Informed consent was obtained from parents of all subjects involved in the study, and assent was obtained from all of the children.

Data Availability Statement: Data used in this study can be obtained from the corresponding author.

Conflicts of Interest: John E. Lochman is the co-developer of the Coping Power program and receives royalties from Oxford University Press for the Coping Power child component implementation guidebook and workbook used in this study. The funders had no role in the design of the study; in the collection, analyses, or interpretation of data; in the writing of the manuscript, or in the decision to publish the results.

References

1. Williams, R.J.; Nowatzki, N.R. Validity of adolescent self report of substance use. *Subst. Use Misuse* **2005**, *40*, 1–13. [CrossRef] [PubMed]
2. Conner, B.T.; Lochman, J.E. Comorbid conduct disorder and substance use disorders. *Clin. Psychol. Sci. Pract.* **2010**, *17*, 337–349. [CrossRef]
3. Marmorstein, N.R.; White, H.R. Comorbidity with substance abuse. In *The Wiley Handbook of Disruptive and Impulse-Control Disorders*; Lochman, J.E., Matthys, W., Eds.; Wiley Blackwell: Hoboken, NJ, USA, 2018; pp. 73–88.
4. Lansford, J.E.; Godwin, J.; McMahon, R.J.; Crowley, M.; Pettit, G.S.; Bates, J.E.; Coie, J.D.; Dodge, K.A. Early Physical Abuse and Adult Outcomes. *Pediatrics* **2021**, *147*, e20200873. [CrossRef]
5. Groenman, A.P.; Janssen, T.; Oosterlaan, J. Childhood Psychiatric Disorders as Risk Factor for Subsequent Substance Abuse: A Meta-Analysis. *J. Am. Acad. Child Adolesc. Psychiatry* **2017**, *56*, 556–569. [CrossRef] [PubMed]
6. Trucco, E.M.; Hicks, B.M.; Villafuerte, S.; Nigg, J.T.; Burmeister, M.; Zucker, R.A. Temperament and externalizing behavior as mediators of genetic risk on adolescent substance use. *J. Abnorm. Psychol.* **2016**, *125*, 565–575. [CrossRef]
7. Tanner-Smith, E.E.; Wilson, S.J.; Lipsey, M.W. The comparative effectiveness of outpatient treatment for adolescent substance abuse: A meta-analysis. *J. Subst. Abus. Treat.* **2013**, *44*, 145–158. [CrossRef]
8. Baldwin, S.A.; Christian, S.; Berkeljon, A.; Shadish, W.R. The Effects of Family Therapies for Adolescent Delinquency and Substance Abuse: A Meta-analysis. *J. Marital Fam. Ther.* **2011**, *38*, 281–304. [CrossRef]
9. Henggeler, S.W.; Borduin, C.M.; Melton, G.B.; Mann, B.J. Effects of multisystemic therapy on drug use and abuse in serious juvenile offenders: A progress report from two outcome studies. *Fam. Dyn. Addict. Q.* **1991**, *1*, 40–51.
10. Letourneau, E.J.; Henggeler, S.W.; Borduin, C.M.; Schewe, P.A.; McCart, M.R.; Chapman, J.E.; Saldana, L. Multisystemic therapy for juvenile sexual offenders: 1-year results from a randomized effectiveness trial. *J. Fam. Psychol.* **2009**, *23*, 89–102. [CrossRef]
11. Timmons-Mitchell, J.; Bender, M.B.; Kishna, M.A.; Mitchell, C.C. An Independent Effectiveness Trial of Multisystemic Therapy with Juvenile Justice Youth. *J. Clin. Child Adolesc. Psychol.* **2006**, *35*, 227–236. [CrossRef]
12. Henggeler, S.W.; McCart, M.R.; Cunningham, P.B.; Chapman, J.E. Enhancing the effectiveness of juvenile drug courts by integrating evidence-based practices. *J. Consult. Clin. Psychol.* **2012**, *80*, 264–275. [CrossRef]
13. Godwin, J.W. The Fast Track intervention's impact on behaviors of despair in adolescence and young adulthood. *Proc. Natl. Acad. Sci. USA* **2020**, *117*, 31748–31753. [CrossRef] [PubMed]
14. Das, J.K.; Salam, R.A.; Arshad, A.; Finkelstein, Y.; Bhutta, Z.A. Interventions for adolescent substance abuse: An overview of systematic reviews. *J. Adolesc. Health* **2016**, *59* (Suppl. 4), S61–S75. [CrossRef]
15. Griffin, K.W.; Botvin, G.J. Evidence-Based interventions for preventing substance use disorders in adolescents. *Child Adolesc. Psychiatr. Clin. N. Am.* **2010**, *19*, 505–526. [CrossRef]
16. Botvin, G.J.; Baker, E.; Dusenbury, L.; Botvin, E.M.; Diaz, T. Long-term Follow-up Results of a Randomized Drug Abuse Prevention Trial in a White Middle-Class Population. *JAMA* **1995**, *273*, 1106–1112. [CrossRef]

17. Dishion, T.J.; Kavanagh, K.; Schneiger, A.; Nelson, S.; Kaufman, N.K. Preventing Early Adolescent Substance Use: A Family-Centered Strategy for the Public Middle School. *Prev. Sci.* **2002**, *3*, 191–201. [CrossRef]
18. Ialongo, N.; Poduska, J.; Werthamer, L.; Kellam, S. The Distal Impact of Two First-Grade Preventive Interventions on Conduct Problems and Disorder in Early Adolescence. *J. Emot. Behav. Disord.* **2001**, *9*, 146–160. [CrossRef]
19. Lochman, J.E.; Wells, K.C. The Coping Power Program for Preadolescent Aggressive Boys and Their Parents: Outcome Effects at the 1-Year Follow-Up. *J. Consult. Clin. Psychol.* **2004**, *72*, 571–578. [CrossRef]
20. Larson, J.; Lochman, J.E. *Helping Schoolchildren Cope with Anger: A Cognitive-Behavioral Intervention*; Guilford Press: New York, NY, USA, 2002.
21. Lochman, J.E. Cognitive-Behavioral intervention with aggressive boys: Three-year follow-up and preventive effects. *J. Consult. Clin. Psychol.* **1992**, *60*, 426–432. [CrossRef]
22. Lochman, J.E.; Wells, K.C.; Lenhart, L.A. *Coping Power: Child Group Program Workbook*; Oxford University Press: New York, NY, USA, 2008.
23. Wells, K.C.; Lochman, J.E.; Lenhart, L.A. *Coping Power: Parent Group Program Workbook*; Oxford University Press: New York, NY, USA, 2008.
24. Lochman, J.E.; Wells, K.C. The Coping Power program at the middle-school transition: Universal and indicated prevention effects. *Psychol. Addict. Behav.* **2002**, *16*, S40–S54. [CrossRef] [PubMed]
25. Lochman, J.E.; Wells, K.C. Effectiveness of the coping power program and of classroom intervention with aggressive children: Outcomes at a 1-year follow-up. *Behav. Ther.* **2003**, *34*, 493–515. [CrossRef]
26. Helander, M.; Lochman, J.; Högström, J.; Ljótsson, B.; Hellner, C.; Enebrink, P. The effect of adding Coping Power Program-Sweden to Parent Management Training-effects and moderators in a randomized controlled trial. *Behav. Res. Ther.* **2018**, *103*, 43–52. [CrossRef]
27. Muratori, P.; Milone, A.; Levantini, V.; Ruglioni, L.; Lambruschi, F.; Pisano, S.; Masi, G.; Lochman, J.E. Six-year outcome for children with ODD or CD treated with the coping power program. *Psychiatry Res.* **2019**, *271*, 454–458. [CrossRef]
28. Muratori, P.; Milone, A.; Manfredi, A.; Polidori, L.; Ruglioni, L.; Lambruschi, F.; Masi, G.; Lochman, J.E. Evaluation of Improvement in Externalizing Behaviors and Callous-Unemotional Traits in Children with Disruptive Behavior Disorder: A 1-Year Follow Up Clinic-Based Study. *Adm. Policy Ment. Health Ment. Health Serv. Res.* **2015**, *44*, 452–462. [CrossRef]
29. Nystrand, C.; Helander, M.; Enebrink, P.; Feldman, I.; Sampaio, F. Adding the Coping Power Programme to parent management training: The cost-effectiveness of stacking interventions for children with disruptive behaviour disorders. *Eur. Child Adolesc. Psychiatry* **2020**, 1–12. [CrossRef]
30. Pullen, S.J.; Horgan, L.; Romanelli, L.H.; Radin, A.; Gardner, K.; Edwards, C.; Crapo, T.; Bolen, B.; Huck, B.; Wells, K.; et al. The effectiveness of training rural mental health clinicians to treat disruptive behavior disorders. *J. Rural. Ment. Health* **2021**. [CrossRef]
31. Cowell, K.; Horstmann, S.; Linebarger, J.; Meaker, P.; Aligne, C.A. A "Vaccine" against violence: Coping Power. *Pediatr. Rev.* **2008**, *29*, 362–363. [CrossRef]
32. Eiraldi, R.; Mautone, J.A.; Khanna, M.S.; Power, T.J.; Orapallo, A.; Cacia, J.; Schwartz, B.S.; McCurdy, B.; Keiffer, J.; Paidipati, C.; et al. Group CBT for Externalizing Disorders in Urban Schools: Effect of Training Strategy on Treatment Fidelity and Child Outcomes. *Behav. Ther.* **2018**, *49*, 538–550. [CrossRef] [PubMed]
33. Jurecska, D.E.; Hamilton, E.B.; Peterson, M.A. Effectiveness of the Coping Power Program in middle-school children with disruptive behaviours and hyperactivity difficulties. *Support Learn.* **2011**, *26*, 168–172. [CrossRef]
34. Lochman, J.E.; Boxmeyer, C.; Powell, N.; Qu, L.; Wells, K.; Windle, M. Dissemination of the Coping Power program: Importance of intensity of counselor training. *J. Consult. Clin. Psychol.* **2009**, *77*, 397–409. [CrossRef] [PubMed]
35. McDaniel, S.C.; Lochman, J.E.; Tomek, S.; Powell, N.; Irwin, A.; Kerr, S. Reducing Risk for Emotional and Behavioral Disorders in Late Elementary School: A Comparison of Two Targeted Interventions. *Behav. Disord.* **2018**, *43*, 370–382. [CrossRef]
36. Peterson, M.A.; Hamilton, E.B.; Russell, A.D. Starting well: Facilitating the middle school transition. *J. Appl. Sch. Psychol.* **2009**, *25*, 286–304. [CrossRef]
37. Cabiya, J.J.; Padilla-Cotto, L.; González, K.; Sanchez-Cestero, J.; Martínez-Taboas, A.; Sayers, S. Effectiveness of a cognitive-behavioral intervention for Puerto Rican children. *Rev. Interam. Psicol.* **2008**, *42*, 195–202.
38. Ludmer, J.A.; Sanches, M.; Propp, L.; Andrade, B.F. Comparing the Multicomponent Coping Power Program to Individualized Parent–Child Treatment for Improving the Parenting Efficacy and Satisfaction of Parents of Children with Conduct Problems. *Child Psychiatry Hum. Dev.* **2017**, *49*, 100–108. [CrossRef]
39. Mushtaq, A.; Lochman, J.E.; Tariq, P.N.; Sabih, F. Preliminary Effectiveness Study of Coping Power Program for Aggressive Children in Pakistan. *Prev. Sci.* **2016**, *18*, 762–771. [CrossRef]
40. Zonnevylle-Bender, M.J.S.; Matthys, W.; Van De Wiel, N.M.H.; Lochman, J.E. Preventive Effects of Treatment of Disruptive Behavior Disorder in Middle Childhood on Substance Use and Delinquent Behavior. *J. Am. Acad. Child Adolesc. Psychiatry* **2007**, *46*, 33–39. [CrossRef]
41. Tremblay, R.E.; Mâsse, L.C.; Vitaro, F.; Dobkin, P.L. The impact of friends' deviant behavior on early onset of deliquency: Longitudinal data from 6 to 13 years of age. *Dev. Psychopathol.* **1995**, *7*, 649–667. [CrossRef]
42. Price, J.; Drabick, D.A.; Ridenour, T.A. Association with Deviant Peers Across Adolescence: Subtypes, Developmental Patterns, and Long-Term Outcomes. *J. Clin. Child Adolesc. Psychol.* **2019**, *48*, 238–249. [CrossRef]

43. Dishion, T.J.; Andrews, D.W. Preventing escalation in problem behaviors with high-risk young adolescents: Immediate and 1-year outcomes. *J. Consult. Clin. Psychol.* **1995**, *63*, 538–548. [CrossRef]
44. Poulin, F.; Dishion, T.J.; Burraston, B. 3-Year Iatrogenic Effects Associated with Aggregating High-Risk Adolescents in Cognitive-Behavioral Preventive Interventions. *Appl. Dev. Sci.* **2001**, *5*, 214–224. [CrossRef]
45. Dishion, T.J.; Tipsord, J.M. Peer Contagion in Child and Adolescent Social and Emotional Development. *Annu. Rev. Psychol.* **2011**, *62*, 189–214. [CrossRef] [PubMed]
46. Lochman, J.E.; Dishion, T.J.; Powell, N.P.; Boxmeyer, C.L.; Qu, L.; Sallee, M. Evidence-Based preventive intervention for preadolescent aggressive children: One-year outcomes following randomization to group versus individual delivery. *J. Consult. Clin. Psychol.* **2015**, *83*, 728–735. [CrossRef] [PubMed]
47. Lochman, J.E.; Glenn, A.L.; Powell, N.P.; Boxmeyer, C.L.; Bui, C.; Kassing, F.; Qu, L.; Romerro, D.E.; Dishion, T. Group versus individual format of intervention for aggressive children: Moderators and predictors of outcomes through 4 years after intervention. *Dev. Psychopathol.* **2019**, *31*, 1757–1775. [CrossRef] [PubMed]
48. Glenn, A.L.; Lochman, J.E.; Dishion, T.; Powell, N.P.; Boxmeyer, C.; Qu, L. Oxytocin Receptor Gene Variant Interacts with Intervention Delivery Format in Predicting Intervention Outcomes for Youth with Conduct Problems. *Prev. Sci.* **2018**, *19*, 38–48. [CrossRef]
49. Glenn, A.L.; Lochman, J.E.; Dishion, T.; Powell, N.P.; Boxmeyer, C.; Kassing, F.; Qu, L.; Romero, D. Toward Tailored Interventions: Sympathetic and Parasympathetic Functioning Predicts Responses to an Intervention for Conduct Problems Delivered in Two Formats. *Prev. Sci.* **2018**, *20*, 30–40. [CrossRef]
50. Lochman, J.E.; Dishion, T.J.; Boxmeyer, C.L.; Powell, N.P.; Qu, L. Variation in Response to Evidence-Based Group Preventive Intervention for Disruptive Behavior Problems: A View from 938 Coping Power Sessions. *J. Abnorm. Child Psychol.* **2017**, *45*, 1271–1284. [CrossRef] [PubMed]
51. Enticott, P.; Ogloff, J.; Bradshaw, J.L. Associations between laboratory measures of executive inhibitory control and self-reported impulsivity. *Personal. Individ. Differ.* **2006**, *41*, 285–294. [CrossRef]
52. Rothbart, M.K. Temperament in childhood: A framework. In *Temperament in Childhood*; Kohnstamm, G.A., Bates, J.E., Rothbart, M.K., Eds.; John Wiley & Sons: Oxford, UK, 1989; pp. 59–73.
53. Barkley, R.A. Behavioral inhibition, sustained attention, and executive functions: Constructing a unifying theory of ADHD. *Psychol. Bull.* **1997**, *121*, 65–94. [CrossRef]
54. Colder, C.R.; Stice, E. A Longitudinal Study of the Interactive Effects of Impulsivity and Anger on Adolescent Problem Behavior. *J. Youth Adolesc.* **1998**, *27*, 255–274. [CrossRef]
55. Sarkisian, K.; Van Hulle, C.; Lemery-Chalfant, K.; Goldsmith, H. Childhood inhibitory control and adolescent impulsivity and novelty seeking as differential predictors of relational and overt aggression. *J. Res. Personal.* **2017**, *67*, 144–150. [CrossRef]
56. Fosco, W.D.; Hawk, L.W.; Colder, C.R.; Meisel, S.N.; Lengua, L.J. The development of inhibitory control in adolescence and prospective relations with delinquency. *J. Adolesc.* **2019**, *76*, 37–47. [CrossRef]
57. Nigg, J.T.; Wong, M.M.; Martel, M.M.; Jester, J.M.; Puttler, L.I.; Glass, J.M.; Adams, K.M.; Fitzgerald, H.E.; Zucker, R.A. Poor Response Inhibition as a Predictor of Problem Drinking and Illicit Drug Use in Adolescents at Risk for Alcoholism and Other Substance Use Disorders. *J. Am. Acad. Child Adolesc. Psychiatry* **2006**, *45*, 468–475. [CrossRef]
58. Tarter, R.E.; Kirisci, L.; Mezzich, A.; Cornelius, J.R.; Pajer, K.; Vanyukov, M.; Gardner, W.; Blackson, T.; Clark, D. Neurobehavioral Disinhibition in Childhood Predicts Early Age at Onset of Substance Use Disorder. *Am. J. Psychiatry* **2003**, *160*, 1078–1085. [CrossRef]
59. Raaijmakers, M.A.J.; Smidts, D.P.; Sergeant, J.A.; Maassen, G.H.; Posthumus, J.A.; Van Engeland, H.; Matthys, W. Executive Functions in Preschool Children with Aggressive Behavior: Impairments in Inhibitory Control. *J. Abnorm. Child Psychol.* **2008**, *36*, 1097–1107. [CrossRef]
60. Utendale, W.T.; Hastings, P.D. Developmental changes in the relations between inhibitory control and externalizing problems during early childhood. *Infant Child Dev.* **2011**, *20*, 181–193. [CrossRef]
61. Oldehinkel, A.J.; Hartman, C.A.; Ferdinand, R.F.; Verhulst, F.C.; Ormel, J. Effortful control as modifier of the association between negative emotionality and adolescents' mental health problems. *Dev. Psychopathol.* **2007**, *19*, 523–539. [CrossRef] [PubMed]
62. Valiente, C.; Eisenberg, N.; Smith, C.L.; Reiser, M.; Fabes, R.A.; Losoya, S.; Guthrie, I.K.; Murphy, B.C. The relations of effortful control and reactive control to children's externalizing problems: A longitudinal assessment. *J. Personal.* **2003**, *71*, 1171–1196. [CrossRef] [PubMed]
63. Pardini, D.; Lochman, J.; Wells, K. Negative Emotions and Alcohol Use Initiation in High-Risk Boys: The Moderating Effect of Good Inhibitory Control. *J. Abnorm. Child Psychol.* **2004**, *32*, 505–518. [CrossRef]
64. Mitchell, Q.P.; Younginer, S.T.; Lochman, J.E.; Vernberg, E.M.; Powell, N.P.; Qu, L. Examining for the Protective Effects of Therapeutic Engagement on Child Aggression. *J. Emot. Behav. Disord.* **2020**. [CrossRef]
65. Ellis, M.L.; Lindsey, M.A.; Barker, E.D.; Boxmeyer, C.L.; Lochman, J.E. Predictors of Engagement in a School-Based Family Preventive Intervention for Youth Experiencing Behavioral Difficulties. *Prev. Sci.* **2013**, *14*, 457–467. [CrossRef]
66. Hogue, A.; Henderson, C.E.; Ozechowski, T.J.; Becker, S.J.; Coatsworth, J.D. Can the group harm the individual? Reviewing potential iatrogenic effects of group treatment for adolescent substance use. *Clin. Psychol. Sci. Pract.* **2019**, *28*, 40–51. [CrossRef]

67. Hill, L.G.; The Conduct Problems Prevention Research Group; Coie, J.D.; Lochman, J.E.; Greenberg, M.T. Effectiveness of Early Screening for Externalizing Problems: Issues of Screening Accuracy and Utility. *J. Consult. Clin. Psychol.* **2004**, *72*, 809–820. [CrossRef]
68. Kassing, F.; Conduct Problems Prevention Research Group; Godwin, J.; Lochman, J.E.; Coie, J.D. Using Early Childhood Behavior Problems to Predict Adult Convictions. *J. Abnorm. Child Psychol.* **2018**, *47*, 765–778. [CrossRef] [PubMed]
69. Dodge, K.A.; Lochman, J.E.; Harnish, J.D.; Bates, J.E.; Pettit, G.S. Reactive and proactive aggression in schoolchildren and psychiatrically impaired chronically assaultive youth. *J. Abnorm. Psychol.* **1997**, *106*, 37–51. [CrossRef] [PubMed]
70. Lindsey, M.A.; Romanelli, M.; Ellis, M.L.; Barker, E.; Boxmeyer, C.L.; Lochman, J.E. The Influence of Treatment Engagement on Positive Outcomes in the Context of a School-Based Intervention for Students with Externalizing Behavior Problems. *J. Abnorm. Child Psychol.* **2019**, *47*, 1437–1454. [CrossRef]
71. Capaldi, D.M.; Rothbart, M.K. Development and Validation of an Early Adolescent Temperament Measure. *J. Early Adolesc.* **1992**, *12*, 153–173. [CrossRef]
72. Reynolds, C.R.; Kamphaus, R.W. *Behavior Assessment System for Children (BASC)*; American Guidance Service: Circle Pines, MN, USA, 1992.
73. Pentz, M.A.; Trebow, E.A.; Hansen, W.B.; MacKinnon, D.P.; Dwyer, J.H.; Johnson, C.A.; Flay, B.R.; Daniels, S.; Cormack, C. Effects of program implementation on adolescent drug use behavior: The Midwestern Prevention Project (MPP). *Eval. Rev.* **1990**, *14*, 264–289. [CrossRef]
74. Shillington, A.; Clapp, J. Self-Report stability of adolescent substance use: Are there differences for gender, ethnicity and age? *Drug Alcohol Depend.* **2000**, *60*, 19–27. [CrossRef]
75. Fite, P.J.; Colder, C.R.; Lochman, J.E.; Wells, K.C. Pathways from proactive and reactive aggression to substance use. *Psychol. Addict. Behav.* **2007**, *21*, 355–364. [CrossRef]
76. Pentz, M.A.; Johnson, C.A.; Dwyer, J.H.; Mackinnon, D.M.; Hansen, W.B.; Flay, B. A Comprehensive Community Approach to Adolescent Drug Abuse Prevention: Effects on Cardiovascular Disease Risk Behaviors. *Ann. Med.* **1989**, *21*, 219–222. [CrossRef]
77. Boxmeyer, C.; Powell, N.P.; Lochman, J.E.; Dishion, T.J.; Wojnaroski, M.; Winter, C. *Cognitive-Behavioral Group Coding System*; University of Alabama: Tuscaloosa, AL, USA, 2015.
78. Raudenbush, S.W.; Bryk, A.S. *Hierarchical Linear Models: Applications and Data Analysis Methods*; Sage Publications: Thousand Oaks, CA, USA, 2002.
79. Johnston, L.D.; Miech, R.A.; O'Malley, P.M.; Bachman, J.G.; Schulenberg, J.E.; Patrick, M.E. *Monitoring the Future Monitoring Survey Results on Drug Use, 1975–2018: 2018 Overview, Key Findings on Adolescent Drug Use*; University of Michigan: Ann Arbor, MI, USA, 2019.
80. Diamond, A. Executive Functions. *Annu. Rev. Psychol.* **2013**, *64*, 135–168. [CrossRef]
81. Pandina, R.J.; Johnson, V.L.; White, H.R. Peer influences on substance use during adolescence and emerging adulthood. In *Handbook of Drug Use Etiology*; Peeters Publishers: Leuven, Belgium, 2009; pp. 383–401.
82. Fite, P.J.; Colder, C.R.; Lochman, J.E.; Wells, K.C. The Relation between Childhood Proactive and Reactive Aggression and Substance Use Initiation. *J. Abnorm. Child Psychol.* **2008**, *36*, 261–271. [CrossRef] [PubMed]
83. Levy, S.; Sherritt, L.; Harris, S.K.; Gates, E.C.; Holder, D.W.; Kulig, J.W.; Knight, J.R. Test-Retest Reliability of Adolescents' Self-Report of Substance Use. *Alcohol. Clin. Exp. Res.* **2004**, *28*, 1236–1241. [CrossRef] [PubMed]
84. Chapman, C.L.; Baker, E.L.; Porter, G.; Thayer, S.D.; Burlingame, G.M. Rating group therapist interventions: The validation of the Group Psychotherapy Intervention Rating Scale. *Group Dyn. Theory Res. Pract.* **2010**, *14*, 15–31. [CrossRef]

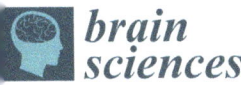

Article

Mindful Coping Power: Comparative Effects on Children's Reactive Aggression and Self-Regulation

Caroline L. Boxmeyer [1,2,*], Shari Miller [3,†], Devon E. Romero [4], Nicole P. Powell [2], Shannon Jones [2], Lixin Qu [2], Stephen Tueller [5] and John E. Lochman [2,6]

1. Department of Psychiatry and Behavioral Medicine, The University of Alabama, Tuscaloosa, AL 35487, USA
2. Center for Youth Development and Intervention, The University of Alabama, Tuscaloosa, AL 35487, USA; npowell@ua.edu (N.P.P.); jones178@ua.edu (S.J.); lxqu@ua.edu (L.Q.); jlochman@ua.edu (J.E.L.)
3. 3605 Moonlight Drive, Chapel Hill, NC 27516, USA; sharipeace@gmail.com
4. Department of Counseling, University of Texas at San Antonio, San Antonio, TX 78249, USA; devon.romero@utsa.edu
5. Division for Applied Justice Research, RTI International, Research Triangle Park, Durham, NC 27709, USA; stueller@rti.org
6. Department of Psychology, The University of Alabama, Tuscaloosa, AL 35487, USA
* Correspondence: boxmeyer@ua.edu; Tel.: +1-205-348-1325
† Formerly at RTI International, Research Triangle Park, Durham, NC 27709, USA.

Abstract: Coping Power (CP) is an evidence-based preventive intervention for youth with disruptive behavior problems. This study examined whether Mindful Coping Power (MCP), a novel adaptation which integrates mindfulness into CP, enhances program effects on children's reactive aggression and self-regulation. A pilot randomized design was utilized to estimate the effect sizes for MCP versus CP in a sample of 102 child participants (fifth grade students, predominantly low-middle income, 87% Black). MCP produced significantly greater improvement in children's self-reported dysregulation (emotional, behavioral, cognitive) than CP, including children's perceived anger modulation. Small to moderate effects favoring MCP were also observed for improvements in child-reported inhibitory control and breath awareness and parent-reported child attentional capacity and social skills. MCP did not yield a differential effect on teacher-rated reactive aggression. CP produced a stronger effect than MCP on parent-reported externalizing behavior problems. Although MCP did not enhance program effects on children's reactive aggression as expected, it did have enhancing effects on children's internal, embodied experiences (self-regulation, anger modulation, breath awareness). Future studies are needed to compare MCP and CP in a large scale, controlled efficacy trial and to examine whether MCP-produced improvements in children's internal experiences lead to improvements in their observable behavior over time.

Keywords: mindfulness; reactive aggression; disruptive behavior; Coping Power; self-regulation; prevention; Mindful Coping Power

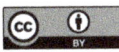

1. Introduction

Coping Power (CP) is an evidence-based preventive intervention for preadolescent children with disruptive behavior problems [1]. Thirteen randomized controlled trials have shown that CP has beneficial effects for children exhibiting elevated levels of aggressive behavior, producing lower rates of children's substance use, aggression, and delinquency in later adolescence compared to children in control groups, and in improving children's social competence and academic functioning (for review, see [1]). Based on a contextual social-cognitive model of risk for aggression and substance use, CP targets mediating child (social cognition, anger coping) and family (parenting) processes [2]. CP's preventive effects on delinquent behavior and substance use are evident four years after intervention [3].

1.1. Reactive Aggression

Despite its strong evidence base, CP's effects have been more mixed on reactive aggression than on proactive aggression. Coping Power had effects on reactive aggression at a three-year follow-up [4], but only had effects on reactive aggression at immediate post-intervention in one of two studies [5,6]. In contrast, Coping Power had significant effects on proactive aggression at both follow-up and immediate post-intervention in these three studies. Reactive aggression is one of two key pathways linking aggression and substance use [7]. Proactive aggression is instrumental, cold-blooded, and unprovoked, whereas reactive aggression is emotionally-driven, impulsive, and hot-blooded [8]. Although children can manifest both forms, factor analytic work consistently finds proactive and reactive aggression to be independent dimensions [9], with unique genetic [10], physiological [11], and social-cognitive processes [12,13]. Proactive and reactive aggression are both important predictors of children's later substance use and delinquency [14]. The current study was undertaken to maximize CP's effects on reactive aggression.

Key characteristics that link reactive aggression and substance use include impulsivity and negative emotionality [15,16]. Youths with high levels of reactive aggression may cope with negative emotionality by self-medicating, consistent with research linking temperamental anger to alcohol use initiation [17]. Reactive aggression is also impulsive in nature, and impulsivity has been associated with substance use [15,16]. The current study sought to enhance the effects of CP by targeting the active mechanisms of reactive aggression.

1.2. Active Mechanisms of Reactive Aggression

Anger arousal and emotional dysregulation. A central mechanism in reactive aggression is emotional dysregulation [18]. Children with reactive aggression experience high levels of anger [19,20], intense emotional arousal [13,21], and negative emotionality [19,22]. Children high on reactive aggression (but not proactive aggression) evidence greater electrodermal reactivity in response to an experimental anger induction task [11].

Impulsivity and behavioral dysregulation. Children high on reactive aggression exhibit deficits in behavioral regulation, particularly poor impulse control (e.g., [19]). When they perceive the slightest threat, they lack behavioral inhibition and respond with angry outbursts and aggression [13,23]. Impulsivity is a symptom of attention-deficit hyperactivity disorder (ADHD) and reactive aggression is more strongly associated with ADHD than proactive aggression [24].

Rumination, perceived threat, and cognitive dysregulation. In ambiguous situations, reactively aggressive children perceive that others have hostile intentions, which leads to angry responses to perceived provocations or threats [9,25]. Anger rumination has been found to be positively associated with reactive aggression in college students [26]. Reactively aggressive children may ruminate about perceived threats and anger-arousing events, which compromises their ability to override tendencies toward aggressive behavior. In an overview of research with adults, this ruminative cognitive style was found to exacerbate anger arousal and create a state of readiness for reactive aggression [27]. Reactive aggression is also linked with deficits in executive function [28].

Attentional capacity. Children high on reactive aggression often exhibit attention difficulties, as reflected by the higher rates of ADHD in children exhibiting reactive aggression [24]. They also have difficulty accurately encoding social cues and recall fewer details of a social situation [29]. Consequently, reactively aggressive children may miss critical information that informs their responses to others. In addition, their attention is selective and biased, and focuses on negative interactions such as rejection, ridicule, and failure [30].

1.3. Rationale for Mindful Coping Power

Improving these active mechanisms is expected to reduce children's reactive aggression and improve their prosocial behavior. In turn, these improvements are expected to disrupt the pathway from reactive aggression to peer rejection, peer delinquency, and substance use. The Mindful Coping Power program (MCP) was developed to maximize program effects on children's reactive aggression and its active mechanisms, with the overarching aim of altering this developmental cascade. Mindfulness is the practice of bringing non-judgmental awareness to the present moment [31]. Mindfulness training was selected to enhance the existing CP program due to the demonstrated benefits of mindfulness on the active mechanisms of reactive aggression, as described below.

Effects of mindfulness on anger arousal and emotion regulation. Mindfulness is associated with improved emotion regulation and decreased aggressive anger expression in adults [32], college students [33], and children [34]. Brain imaging research with adults and college students indicates that mindfulness training yields improvements in brain regions associated with emotion regulation [35,36]. In studies with youths, mindfulness training has been found to decrease emotional arousal and increase self-efficacy in emotional regulation [34,37].

Effects of mindfulness on impulse control and behavioral regulation. Mindfulness training has been found to improve both impulsivity and aggressive behavior in youths with classroom behavior difficulties [38]. A mindfulness-based school program led to improvements in children's prosocial behavior, aggression, and peer acceptance [39]. Children with ADHD [40,41], children with co-existing ADHD and oppositional defiant disorder [42], and adolescents with disruptive behavior disorders [43] exhibit behavioral improvements following mindfulness training, including reduced hyperactivity and impulsivity.

Effects of mindfulness on rumination and cognitive regulation. Mindfulness training has demonstrated benefits for several aspects of cognitive regulation. It decreases rumination in adolescents [43,44]. In an electroencephalogram study, mindfulness was inversely associated with rumination [45]. The non-judgment component of mindfulness training appears to be relevant for the negative relation between mindfulness and rumination in research with adult participants [46]. Mindfulness training also improves cognitive flexibility with adults [35,47], and with children when implemented in school settings [39].

Effects of mindfulness on attention regulation. Prior adult studies have shown benefits of mindfulness training on attention (e.g., [48]), including intensive [49] and shorter-term [33] meditation training. Mindfulness improves electrophysiological markers of attentional control [50] and functional connectivity in brain regions important to attention [51] for adults. Important to the current study, Schonert-Reichl and colleagues [39] found that a mindfulness-based school program had positive effects on several behavioral measures of children's attention and executive function. Further, in two studies of children with ADHD, mindfulness training improved children's attention [41,42].

School-based mindfulness intervention. Although schools can represent an optimal setting for providing mindfulness intervention to a broad range of children, concerns have been raised that the implementation of mindfulness-based interventions is proceeding faster than the current evidence base for school-based implementation documents [52–54]. Reviews of the rapidly growing research literature on school-based mindfulness interventions indicate promising effects on attention control, coping with stressors, and, in some cases, on anxiety, but there have been noted concerns about study quality and implementation acceptability (e.g., [55,56]). A systematic review of school-based mindfulness studies concluded that there was insufficient attention to intervention integrity and to feasibility of mindfulness of interventions in school settings [53]. In sum, there is a research base indicating that mindfulness training can lead to improvements in the active mechanisms for reactive aggression in children. The present study was the first to test a school-based mindfulness enhancement of an existing, evidence-based preventive intervention with children with high levels of reactive aggression, with special attention to intervention integrity and to the feasibility and acceptability of the intervention according to intervention providers, children, and parents.

1.4. Current Study

The current study examined whether optimizing CP by infusing it with mindfulness enhances program effects over and above standard CP on children's reactive aggression and its active mechanisms. A randomized comparative effectiveness trial design [57] was employed to test a previously established "best practice" (CP) against a novel intervention (MCP). The primary study aim was to estimate effect sizes comparing MCP and CP, in preparation for a large-scale efficacy trial. The study had the following a priori hypotheses: (1) MCP will yield greater decreases in children's reactive aggression than CP; (2) MCP will yield stronger effects than CP on the active mechanisms of reactive aggression, including: decreased child anger arousal and emotional reactivity, increased impulse control and behavioral regulation, decreased anger rumination and cognitive dysregulation, and increased child attentional capacity; (3) MCP will yield greater improvements in children's social skills than CP, including increased prosocial behavior and decreased externalizing behavior problems.

2. Materials and Methods

2.1. Participants

Participating schools. Five elementary schools from a public-school system in urban and suburban areas in Alabama were recruited to participate in this study. All schools agreed to participate. The five participating schools varied on sociodemographic measures, including percent of children from economically disadvantaged households (which ranged from 76% to 32%) and child race (Black or African American was most prevalent and ranged from 92% to 32%). Random assignment to condition occurred within school to control for sociodemographic variation.

Child and parent participants. This study included a sample of 102 children with elevated levels of reactive aggression, and their parents and teachers. This sample size was selected because it was the maximal number of participants who could be assessed and treated within the project's grant budget as a pilot and feasibility trial. Power to detect statistically significant differences between the two active interventions was limited. A priori power estimates ranged from 0.21 to 0.62 for small (0.2) to moderate (0.4) effects. This sample size was adequate for the primary aim of estimating the comparative effects of MCP and CP in preparation for a large-scale prevention trial.

Child participants were identified at the end of fourth grade and participated in the intervention during fifth grade. CP was designed to provide skills-training prior to the middle school transition, when risk for substance use initiation increases (e.g., [58]). To identify children with elevated levels of reactive aggression, fourth grade teachers completed the 3-item reactive aggression scale from the Teacher Report of Reactive and Proactive Aggression [8] on all students in their classroom. Detailed information about this measure is provided below. Screening occurred at the end of fourth grade when teachers were very familiar with children's behavior. This also allowed families to be recruited and assessed near the start of fifth grade.

Ratings were compiled across the participating schools to identify an empirical cut-off score reflecting the top quartile of fourth grade students on reactive aggression. A cut-off score of 8 was used. This is consistent with prior studies of CP, in which children with teacher-rated reactive aggression above 8.5 had parent-rated externalizing problems in the at-risk or clinical range on the Behavior Assessment Scale for Children [59]. Thus, teacher screener scores at or above this level are indicative of a child's risk status from both teacher and parent perspectives [60,61]. Parent participants were the primary caregiver(s) of each child enrolled in the study.

A total of 638 fourth grade students were screened for study participation. Of those, 428 scored below the empirical cut-off for teacher-rated reactive aggression. One child with an eligible screener score was excluded due to a language barrier that could not be addressed with local resources. The remaining families were contacted in random order until the total number of intervention slots at each school had been filled. Six families declined study participation (the most common reasons were that the child already received services elsewhere, or lack of perceived need). These children did not significantly differ on baseline characteristics from those enrolled. One hundred and eight children were initially enrolled in the study. Five of these children moved to different schools prior to starting fifth grade. The remaining 103 participants were randomly assigned to MCP or CP in yoked pairs, as described below. One child withdrew from the study after participating in one session (due to perceived lack of need and social concerns), which resulted in a total sample of 102 child participants, as well as their parents and teachers. Participants were recruited in two annual cohorts (n = 44 in Cohort 1 and n = 58 in Cohort 2).

Table 1 summarizes the demographic characteristics of the study sample. Sixty-one percent of the recruited children were male (n = 62) and 39% (n = 40) were female. Child age ranged from 9 to 11 (M = 9.97, SD = 0.48). The parent-reported racial composition of the sample was 87.3% Black or African American (n = 89), 5.9% White or Caucasian (n = 6), 3.9% more than one race (n = 4), and 2.9% Unknown or not reported (n = 3). At one of the five schools, the percent of Black or African American children enrolled in the study (70%) was significantly higher than the percent in fifth grade at that school (32%). For family income, 33.4% of parents reported an annual household income of less than USD 15,000, 29.4% reported USD 15,000 to USD 29,999, 21.5% reported USD 30,000 to USD 49,999, 13.8% reported annual family income of more than USD 50,000, and 1.9% did not provide information about annual family income.

Table 1. Participant characteristics at time of recruitment.

Demographic variable	Overall Sample (n = 102)	MCP Condition (n = 52)	CP Condition (n = 50)
	M (SD)	M (SD)	M (SD)
Child age	9.97 (0.48)	10 (0.49)	9.94 (0.47)
Child 4th grade reactive aggression	11.18 (2.37)	11.17 (2.39)	11.18 (2.37)
	n (%)	n (%)	n (%)
Child gender			
Male	62 (60.8%)	33 (63.5%)	29 (58.0%)
Female	40 (39.2%)	19 (36.5%)	21 (42.0%)
Child ethnicity			
Hispanic or Latino	3 (2.9%)	1 (1.9%)	2 (4.0%)
Not Hispanic or Latino	92 (90.2%)	47 (90.4%)	45 (90.0%)
Unknown or not reported	7 (6.9%)	4 (7.7%)	3 (6.0%)
Child race			
Black or African American	89 (87.3%)	47 (90.4%)	42 (84.0%)
White or Caucasian	6 (5.9%)	2 (3.8%)	4 (8.0%)
More than one race	4 (3.9%)	1 (1.9%)	3 (6.0%)
Unknown or not reported	3 (2.9%)	2 (3.8%)	1 (2.0%)
Child repeated grade	18 (17.5%)	9 (17.3%)	9 (18.0%)
Caregiver relation to child			
Biological parent	85 (82.5%)	44 (84.6%)	41 (82%)
Adoptive parent	5 (4.9%)	3 (5.8%)	2 (3.8%)
Grandparent	7 (6.8%)	2 (3.8%)	5 (10%)
Other	5 (4.9%)	3 (5.8%)	2 (3.8%)
Annual family income			
Less than USD 15,000	34 (33.4%)	17 (32.7%)	17 (34.0%)
USD 15,000 to <29,999	30 (29.4%)	13 (25.0%)	17 (34.0%)
USD 30,000 to <49,999	22 (21.5%)	14 (26.9%)	8 (16.0%)
More than USD 50,000	14 (13.8%)	7 (13.5%)	7 (14.0%)
Unknown or not reported	2 (1.9%)	1 (1.9%)	1 (2.0%)

Teachers. Children's fourth grade teachers provided initial child behavioral screening data. Children's fifth grade teachers completed pre- and post-intervention assessments regarding children's academic and behavioral functioning. The pre-intervention assessment occurred at least four to six weeks after the beginning of fifth grade, to allow time for teachers to get to know the children well. The post-intervention assessment occurred at the end of fifth grade, after the intervention was complete. Teachers were blind to intervention condition (CP or MCP). They only knew that specific children were participating in one of two Coping Power groups being offered at their school (e.g., the Wednesday group or the Friday group). The only other overt difference was that yoga mats were used in MCP but not CP. The yoga mats were stored in a separate meeting room throughout the year, then given to children to keep after all intervention and assessments had been completed. It is possible that children in MCP discussed some of the unique program elements (e.g., yoga stretches, mindfulness practices) with their teachers, but this was not directly evaluated.

Coping Power leaders. There were five primary group leaders. Each implemented both versions of the intervention (MCP and CP). These leaders were doctoral ($n = 2$) or master's ($n = 3$) level clinicians with considerable experience implementing Coping Power (three of the five were licensed clinicians, each with more than twelve years of experience running CP groups; two were advanced doctoral students with prior experience leading or co-leading CP groups). Four of the leaders were female and one male. Four of the leaders were Caucasian and one identified as more than one race. All of the primary leaders completed Mindfulness-Based Stress Reduction training prior to the start of the study. They also committed to maintaining a regular mindfulness practice of at least ten minutes a day throughout the study and participated in weekly group supervision meetings that included group mindfulness practice and discussion. Master's and advanced undergraduate students served as group co-leaders, to provide additional group oversight and behavior support. These co-leaders participated in CP and mindfulness training workshops prior to program implementation and committed to maintaining a regular personal mindfulness practice.

2.2. Procedure

The University of Alabama Institutional Review Board approved all study procedures and conducted continuing review throughout study administration.

Random assignment to condition. Children with scores of 8 or higher on the teacher-rated reactive aggression screener items were considered eligible for participation. The participating schools varied in the number of children who fell within the eligible range. A random calling order was created for eligible children from each school and families were contacted according to their placement on this list until twelve children were enrolled at each school. Once recruited into the study, children were randomly assigned to one of the two active conditions: CP ($n = 50$) or MCP ($n = 52$). Random assignment occurred within each school. Yoked pairs of students with similar reactive aggression scores and demographic characteristics (i.e., gender and race) were randomly assigned to either the CP or MCP group at that school. The CP and MCP groups were equivalent on teacher-reported reactive aggression at the end of fourth grade (as shown in Table 1).

Pre-intervention data (Time 1) were gathered from parents and children near the start of fifth grade and from teachers four to six weeks into the school year. This allowed time to enroll participants while fifth grade teachers were becoming familiar with the children's behavior (beyond any honeymoon period). The intervention began after all Time 1 assessments were completed. Post-intervention data (Time 2) were collected from teachers in late spring of fifth grade and from parents and children in late spring-early summer after fifth grade. Research staff members who administered the parent and child assessments were blind to condition. Teachers received USD 10 for each child assessed. Parents received USD 50 and child participants received USD 10 at each assessment time point.

Intervention. Two active preventive interventions were compared in this study. CP and MCP both included the same number of sessions (25 child group sessions, 10 parent group sessions) and utilized curriculum manuals with specific objectives for each session. Child group sessions were conducted in a private meeting space during the regular school day and lasted approximately 45 min each. Parent group sessions were held in the morning or evening (both options were offered in each condition) in a location central to the participating schools. Parent group sessions lasted $1-1\frac{1}{2}$ hours each. Sessions were spaced to provide the content in one school year (about 7–8 months). Child groups met weekly and parent groups met 1–2 times per month.

Coping Power. CP is an evidence-based preventive intervention for youths with or at risk for disruptive behavior disorders [1]. CP draws upon a cognitive-behavioral framework to teach children social and emotional coping skills and to teach parents positive parenting and self-care skills. Topics covered in the child program include: personal goal setting, identification of feelings, coping with anger, perspective-taking, problem-solving, affiliating with prosocial peers, and resisting peer pressure. Topics covered in the parent program include: supporting children's academic learning, strengthening the parent–child relationship and family cohesion, managing the stress of parenting, setting household rules and expectations, praise, ignoring, effective discipline techniques, family problem-solving, and planning for the future.

Mindful Coping Power. MCP is a novel adaptation of CP in which mindfulness practices were integrated with the existing cognitive-behavioral elements. All of the core content from the CP child and parent components was retained in MCP. Mindfulness practices were integrated into CP in three ways: (a) mindfulness-only sessions (several sessions were added to the MCP child and parent programs to introduce mindfulness theory and practice); (b) mindfulness in every session (each MCP child and parent session began and ended with a series of mindfulness practices, including the ringing of a chime, a breath awareness practice, yoga poses, and a compassion practice); (c) integration of mindfulness into existing Coping Power activities (e.g., an existing component on identifying early physiological cues of anger was enhanced through regular body awareness practices; compassion practices informed activities designed to help children and parents see situations from others' perspectives; thought awareness practices helped children and parents allow angry thoughts to 'pass on by' rather than clinging to them as facts). For further detail about the integration of mindfulness into CP, including the comprehensive theoretical model for MCP and sample sessions highlighting the differences between MCP and CP, see Miller and colleagues [62].

Every child and parent intervention session (CP and MCP) was video recorded. Group leaders received monthly individualized feedback as well as weekly group supervision from the principal investigators. To ensure high fidelity to the new program elements, leaders received feedback on every mindfulness-only session held. Leaders were trained to ensure that they did not incorporate mindfulness-specific language or practices into CP sessions. CP did not have any intervention content that was not also in MCP. Effort was made to keep the length of sessions consistent across the two conditions. Due to the added mindfulness practices in MCP, leaders were able to spend more time on some program elements during CP sessions than MCP sessions (e.g., reviewing progress toward weekly personal goals and setting new goals; personal sharing related to intervention topics; opportunities to practice new skills in session; summarizing key points at the end of sessions). There were a total of 18 unique child groups (9 MCP, 9 CP) and 8 unique parent groups (4 MCP, 4 CP). Four schools participated in Cohort 1 and a fifth school was added for Cohort 2. The same leader ran both the MCP and CP groups at each school each year.

2.3. Measures

Teacher Report of Reactive and Proactive Aggression (TRRPA) [8]. To identify students with moderate to high levels of reactive aggression, fourth grade teachers completed the 6-item TRRPA for all of the children in their class. This instrument consisted of three items assessing reactive aggression ("overreacts angrily to accidents," "strikes back when teased," and "blames others in fights") and three items assessing proactive aggression ("gets others to gang up on a peer," "uses physical force to dominate," and "threatens and bullies others"). Each item was rated on a 5-point scale (1 = *Never* to 5 = *Almost Always*). Children's scores on the 3-item teacher-reported reactive aggression scale were used to determine study eligibility (scores can range from 3 to 15, with higher scores reflecting greater reactive aggression). Teachers also completed this measure pre- and post-intervention to assess for change. In the current sample, Cronbach's alpha for teacher-rated reactive aggression was 0.91.

Abbreviated Dysregulation Inventory (ADI) [63]. The 31-item ADI includes three subscales: affective dysregulation (arousability, weak emotional control, and irritability); behavioral dysregulation (impulsivity, inattention, and hyperactivity); cognitive dysregulation (poor problem-solving and planning, inability to learn from experience, and cognitive inflexibility). Students rated how true each statement was in the past month on a Likert-type scale from 1 (*never true*) to 4 (*always true*). Total dysregulation was calculated by averaging the scores for all three subscales, with higher scores reflecting greater overall dysregulation. Five of the affective dysregulation items comprise the Anger Scale (e.g., "I have trouble controlling my temper," "when I am angry I lose control over my actions," "I get so frustrated that I often feel like a bomb ready to explode), with higher scores indicating greater difficulty regulating anger. This well-established instrument has been used with children and adults and is used to assess risk for substance use disorders. In the current sample, Cronbach's alpha was 0.81 for total dysregulation and 0.74 for the anger scale.

Early Adolescent Temperament Questionnaire (EATQ) [64]. The EATQ is a self-report measure that assesses various aspects of adolescent temperament [64]. The inhibitory control subscale of the EATQ was administered as a child self-report measure of behavioral self-regulation. This subscale consists of five items (e.g., "when someone tells me to stop doing something, it is easy for me to stop"). Higher mean scores reflect a greater capacity to plan and suppress inappropriate responses. Cronbach's alpha for the EATQ inhibitory control subscale was 0.63 in the current sample. The attention subscale of the EATQ-Revised Parent Report (EATQ-R) [65] was administered as a parent-report measure of children's attentional capacity. This subscale consists of six items (e.g., "my child finds it really easy to concentrate on a problem," "my child is good at keeping track of several different things that are happening around him/her"). Higher mean scores reflect better child attentional capacity. Cronbach's alpha for the EATQ-R attention subscale was 0.73 in the current sample.

Behavior Assessment System for Children (BASC) [59]. Child externalizing behavior problems and social skills were assessed using the Parent Rating Scale (PRS) and Teacher Rating Scale (TRS) of the BASC. Items of the PRS and TRS were rated on a 4-point scale (e.g., "Mean to others," "Sudden changes in mood or feelings"; 0 = *Never* to 3 = *Almost Always*). The child version (appropriate for ages 6–11) was used for both the TRS and PRS. Teachers and parents completed the BASC at pre- and post-intervention time points.

Program effects on children's aggressive and disruptive behavior were measured using the externalizing problems composite, which consists of subscales measuring aggression, conduct problems, and hyperactivity. Higher composite scores reflect worse child externalizing problems. Cronbach's alpha for the externalizing problems scale was 0.89 for the PRS and 0.96 for the TRS in the current sample. The social skills subscale was also included as a measure of program effects on children's prosocial behavior. Sample items include "offers to help others," "shows interest in others' ideas," and "tries to bring out the best in others." Higher scores reflect better child social skills. Cronbach's alpha for the social skills subscale was 0.89 for the PRS and 0.92 for the TRS. Parent and teacher reports of children's externalizing behavior problems ($r = 0.34$) and social skills ($r = 0.20$) were significantly correlated but represent unique perspectives, thus were considered separately in analyses.

Scale of Body Connection (SBC) [66]. Breath awareness was examined as a measure of mindfulness. Four items assessing children's breath awareness were adapted based on the SBC [61], which includes a range of items measuring body awareness and bodily dissociation. Items were rated on a 1 (*not at all*) to 5 (*all of the time*) Likert scale. Sample items included "I can feel my breath travel through my body" and "I notice how my breath changes when I am tense or nervous." Higher mean scores reflect greater child awareness of their breath. Cronbach's alpha for the breath awareness scale in the current sample was 0.65.

Program Implementation. Child and parent group leaders documented program implementation in several ways. For each CP and MCP session, they documented participant attendance, level of engagement, and completion of in- and out-of-session activities. They also documented the duration of each session and completion of the planned objectives. Supervisors also rated leaders' implementation fidelity and quality using program-specific measures (assessing completion of planned program objectives and constructs such as: ability to engage participants in the intervention, effective instructional style, and consistency with guiding theoretical principles).

Program Feasibility, Acceptability, and Impact. Participants provided feedback on MCP and CP acceptability and impact after every 5 child group sessions and every 2 parent group sessions, and provided overall feedback at post-intervention. Group leaders provided feedback on the feasibility and impact of each MCP and CP session and overall feedback at post-intervention.

2.4. Data Analyses

Latent Change Score (LCS) analyses were conducted to compare CP and MCP intervention effects on the primary child outcome measures. LCS is a structural equation model (SEM) that can be used to fit the paired *t*-test model in a way that is more flexible than the usual paired *t*-test [67]. For the current data, this allowed multiple group *t*-tests to be fit and to examine whether there were pre–post outcome changes within the standard and mindful Coping Power groups, and whether the amount of change differed between the CP and MCP groups (this can be seen as an SEM implementation of the difference-in-differences estimator).

The multiple group latent change scores were fit using the lavaan [68] R package [69]. Models were fit such that pre-test values predicted the latent change score, which allows for the likely possibility of imperfect test-retest reliability [67]. The LCS approach also has better missing data handling than the paired *t*-test since it assumes data are missing at random (MAR) conditional on other variables in the model instead of the missing completely at random (MCAR) assumption made by the *t*-test, which excludes all participants with any missing data. For a review of these missing data concepts, see Enders [70]. Full information maximum likelihood estimation was used to address missing data so that all participants were retained in the analyses. All participants with an observation for at least one time point are retained. At pre-intervention, 1 of 52 MCP participants and 1 of 50 CP participants were missing data on variable(s) of interest. At post-intervention, 3 MCP and 8 CP participants were missing data on variable(s) of interest. Before conducting LCS analyses, *t*-tests were run to compare MCP and CP for baseline equivalence on each of the primary child outcome measures. The distribution of scores on each measure was also examined for skewness and kurtosis.

The focus of the analyses was on estimating effect sizes in MCP and CP to inform power analyses for a future, large-scale efficacy trial. It was expected that preliminary support for MCP would be evidenced by at least small to moderate effect sizes relative to CP on the primary outcomes ($d = 0.2$ or larger), which would warrant further evaluation of MCP in a large-scale efficacy trial.

3. Results

LCS analyses compared the effects of the new MCP preventive intervention to the effects of the existing, evidence-based CP program on reactive aggression and its active mechanisms. Table 2 summarizes the findings observed. Results are presented by informant group, with a focus on the effect size estimates observed.

Table 2. Comparative effects of standard Coping Power (CP) and Mindful Coping Power (MCP) on child outcomes in a pilot randomized trial.

	Means				Latent Change Score (LCS)				Group Differences in LCS	
	Standard Coping Power		Mindful Coping Power		Standard Coping Power		Mindful Coping Power			
	Pre	Post	Pre	Post	Estimate	p	Estimate	p	Cohen's d (95% CI)	p
				Child-reported outcomes						
Total Dysregulation (ADI) [a]	1.05	1.13	1.13	0.96	0.07	0.248	−0.18	0.000	−0.76 (−1.40, −0.10)	0.001
Anger Scale (ADI) [a]	1.02	1.09	1.07	0.80	0.08	0.540	−0.28	0.010	−0.45 (−0.70, −0.03)	0.033
Inhibitory Control (EATQ) [b]	3.64	3.56	3.57	3.77	−0.07	0.558	0.20	0.043	0.37 (−0.03, 0.58)	0.081
Breath Awareness (SBC) [b]	3.33	3.37	3.11	3.64	0.07	0.702	0.53	0.008	0.31 (−0.07, 0.99)	0.090
				Parent-reported outcomes						
Attention (EATQ) [b]	3.28	3.16	3.08	3.23	−0.09	0.326	0.16	0.228	0.32 (−0.07, 0.58)	0.121
Social Skills T-score (BASC) [b]	53.78	52.05	51.06	51.63	−1.77	0.149	0.65	0.593	0.30 (−0.96, 5.79)	0.161
Externalizing Problems T-score (BASC) [a]	52.57	49.80	51.98	53.18	−2.81	0.104	1.11	0.422	0.36 (−0.42, 8.25)	0.077
				Teacher-reported outcomes						
Reactive Aggression (TRRPA) [a]	9.40	10.08	9.80	10.56	0.69	0.215	0.87	0.029	0.13 (−1.17, 1.51)	0.802
Social Skills T-score (BASC) [b]	41.16	44.14	39.87	42.00	2.81	0.013	2.06	0.019	−0.02 (−3.55, 2.04)	0.598
Externalizing Problems T-score (BASC) [a]	57.78	61.59	58.58	60.74	4.12	0.001	2.13	0.021	−0.04 (−5.61, 1.62)	0.279

[a] Lower scores reflect positive outcomes. [b] Higher scores reflect positive outcomes.

3.1. Child Self-Report Outcomes

Children in MCP exhibited a significantly greater reduction in total dysregulation on the ADI compared to children in CP, yielding a moderate–large effect size (Cohen's $d = -0.76$, 95% CI $[-1.40, -0.10]$, $p = 0.001$). Figure 1 depicts this finding.

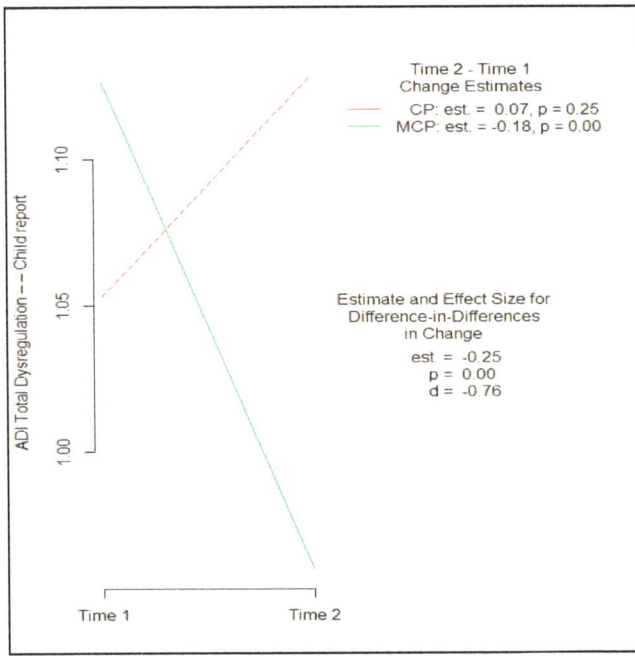

Figure 1. Comparative effects of Coping Power and Mindful Coping Power on children's total dysregulation (affective, behavioral, cognitive) on the Abbreviated Dysregulation Inventory.

Moderate effect sizes favoring MCP were observed on the affective dysregulation (Cohen's $d = -0.42$, 95% CI $[-0.53, -0.003]$, $p = 0.048$) and behavioral dysregulation (Cohen's $d = -0.41$, 95% CI $[-0.52, 0.001]$, $p = 0.051$) subscales of the ADI. A smaller effect size was observed on the cognitive dysregulation subscale (Cohen's $d = -0.33$, 95% CI $[-0.47, 0.04]$, $p = 0.102$), also favoring MCP. Only the effect on affective dysregulation was statistically significant in this feasibility sample. Children in MCP exhibited a significantly greater reduction on the ADI Anger Scale than children in CP, yielding a moderate effect size (Cohen's $d = -0.45$, 95% CI $[-0.70, -0.03]$, $p = 0.033$).

A small to moderate effect size favoring MCP was observed for child-reported inhibitory control on the EATQ (Cohen's $d = 0.37$, 95% CI $[-0.03, 0.58]$, $p = 0.081$). This finding is depicted in Figure 2. Breath awareness, a measure of child mindfulness, also yielded a small to moderate effect size favoring MCP (Cohen's $d = 0.31$, 95% CI $[-0.07, 0.99]$, $p = 0.090$). These effects were not statistically significant in this feasibility sample.

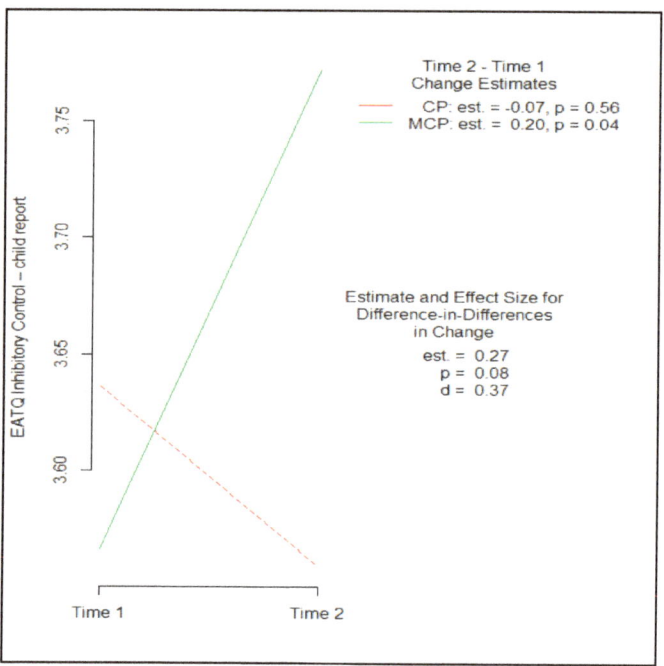

Figure 2. Comparative effects of Coping Power and Mindful Coping Power on children's inhibitory control on the Early Adolescent Temperament Questionnaire.

3.2. Parent-Report Outcomes

Small to moderate effect sizes favoring MCP were observed for parent-reported improvements in child attention on the EATQ (Cohen's d = 0.32, 95% CI [−0.07, 0.58], p = 0.121) and children's social skills on the BASC (Cohen's d = 0.30, 95% CI [−0.96, 5.79], p = 0.161). In contrast, there was a small to moderate effect favoring CP for reduction in parent-reported BASC externalizing problems (Cohen's d = 0.36, 95% CI [−0.42, 8.25], p = 0.077). No parent-reported outcome effects were statistically significant in this feasibility sample.

3.3. Teacher-Report Outcomes

On teacher-rated child reactive aggression, a key outcome of interest, the difference between MCP and CP was small and non-significant (Cohen's d = 0.13, 95% CI [−1.17, 1.51], p = 0.802). Negligible differences between MCP and CP were also observed on the two other teacher-reported outcomes, child externalizing problems on the BASC (Cohen's d = −0.04, 95% CI [−5.61, 1.62], p = 0.279) and child social skills on the BASC (Cohen's d = −0.02, 95% CI [−3.55, 2.04], p = 0.598).

3.4. Implementation Fidelity and Quality

Supervisors who observed video-recorded sessions provided overall ratings of leaders' implementation fidelity and quality, with scores ranging from 1 (low) to 10 (high). Mean supervisor-rated effective completion of session objectives was 8.33 (SD = 0.89) for CP and 8.44 (SD = 0.99) for MCP. Mean supervisor-rated effective engagement of participants was 8.67 (SD = 0.89) for CP and 9.00 (SD = 1.78) for MCP. Supervisors also rated MCP leaders' ability to articulate mindfulness theory clearly and accurately, yielding a mean score of 8.78 (SD = 1.23) and ability to implement mindfulness practices effectively, yielding a mean score of 8.44 (SD = 1.75).

3.5. School and Leader Effects

Exploratory analyses assessed for school-level effects. No significant effects were observed at the school level. Leader effects were on the same level, since random assignment to condition occurred within schools (i.e., the same leader implemented both the CP and MCP groups at each school). No significant effects at this level were observed.

3.6. Feasibility and Participant Satisfaction

Leaders provided feedback on the comparative feasibility of MCP and CP at post-intervention. On a scale ranging from 0 (not at all) to 10 (very much), the mean score for how feasible the MCP child program was to implement was 7.29 ($SD = 0.76$) and the mean score for how well the leader was able to cover the core skills from standard CP during MCP child sessions was 7.71 ($SD = 1.28$). When asked to rate which program was easier to implement, the mean score was 4.57 ($SD = 2.30$), on a scale ranging from 0 (CP) to 5 (equal) to 10 (MCP). The following quote summarizes the most prevalent themes in the leader feedback regarding the comparative feasibility of MCP versus CP: "CP had fewer topics to cover in each session, so it was easier to implement in that way. However, as the program went on, the MCP group became calmer and easier to manage. So, even though there was more to cover in any given session, it became somewhat easier to implement overall."

On post-intervention feedback surveys, children rated how helpful the MCP or CP program was to their life. Children's mean rating for MCP was 3.5 ($SD = 0.7$) compared to 3.3 ($SD = 1.2$) for CP on a 4-point Likert scale ranging from 1 (Not at all) to 4 (Very much). Children rated how well they liked being in the program on the same scale, which yielded a mean score of 3.6 ($SD = 0.5$) for MCP compared to 3.3 ($SD = 1.1$) for CP. Some of the children's comments about what they liked best about MCP were: "everything," "it helps you work on your friendships and stuff," "MCP helps you with your heart," "we learn things that help us take care of our problems," "the mindful stuff," "being normal and calm," "it helps me handle my feelings," "PTP and Take 2," "it teaches you to respond not react," and "I liked doing Feel and Spread the Good Vibes." Some of the children's suggested changes to improve MCP were "nothing," "that we have more time," "do it every day," "to add more people to the group," "stay longer," "do more fun stuff," "the timing [of group meetings at school]," and "get more points and prizes."

Without the same time constraints for the parent group meetings, leaders found the MCP parent group to be equally feasible to implement as CP, with a mean score of 5.00 ($SD = 0$) on a scale ranging from 0 (CP) to 5 (equal) to 10 (MCP). Leaders reported that it was very feasible to implement the MCP parent group, with a mean rating of 9.5 out of 10 ($SD = 0.58$). They also reported that they were readily able to cover the standard CP topics in the parent MCP group, with a mean of 10.0 ($SD = 0$).

Parents who participated in MCP parent meetings were very receptive to the program. The following quotes represent common feedback from parents about the MCP parent program: "parents and children should participate to learn how to handle situations by thinking before they react and pay attention to how they cope with different situations;" "I really enjoyed each session because every session was growth and knowledge about solving problems effectively, communicating more calmly, and becoming aware of how to deal with certain situations." Recommended improvements focused on maintaining the supportive community, e.g., "we should have a dinner or picnic," and "we should stay in touch and keep supporting each other" as well as practical scheduling matters.

4. Discussion

This comparative effectiveness study examined whether MCP leads to greater improvements in child reactive aggression and its active mechanisms than CP, with the primary goal of estimating effect sizes in advance of a large-scale efficacy trial. CP is an evidence-based preventive intervention for children with disruptive behavior problems. Thus, the effect-size estimates observed provide valuable information regarding potential enhancing effects of MCP for children with disruptive behavior problems. Findings varied by informant group, as discussed below.

4.1. Child Self-Report Findings

MCP yielded stronger effects than CP on children's self-reported total dysregulation on the ADI, as well as on each of the ADI's subscales (emotional, behavioral and cognitive dysregulation). This is noteworthy for several reasons. First, it provides support for the hypothesis that integrating mindfulness into CP would strengthen program effects on the active mechanisms of reactive aggression, including anger arousal and emotion regulation, impulsivity and behavior regulation, and anger rumination and cognitive regulation. This is also important because past studies have shown that children's scores on the ADI during preadolescence account for a significant proportion of the variance in substance use at later ages [71]. Given the important role of anger arousal in reactive aggression, scores on the ADI anger scale were examined separately. Despite limited statistical power in this feasibility trial, MCP produced significantly greater improvements in children's anger modulation on the ADI than CP. Improved anger modulation is also expected to contribute to longer-term beneficial effects across the developmental cascade.

Other child self-report outcomes provided further support for the study hypotheses. Small to moderate effect sizes favoring MCP were also observed on children's self-reported inhibitory control and breath awareness. EATQ inhibitory control was included as a separate measure of behavioral self-regulation, which is often deficient in children who exhibit high levels of reactive aggression. Thus, MCP was found to strengthen CP's effects across two different child-report measures of inhibitory control, the ADI and EATQ.

Breath awareness was included as a measure of children's present moment and embodied mindful awareness. In MCP, there was especially good uptake of a specific breath awareness practice called "Press the Pause and Take Two Breaths" (PTP and Take 2). Once this brief breath awareness practice was introduced, children in MCP were readily able to recall and practice it on their own. They shared real life situations in which they noticed a need for a calming, centering activity and opted on their own to practice PTP and Take 2. Breath-centered meditation practices have many health benefits, which Melnychuk and colleagues [72] attribute to the coupling of respiration and attention. Specifically, focusing on and regulating breathing can optimize attention, and likewise, focusing one's attention leads breathing to become more synchronized.

4.2. Parent-Report Findings

Parent-report outcomes yielded mixed results. Small to moderate effect sizes favoring MCP were observed on two parent reported outcomes. The first was child attention, as measured on the EATQ. This finding supports the hypothesis that adding mindfulness to CP would enhance program effects on the active mechanisms of reactive aggression, including children's attentional capacity. As described above, reactive aggression is more strongly associated with attentional difficulties than proactive aggression, including the diagnosis of ADHD [24]. The current findings indicate that incorporating mindfulness into CP has a small to moderate enhancing effect on attentional capacity in children with reactive aggression (based on parent observations). Better present moment awareness and attentional control may help children encode social cues more accurately and relate better with others.

A small to moderate effect size favoring MCP was also observed for children's social skills, as measured by parent-report on the BASC. Children with reactive aggression often have both attentional and social difficulties, which are interrelated. Children with reactive aggression have difficulty accurately encoding social cues and recall fewer details of a social situation [29]. Consequently, reactively aggressive children may miss critical information that informs their responses to others. In addition, their attention is selective and biased, and focuses on negative interactions such as rejection, ridicule, and failure [30] and perceived threats. The current findings indicate that MCP enhances CP's effects on children's social skills (based on parent observation). Future research can explore the extent to which social skill improvements are related to interpersonal skills taught in the program versus improved attention.

One of the mindfulness enhancements in MCP was the practice of extending compassion to self and others. This practice, Feel and Spread the Good Vibes, was repeated at the end of every MCP session (and was not included in CP). The addition of repeated compassion practices may have contributed to MCP's enhanced effects on children's prosocial behavior. Reactive aggression is linked to substance use through a complex mediational chain, in which reactive aggression leads to peer rejection, peer rejection leads to peer delinquency, and peer delinquency leads to substance use [7]. Improving children's social skills may disrupt this trajectory by reducing peer rejection and delinquency. Thus, it is important to maximize program effects on children's social skills and peer acceptance. Long-term follow-up is needed to assess the impact of MCP across this developmental cascade.

An unexpected finding was a small to moderate effect size favoring CP for parent-reported child externalizing problems on the BASC. Although the opposite effect was hypothesized, there are some possible explanations for this finding. In an effort to balance the amount of home practice in MCP and CP, daily home behavior goals were added to CP (the original CP program only includes school behavior goals). Children in CP set a personal home behavior goal every week (e.g., complete my chores with a positive attitude, get along better with my sister, follow directions the first time) and earned points for completing these goals. Many children in CP put considerable effort into accomplishing these home behavior goals. This may have been a more "active ingredient" than anticipated, contributing to more observable behavioral improvement at home in CP at post-intervention, relative to the corresponding home mindfulness practices completed by children in MCP.

The MCP and CP conditions may have also differed (unintentionally) in the amount of time spent on discussion and practice of cognitive-behavioral skills. MCP was designed to include all of the same cognitive-behavioral topics as CP, plus additional opening and closing mindfulness practices. Child session content was planned for 50–60 min; however, many schools asked for the child groups to be held over lunch, which allowed for sessions lasting closer to 35–45 min (for both CP and MCP). In MCP, it was important for the mindfulness practices at the beginning and end of each session to be led in an unhurried way. This left less time in the middle of some MCP sessions for discussion and practice of new cognitive-behavioral skills. Leaders reported that they were able to cover all of the core intervention content in MCP, but had more limited opportunities to discuss and practice new cognitive-behavioral skills than in CP. It is possible that this diminished MCP effects on observable child behavioral outcomes. This can be addressed in the future by holding sessions that last the full 50–60 min (as planned), or by modifying the content to be offered in a larger number of sessions that meet for 35–45 min each, which may work better in school settings.

4.3. Teacher-Report Findings

Teacher-report data yielded no effect sizes in the small ($d = 0.20$) or larger range that differentiated the outcomes observed in MCP and CP. This included teacher-rated reactive aggression, which was a primary outcome variable of interest (and the measure upon which children were screened for the intervention). This also included teacher-rated child externalizing problems and social skills on the BASC. Thus, the hypothesis that MCP would enhance the effects of CP on reactive aggression and other teacher-reported child behavioral outcomes was not supported. Teachers are valuable informants given their experience interacting with a wide range of children and the frequent opportunities they have to observe children's behavior and social interactions throughout the school day.

Of note, children's teacher-reported BASC externalizing problems worsened from pre- to post-intervention in both MCP and CP. This may relate to the timing of the pre- and post-intervention assessments, which were collected near the beginning and end of the school year, in contrast to the typical format of prior Coping Power studies where the pre-intervention assessment has been collected one spring and post-intervention the following spring. Teachers may have less information about children's problems in a fall assessment. A prior CP adaptation study with the same fall-to-spring assessment schedule also found that children in both the intervention and control groups had increases in teacher-rated behavior problems from fall-to-spring. However, the children in CP had significantly less increase in conduct problems than control children [73]. This pattern can be better examined in study designs with a no-treatment comparison condition, which the current study did not include. Designs with no-treatment control conditions also help measure whether preventive interventions attenuate increases in behavioral and academic problems across the transition to adolescence in at-risk youths, even if they do not lead to overall net improvements. Although prior research found that CP yielded teacher-rated behavioral improvement for children in comparison to an untreated randomized control group, CP did not influence more trait-like dysregulation scores on the ADI [5]. Thus, MCP has the potential advantage of producing broader generalized changes in children's ability to self-regulate their behavior and affect relative to CP and no treatment. These are important opportunities for future research.

4.4. Implementation Findings

This study addresses the need for school-based mindfulness studies with rigorous attention to intervention integrity and to assessing the feasibility of mindfulness interventions in school settings [53]. A rigorous approach was taken in this study to maintain intervention integrity and to assess comparative feasibility from multiple stakeholders' perspectives. The study provides strong support for the feasibility and uptake of the MCP child and parent programs overall. As described above, modifications can be made to the reduce the amount of content in each MCP child session, to better match the school schedule and improve program feasibility.

4.5. Limitations and Future Research

The current study's comparative effectiveness design was rigorous in that it compared two active interventions in a randomized design. CP is a well-established preventive intervention that has exhibited positive effects in 13 randomized trials, including long-term follow-up. Thus, improving upon CP's effects in targeted areas is noteworthy. Given the feasibility nature of this study, statistical power was only sufficient to detect effects in the medium to large range. Overall, the current study met its aim of generating effect size estimates to inform a future large-scale efficacy study comparing MCP and CP.

Participants in the current sample were predominantly Black and low-to-middle income, reflecting the region in which the study was conducted. This is both a strength, in that this study adds to our understanding of the effects of mindfulness-based interventions in racially and economically disadvantaged samples, and a limitation, because future studies are needed to understand the generalizability of this study's findings in more diverse samples. A specific concern in this study is that there may have been bias in the teacher behavior ratings used to identify at-risk students, particularly at one school in which Black/African American students were overrepresented relative to the overall school population. Screening procedures should account for possible teacher bias, such as by including a second parent-gate screening.

Future studies would also benefit from collecting long-term follow-up data to examine whether program benefits are sustained beyond post-intervention and impact later outcomes in the developmental cascade, including peer delinquency and substance use. Despite the benefits of MCP on several child-reported outcomes, neither parent- nor teacher-report outcomes yielded the hypothesized enhancing effects of MCP on child aggression or externalizing behavior. One explanation for this pattern of results is that it may take time for the improvements in MCP children's internal experiences of emotional, behavioral, and cognitive self-regulation to manifest into improvements in aggression and externalizing behavior that are clearly discernable to parents and teachers. In the future, it would be beneficial to conduct longer-term follow-up assessments to assess for this. It would also be valuable to include direct child behavioral assessments to complement child self-report data.

Since parents were also direct participants in MCP and CP, it will be important to examine program effects on parent-specific outcomes. Innovative study designs could also unpack the relative contributions of various skill-training components included in the comprehensive MCP and CP interventions for children and parents (i.e., attention training, compassion training, goal setting, emotional awareness, thought awareness, problem-solving, assertive communication, mindful parenting, and mindful communication). A precision medicine approach could be applied to identify specific subgroups who would benefit most from specific skill-training components.

Other important questions in the mindfulness literature are how much practice (frequency, quantity) is needed to yield meaningful benefits, and whether secularized forms of mindfulness practice (such as those that can be taught within public-school settings) have as much benefit as traditions in which these practices are couched within a broader lifestyle and ethic. The overarching principles taught in CP are that everyone experiences difficult emotions and difficult situations, and it is important to be aware of these experiences and to practice ways of coping with them that are compassionate toward oneself and others. While this was consistent across both MCP and CP, the MCP program offered more first-person, in-depth learning opportunities. Future studies can examine whether dosage of practice (both in and out of sessions) and leader embodiment of mindfulness impact short- and long-term program effects.

5. Conclusions

This study provides a valuable contribution to the literature by estimating the comparative effects of MCP, a mindfulness-enhanced adaptation of the Coping Power preventive intervention, to standard CP in a rigorous randomized trial. MCP had the strongest comparative effects on child-reported self-regulation and anger modulation, varied effects on parent-reported outcomes, and minimal effects on teacher-reported outcomes (including child reactive aggression).

Author Contributions: Contributions to the project and manuscript are summarized as follows: Conceptualization C.L.B., S.M. and J.E.L.; methodology, C.L.B., S.M., J.E.L., L.Q. and S.T.; software, L.Q., S.T., C.L.B. and D.E.R.; validation, L.Q., S.T. and C.L.B.; formal analysis, L.Q., S.T., C.L.B. and D.E.R.; investigation, C.L.B., S.M., D.E.R. and J.E.L.; resources, C.L.B., D.E.R., S.J., N.P.P. and J.E.L.; data curation, D.E.R., C.L.B., S.J. and L.Q.; writing—original draft preparation, C.L.B., S.M., D.E.R. and S.T.; writing—review and editing, C.L.B., S.M., J.E.L., D.E.R., S.T., L.Q., N.P.P. and S.J.; visualization, C.L.B. and S.T.; supervision, C.L.B., S.M. and D.E.R.; project administration, C.L.B., S.M. and D.E.R.; funding acquisition, C.L.B., S.M., J.E.L. and N.P.P. All authors have read and agreed to the published version of the manuscript.

Funding: This research was funded by the National Institute on Drug Abuse, National Institutes of Health, through grant number R34 DA035946.

Institutional Review Board Statement: The study was conducted according to the guidelines of the Declaration of Helsinki and approved by the Institutional Review Board of The University of Alabama (protocol number 19-05-2365, approved 11/14/14 with continuing review thereafter).

Informed Consent Statement: Informed consent was obtained from all subjects involved in the study.

Data Availability Statement: The data presented in this study are available upon request from the corresponding author. The data will be made publicly available after all planned grant analyses have been published.

Conflicts of Interest: John E. Lochman is the co-developer of the Coping Power program and receives royalties from Oxford University Press for the Coping Power child component implementation guidebook and workbook. The funders had no role in the design of the study; in the collection, analyses, or interpretation of data; in the writing of the manuscript, or in the decision to publish the results.

References

1. Powell, N.P.; Lochman, J.E.; Boxmeyer, C.L.; Barry, T.D.; Pardini, D.A. The Coping Power Program for aggressive behavior in children. In *Evidence-Based Psychotherapies for Children and Adolescents*, 3rd ed.; Weisz, J.R., Kazdin, A.E., Eds.; Guilford Press: New York, NY, USA, 2017; pp. 159–176. Available online: https://psycnet.apa.org/record/2017-25888-010 (accessed on 1 June 2021).
2. Lochman, J.E.; Wells, K.C. Contextual social-cognitive mediators and child outcome: A test of the theoretical model in the Coping Power Program. *Dev. Psychopathol.* **2002**, *14*, 971–993. [CrossRef]
3. Zonnevylle-Bender, M.J.; Matthys, W.; van de Wiel, N.M.; Lochman, J.E. Preventive effects of treatment of disruptive behavior disorder in middle childhood on substance use and delinquent behavior. *J. Am. Acad. Child Adolesc. Psychiatry* **2007**, *46*, 33–39. [CrossRef] [PubMed]
4. Lochman, J.E.; Baden, R.E.; Boxmeyer, C.L.; Powell, N.P.; Qu, L.; Salekin, K.L.; Windle, M. Does a booster intervention augment the preventive effects of an abbreviated version of the Coping Power Program for aggressive children? *J. Abnorm. Child Psychol.* **2014**, *42*, 367–381. [CrossRef]
5. Lochman, J.E.; Wells, K.C. The Coping Power Program at the middle school transition: Universal and indicated prevention effects. *Psychol. Addict. Behav.* **2002**, *16*, S40–S54. [CrossRef]
6. Mushtaq, A.; Lochman, J.E.; Tariq, P.N.; Sabih, F. Preliminary effectiveness study of Coping Power program for aggressive children in Pakistan. *Prev. Sci.* **2017**, *18*, 762–771. [CrossRef]
7. Fite, P.J.; Colder, C.R.; Lochman, J.E.; Wells, K.C. Pathways from proactive and reactive aggression to substance use. *Psychol. Addict. Behav.* **2007**, *21*, 355–364. [CrossRef]
8. Dodge, K.A.; Coie, J.D. Social-information-processing factors in reactive and proactive aggression in children's peer groups. *J. Personal. Soc. Psychol.* **1987**, *53*, 1146–1158. [CrossRef]
9. Fite, P.J.; Colder, C.; Pelham, W. A factor analytic approach to distinguish pure and co-occurring dimensions of proactive and reactive aggression. *J. Clin. Child Adolesc. Psychol.* **2006**, *35*, 578–582. [CrossRef]
10. Bezdjian, S.; Raine, A.; Baker, L.A.; Lyman, D.R. Psychopathic personality in children: Genetic and environmental contributions. *Psychol. Med.* **2011**, *41*, 589–600. [CrossRef] [PubMed]
11. Hubbard, J.A.; Smithmyer, C.M.; Ramsden, S.R.; Parker, E.H.; Flanagan, K.D.; Dearing, K.F.; Simons, R.F. Observational, physiological, and self–report measures of children's anger: Relations to reactive versus proactive aggression. *Child Dev.* **2002**, *73*, 1101–1118. [PubMed]
12. Bierman, K.L.; Coie, J.; Dodge, K.; Greenberg, M.; Lochman, J.; McMahon, R.; Pinderhughes, E.; CPPRG. School outcomes of aggressive-disruptive children: Prediction from kindergarten risk factors and impact of the fast track prevention program. *Aggress. Behav.* **2013**, *39*, 114–130. [CrossRef]
13. Ellis, M.L.; Weiss, B.; Lochman, J.E. Executive functions in children: Associations with aggressive behavior and appraisal processing. *J. Abnorm. Child Psychol.* **2009**, *37*, 945–956. [CrossRef]
14. Fite, P.J.; Raine, A.; Stouthamer-Loeber, M.; Loeber, R.; Pardini, D.A. Reactive and proactive aggression in adolescent males: Examining differential outcomes 10 years later in early adulthood. *Crim. Justice Behav.* **2009**, *37*, 141–157. [CrossRef]
15. Acton, G.S. Measurement of impulsivity in a hierarchical model of personality traits: Implications for substance use. *Subst. Use Misuse* **2003**, *38*, 67–83. [CrossRef]
16. Moeller, F.G.; Dougherty, D.M. Impulsivity and substance abuse: What is the connection? *Addict. Disord. Treat.* **2002**, *1*, 3–10. [CrossRef]
17. Pardini, D.; Lochman, J.; Wells, K. Negative emotions and alcohol use initiation in high-risk boys: The moderating effect of good inhibitory control. *J. Abnorm. Child Psychol.* **2004**, *32*, 505–518. [CrossRef] [PubMed]
18. Marsee, M.A.; Frick, P.J. Exploring the cognitive and emotional correlates to proactive and reactive aggression in a sample of detained girls. *J. Abnorm. Child Psychol.* **2007**, *35*, 969–981. [CrossRef] [PubMed]
19. Barry, T.D.; Thompson, A.; Barry, C.T.; Lochman, J.E.; Adler, K.; Hill, K. The importance of narcissism is predicting proactive and reactive aggression in moderately to highly aggressive children. *Aggress. Behav.* **2007**, *33*, 185–197. [CrossRef]
20. Eisenberg, N.; Fabes, R.A.; Nyman, M.; Bernzweig, J.; Pinuelas, A. The relations of emotionality and regulation to children's anger-related reactions. *Child Dev.* **1994**, *65*, 109–128. [CrossRef] [PubMed]
21. Cummings, E.M.; Iannotti, R.J.; Zahn-Waxler, C. Influence of conflict between adults on the emotions and aggression of young children. *Dev. Psychol.* **1985**, *21*, 495–507. [CrossRef]
22. Vitaro, F.; Brendgen, M.; Tremblay, R.E. Reactively and proactively aggressive children: Antecedent and subsequent characteristics. *J. Child Psychol. Psychiatry* **2002**, *43*, 495–506. [CrossRef]
23. Dodge, K.A. The structure and function of reactive and proactive aggression. In *The Development and Treatment of Childhood Aggression*; Pepler, D.J., Rubin, K.H., Eds.; Lawrence Erlbaum Associates, Inc.: Hillsdale, NJ, USA, 1991; pp. 201–218.
24. Murray, A.L.; Obsuth, I.; Zirk-Sadowsklli, J.; Ribeaud, D.; Eisner, M. Developmental relations between ADHD symptoms and reactive versus proactive aggression across childhood and adolescence. *J. Atten. Disord.* **2016**, *10*, 1701–1710. [CrossRef] [PubMed]
25. De Castro, B.O.; Merk, W.; Koops, W.; Veerman, J.W.; Bosch, J.D. Emotions in social information processing and their relations with reactive and proactive aggression in referred aggressive boys. *J. Clin. Child Adolesc. Psychol.* **2005**, *34*, 105–116. [CrossRef]
26. White, B.A.; Turner, K.A. Anger rumination and effortful control: Mediation effects on reactive but not proactive aggression. *Personal. Individ. Differ.* **2014**, *56*, 186–189. [CrossRef]
27. Denson, T.F.; De Wall, C.N.; Finkel, E.J. Self-control and aggression. *Curr. Dir. Psychol. Sci.* **2012**, *21*, 20–25. [CrossRef]

28. Rohlf, H.L.; Holl, A.K.; Kirsch, F.; Krahé, B.; Elsner, B. Longitudinal links between executive function, anger, and aggression in middle childhood. *Front. Behav. Neurosci.* **2018**, *12*, 27. [CrossRef] [PubMed]
29. Dodge, K.A.; Lochman, J.E.; Harnish, J.D.; Bates, J.E.; Pettit, G.S. Reactive and proactive aggression in school children and psychiatrically impaired chronically assaultive youth. *J. Abnorm. Psychol.* **1997**, *106*, 37–51. [CrossRef]
30. Schippel, P.L.; Vasey, M.W.; Cravens-Brown, L.M.; Bretveld, R.A. Suppressed attention to rejecction, ridicule, and failure cues: A unique correlate of reactive but not proactive aggression in youth. *J. Clin. Child Adolesc. Psychol.* **2003**, *32*, 40–55. [CrossRef]
31. Kabat-Zinn, J. Mindfulness-based interventions in context: Past, present, and future. *Clin. Psychol. Sci. Pract.* **2003**, *10*, 144–156. [CrossRef]
32. Jha, A.P.; Stanley, E.A.; Kiyonaga, A.; Wong, L.; Gelfand, L. Examining the protective effects of mindfulness training on working memory capacity and affective experience. *Emotion* **2010**, *10*, 54–64. [CrossRef]
33. Tang, Y.; Ma, Y.; Wang, J.; Fan, Y.; Feng, S.; Lu, Q.; Posner, M.I. Short-term meditation training improves attention and self-regulation. *Proc. Natl. Acad. Sci. USA* **2007**, *104*, 17152–17156. [CrossRef]
34. Metz, S.M.; Frank, J.L.; Reibel, D.; Cantrell, T.; Sanders, R.; Broderick, P.C. The effectiveness of the Learning to BREATHE Program on adolescent emotion regulation. *Res. Hum. Dev.* **2013**, *10*, 252–272. [CrossRef]
35. Holzel, B.K.; Carmody, J.; Vangel, M.; Congleton, C.; Yerramsetti, S.M.; Lazar, S.W. Mindfulness practice leads to increases in regional brain gray matter density. *Psychiatry Res.* **2011**, *191*, 36–43. [CrossRef] [PubMed]
36. Tang, Y.Y.; Tang, R.; Posner, M. Mindfulness meditation improves emotion regulation and reduces drug abuse. *Drug Alcohol Depend.* **2016**, *163*, 13–18. [CrossRef]
37. Mendelson, T.; Greenberg, M.T.; Dariotis, J.K.; Gould, L.F.; Rhoades, B.L.; Leaf, P.J. Feasibility and preliminary outcomes of a school-based mindfulness intervention for urban youth. *J. Abnorm. Child Psychol.* **2010**, *38*, 985–994. [CrossRef]
38. Franco, C.; Amutio, A.; López-González, L.; Oriol, X.; Martínez-Taboada, C. Effect of a mindfulness training program on the impulsivity and aggression levels of adolescents with behavioral problems in the classroom. *Front. Psychol.* **2016**, *7*, 1385. [CrossRef] [PubMed]
39. Schonert-Reichl, K.A.; Oberle, E.; Lawlor, M.S.; Abbott, D.; Thomson, K.; Oberlander, T.F.; Diamond, A. Enhancing cognitive and social-emotional development through simple-to-administer mindfulness-based school program for elementary school children: A randomized controlled trial. *Dev. Psychol.* **2015**, *51*, 52–66. [CrossRef]
40. Singh, N.N.; Singh, A.N.; Lancioni, G.E.; Singh, J.; Winton, A.S.W.; Adkins, A.D. Mindfulness training for parents and their children with ADHD increases the children's compliance. *J. Child Fam. Stud.* **2010**, *19*, 157–166. [CrossRef]
41. van der Oord, S.; Bögels, S.M.; Peijnenburg, D. The effectiveness of mindfulness training for children with ADHD and mindful parenting for their parents. *J. Child Fam. Stud.* **2012**, *21*, 139–147. [CrossRef] [PubMed]
42. Muratori, P.; Conversano, C.; Levantini, V.; Masi, G.; Milone, A.; Villani, S.; Bögels, S.; Gemignani, A. Exploring the Efficacy of a Mindfulness Program for Boys with Attention-Deficit Hyperactivity Disorder and Oppositional Defiant Disorder. *J. Atten. Disord.* **2020**, *25*, 1544–1553. [CrossRef]
43. Bögels, S.; Hoogstad, B.; van Dun, L.; de Schutter, S.; Restifo, K. Mindfulness training for adolescents with externalizing disorders and their parents. *Behav. Cogn. Psychother.* **2008**, *36*, 193–209. [CrossRef]
44. Sibinga, E.; Perry-Parrish, C.; Chung, S.E.; Johnson, S.B.; Smith, M.; Ellen, J.M. School-based mindfulness instruction for urban male youth: A small randomized controlled trial. *Prev. Med.* **2013**, *57*, 799–801. [CrossRef]
45. Keune, P.M.; Bostanov, V.; Kotchoubey, B.; Hautzinger, M. Mindfulness versus rumination and behavioral inhibition: A perspective from research on frontal brain asymmetry. *Personal. Individ. Differ.* **2012**, *53*, 323–328. [CrossRef]
46. Evans, D.R.; Segerstrom, S.C. Why do mindful people worry less? *Cogn. Ther. Res.* **2010**, *35*, 505–510. [CrossRef]
47. Moore, A.; Malinowski, P. Meditation, mindfulness and cognitive flexibility. *Conscious. Cogn.* **2009**, *18*, 175–186. [CrossRef] [PubMed]
48. Jha, A.; Krompinger, J.; Baine, M.J. Mindfulness training modifies subsystems of attention. *Cogn. Affect. Behav. Neurosci.* **2007**, *7*, 109–119. [CrossRef] [PubMed]
49. MacLean, K.A.; Ferrer, E.; Aichele, S.R.; Bridwell, D.A.; Zanesco, A.P.; Jacobs, T.L.; Saron, C.D. Intensive meditation training improves perceptual discrimination and sustained attention. *Psychol. Sci.* **2010**, *21*, 829–839. [CrossRef]
50. Moore, A.; Gruber, T.; Derose, J.; Malinowski, P. Regular, brief mindfulness meditation practice improves electrophysiological markers of attentional control. *Front. Hum. Neurosci.* **2012**, *6*, 18. [CrossRef]
51. Creswell, J.D.; Taren, A.A.; Lindsay, E.K.; Greco, C.M.; Gianaros, P.J.; Fairgrieve, A.; Marsland, A.L.; Brown, K.W.; Way, B.M.; Rosen, R.K.; et al. Alterations in resting-state functional connectivity link mindfulness meditation with reduced Interleukin-6: A randomized controlled trial. *Biol. Psychiatry* **2016**, *80*, 53–61. [CrossRef]
52. Crane, R.S.; Kuyken, W.; Williams, J.M.G.; Hastings, R.P.; Cooper, L.; Fennell, M.J. Competence in teaching mindfulness-based courses: Concepts, development and assessment. *Mindfulness* **2012**, *3*, 76–84. [CrossRef]
53. Emerson, L.; de Diaz, N.N.; Sherwood, A.; Waters, A.; Farrell, L. Mindfulness interventions in schools: Integrity and feasibility of implementation. *Int. J. Behav. Dev.* **2020**, *44*, 62–75. [CrossRef]
54. Greenberg, M.T.; Harris, A.R. Nurturing mindfulness in children and youth: Current state of research. *Child Dev. Perspect.* **2012**, *6*, 161–166. [CrossRef]
55. McKeering, P.; Hwang, Y.S. A systematic review of mindfulness-based school interventions with early adolescents. *Mindfulness* **2019**, *10*, 593–610. [CrossRef]

56. Zenner, C.; Herrnleben-Kurz, S.; Walach, H. Mindfulness-based interventions in schools—A systematic review and meta-analysis. *Front. Psychol.* **2014**, *5*, 603–623. [CrossRef] [PubMed]
57. Shegog, R.; Markham, C.M.; Peskin, M.F.; Johnson, K.; Cuccaro, P.; Tortolero, S.R. It's Your Game. Keep It Real: Can innovative public health prevention research thrive within a comparative effectiveness research framework? *J. Prim. Prev.* **2013**, *34*, 89–108. [CrossRef] [PubMed]
58. Johnston, L.D.; O'Malley, P.M.; Bachman, J.G.; Schulenberg, J.E. *Monitoring the Future: National Survey Results on Drug Use*; Institute for Social Research: Ann Arbor, MI, USA, 2011; pp. 1975–2010.
59. Reynolds, C.R.; Kamphaus, R.W. *Behavior Assessment System for Children*; American Guidance Service: Circle Pines, MN, USA, 1992.
60. Lochman, J.E.; Wells, K.C. Effectiveness study of Coping Power and classroom intervention with aggressive children: Outcomes at a one-year follow-up. *Behav. Ther.* **2003**, *34*, 493–515. [CrossRef]
61. Lochman, J.E.; Wells, K.C. The coping power program for preadolescent aggressive boys and their parents: Outcome effects at the 1-year follow-up. *J. Consult. Clin. Psychol.* **2004**, *72*, 571–578. [CrossRef]
62. Miller, S.; Boxmeyer, C.; Romero, D.E.; Powell, N.; Jones, S.; Lochman, J.E. Theoretical model of Mindful Coping Power: Optimizing a cognitive behavioral program for high risk children and their parents by integrating mindfulness. *Clin. Child Fam. Psychol. Rev.* **2020**, *23*, 393–406. [CrossRef]
63. Mezzich, A.C.; Tarter, R.E.; Giancola, P.R.; Lu, S.; Kirisci, L.; Parks, S. Substance use and risky sexual behavior in female adolescents. *Drug Alcohol Depend.* **1997**, *44*, 157–166. [CrossRef]
64. Capaldi, D.M.; Rothbart, M.K. Development and validation of an early adolescent temperament measure. *J. Early Adolesc.* **1992**, *12*, 153–173. [CrossRef]
65. Ellis, L.K.; Rothbart, M.K. Revision of the Early Adolescent Temperament Questionnaire. In Proceedings of the 2001 Biennial Meeting of the Society for Research in Child Development, Minneapolis, MI, USA, 2001. Available online: https://research.bowdoin.edu/rothbart-temperament-questionnaires/files/2016/09/lesa-ellis-srcd-poster-reprint.pdf (accessed on 1 June 2018).
66. Price, C.J.; Thompson, E.A.; Cheng, S.C. Scale of Body Connection: A multi-sample construct validation study. *PLoS ONE* **2017**, *12*, e0184757. [CrossRef]
67. Coman, E.N.; Pichu, K.; McArdle, J.J.; Villagra, V.; Dierker, L.; Iordache, E. The paired t-test as a simple latent change score model. *Front. Psychol.* **2013**, *4*, 738. [CrossRef]
68. Rosseel, Y. lavaan: An R Package for Structural Equation Modeling. *J. Stat. Softw.* **2012**, *48*, 1–36. [CrossRef]
69. R Core Team. *R: A Language and Environment for Statistical Computing*; R Foundation for Statistical Computing: Vienna, Austria, 2017; Available online: https://www.R-project.org/ (accessed on 15 June 2018).
70. Enders, C.K. *Applied Missing Data Analysis*; Guilford Press: New York, NY, USA, 2010.
71. Mezzich, A.C.; Tarter, R.E.; Giancola, P.R.; Kirisci, L. The Dysregulation Inventory: A new scale to assess the risk for substance use disorder. *J. Child Adolesc. Subst. Abus.* **2001**, *10*, 35–43. [CrossRef]
72. Melnychuk, M.C.; Dockree, P.M.; O'Connell, R.G.; Murphy, P.R.; Balsters, J.H.; Robertson, I.H. Coupling of respiration and attention via the locus coeruleus: Effects of meditation and pranayama. *Psychophysiology* **2018**, *55*, e13091. [CrossRef] [PubMed]
73. Lochman, J.E.; Boxmeyer, C.L.; Jones, S.; Qu, L.; Ewoldsen, D.; Nelson, W.M., III. Testing the feasibility of a briefer school-based preventive intervention with aggressive children: A hybrid intervention with face-to-face and internet components. *J. Sch. Psychol.* **2017**, *62*, 33–50. [CrossRef] [PubMed]

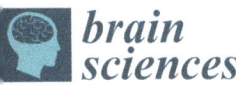

Article

A Comparison between Severe Suicidality and Nonsuicidal Self-Injury Behaviors in Bipolar Adolescents Referred to a Psychiatric Emergency Unit

Gabriele Masi *, Ilaria Lupetti, Giulia D'Acunto, Annarita Milone, Deborah Fabiani, Ursula Madonia, Stefano Berloffa, Francesca Lenzi and Maria Mucci

IRCCS Stella Maris, Scientific Institute of Child Neurology and Psychiatry, Calambrone, 56128 Pisa, Italy; ilariaL89@otmail.it (I.L.); gdacunto@fsm.unipi.it (G.D.); annarita.milone@fsm.unipi.it (A.M.); deborah.fabiani@gmail.com (D.F.); madoniau@mail.com (U.M.); stefano.berloffa@fsm.unipi.it (S.B.); francesca.lenzi@fsm.unipi.it (F.L.); maria.mucci@fsm.unipi.it (M.M.)
* Correspondence: gabriele.masi@fsm.unipi.it

Abstract: Background: Severe suicide ideation or attempts and non-suicidal self-injury (NSSI) present both differences and relevant overlaps, including frequent co-occurrence and shared risk factors. Specific categorical diagnoses, namely bipolar disorder (BD), may affect clinical features and natural histories of suicidal or not suicidal self-harm behaviour. Our study aimed to compare suicidality (severe suicidal ideation or suicidal attempts) and NSSI in referred bipolar adolescents. Methods: The sample included 95 bipolar adolescents (32 males, 63 females) aged 11 to 18 years. Thirty adolescents with suicide attempts/suicidal ideation and BD (SASIB) were compared with structured measures to 35 adolescents with NSSI and BD, without suicidal ideation or attempts (NSSIB), and to 30 adolescents with BD, without suicidal ideation or attempts or NSSI (CB). Results: Compared to CB, suicidality and NSSI were both associated with female sex, borderline personality disorder and self-reported internalizing disorders, anxiety/depression and thought disorders. The NSSI were specifically associated with somatic problems. Severe suicidal ideation and suicide attempts were associated with adverse life events, immigration, bullying, eating disorders, social problems, depressive feelings, performance and social anxiety, and feelings of rejection. Conclusions: Both shared and differential features between suicidal and not suicidal adolescents may represent possible targets for diagnostic and preventative interventions.

Keywords: suicidality; non-suicidal self-injuries; bipolar disorder

1. Introduction

Suicide is a global health problem, with at least 800,000 people dying by suicide each year; among 15–29 years old, it is the second leading cause of death [1]. Suicide attempt is defined as a nonfatal, self-directed, potentially injurious behavior with an intent to die, even if it does not result in injury, whereas suicidal ideation is thinking about, considering, or planning suicide. Nonsuicidal self-injury (NSSI) is the deliberate destruction of one's own body without suicidal intent [2]. This category has been included in Section 3 of the Diagnostic and Statistical Manual of Mental Disorders-fifth edition (DSM-5) as a "condition for further study" [3].

The fundamental criterion for distinguishing between non-suicidal self-destructive behaviors and suicide is the intention of death [4]. Other important differences have been identified between suicide attempt and NSSI, including prevalence, frequency, lethality of methods, and attitudes towards life and death [5]. Although these differences led to the classification of NSSI and suicidal behavior as distinct clinical phenomena in the DSM-5 [3], the overlaps between self-harm with and without suicidal intent are relevant, including that many individuals engage in both behaviors [6]. This notion has led to argue that they

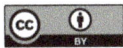

are best conceptualised along a continuum [7], supported by growing evidence suggesting that NSSI is one of the strongest predictors of suicide attempts, above and beyond previous suicidal behavior [8]. The "continuum" model is supported by studies reporting on shared risk factors for both NSSI and suicidal behavior, including depression and borderline personality disorder [9], physical or sexual abuse [10], externalizing behaviors [9], impulsivity [11], and problems in the family [12].

Studies comparing individuals who engaged in both NSSI and suicidal behavior to individuals who engaged in NSSI, but not suicidal behavior have found that individuals who engaged in both NSSI and suicidal behavior presented more severe symptoms of psychopathology and greater psychosocial impairment than individuals who engaged only in NSSI [13,14]. Inpatient adolescents who engaged in NSSI and had attempted suicide reported greater depression, hopelessness and impulsivity [15] and greater family conflict [14] than adolescents who engaged in NSSI alone.

A study comparing youth who engaged in NSSI and suicidal behavior with those who engaged only in suicidal behavior reported that youth suicide attempters with NSSI presented more depressed symptoms, hopelessness, internalized anger, risky behaviors, loneliness than youth suicide attempters without NSSI [16]. On the contrary, other studies have found that individuals who engaged in NSSI and suicidal behavior did not report significantly greater symptoms of psychopathology than individuals who engaged in suicidal behavior but not NSSI [17,18].

Finally, few studies included comparisons between individuals who engaged in NSSI only and individuals who had made at least one suicidal attempt with unknown NSSI histories. According to these studies, individuals who had made a suicidal attempt reported more depression [19], stressful life events and more help-seeking previous the suicide attempt than individuals engaged in NSSI only [20].

Most of these studies included patients with NSSI and/or suicide attempt, irrespective of the categorical psychiatric diagnosis. It may be argued that specific psychiatric diagnoses (i.e., unipolar depression versus bipolar disorders) may strongly affect the clinical features and the natural histories of suicidal or not suicidal self-injurious behaviors. Among psychiatric disorders, bipolar disorder (BD) is characterized by the highest suicide risk [21]. Pediatric BD disrupts a child's developmental and emotional growth, causing school failure, high-risk behaviors, substance abuse, disturbed interpersonal relationships, and hospitalizations [22]. According to the World Health Organization, BD is the fourth most burdensome illness affecting individuals between 10–24 years of age [23].

The aim of our study was to assess similarities and differences between severe suicidal ideation or suicide attempt and NSSI in a sample of bipolar adolescents, hypothesizing that different clinical and psychological features may distinguish suicidal patients from patients with NSSI.

2. Materials and Methods

Sample

This was a retrospective study based on a clinical database of 95 adolescents (32 males, 63 females) aged between 11 and 18 years (mean age 14.8 ± 1.8 years), referred as inpatients to the Psychiatric Emergency Unit of our hospital between January 2018 and January 2020. Inclusion criteria were the presence of a diagnosis of BD and an IQ above 70, based on the Wechsler Intelligence Scale for Children-Fourth Edition (WISC-IV) [24]. The diagnosis of BD was based on DSM-5 criteria and a diagnostic interview, the Kiddie Schedule for Affective Disorders and Schizophrenia for School-Aged Children-Present and Lifetime Version (K-SADS-PL) [25], administered to the patient and at least one parent.

The sample was divided into three groups:
- Suicidal attempt or suicidal ideation bipolar (SASIB) group: 30 individuals (22 females, eight males, mean age 14.8 ± 1.9 years) with severe suicidal ideation (score 3 or above according to the Columbia-Suicide Severity Rating Scale (CSSRS) [26] without prior

suicidal attempts, or at least one previous suicide attempt, regardless of the level of suicidal ideation;
- Nonsuicidal self-injury bipolar (NSSIB) group: 35 individuals (29 females, six males, mean age 15.0 ± 1.6 years) with NSSI, suicidal ideation absent or low (score below 3 at the CSSRS), and without prior suicide attempts. These individuals were required to meet DSM-5 criteria for NSSI disorder, in that they engaged in NSSI on at least 5 days within the past year [3];
- Control bipolar (CB) group: 30 individuals (12 females, 18 males, mean age 14.5 ± 1.9 years) without suicidal ideation and without prior suicide attempts and without NSSI.

3. Measures

Categorical diagnosis was assessed using the K-SADS-PL, a semi-structured interview administered by trained child psychiatrists, to diagnose BD and comorbidities, It provides a reliable and valid measurement of DSM-IV Axis I psychopathology in children and adolescents. The K-SADS-PL is administered to the parent first and then to the child. Both parties may be re-interviewed to resolve informant discrepancies. Test-retest reliability and kappa coefficients are in the good to excellent range across diagnoses [25] Clinical severity was assessed with the Clinical Global Impression Severity (CGI-S) [27] and the functional impairment with the Child Global Assessment Scale (C-GAS) [28].

CGI-S is a 7-point scale that requires the clinician to rate the severity of the patient's illness at the time of assessment; the score ranges from 1 (normal, not at all ill) to 7 (among the most extremely ill patients).

C-GAS provides a global measure of level of functioning; the score ranges from 0 (needs constant supervision) to 100 (superior functioning). The threshold of normality is defined for scores higher than 70.

Information about the presence of familial psychiatric disorders, familial attempted or completed suicides, and familial mood disorders, was retrospectively collected using a specific questionnaire. Adverse Childhood Experiences (ACE), parental separation/divorce, bullying, family mourning and second generation immigration were assessed with an unstructured checklist.

The Columbia–Suicide Severity Rating Scale (C-SSRS) was used for the assessment of the severity of suicidal risk. This scale defines five levels of suicidal ideation:

- Level 1: Wish to be dead;
- Level 2: Non-Specific Active Suicidal Thoughts;
- Level 3: Active Suicidal Ideation with Any Methods (Not Plan) without Intent to Act;
- Level 4: Active Suicidal Ideation with Some Intent to Act, without Specific Plan;
- Level 5: Active Suicidal Ideation with Specific Plan and Intent.

According to the definition of this scale an actual suicidal attempt is a potentially self-injurious act committed with at least some wish to die, as a result of act. Intent does not have to be 100%. If there is any intent/desire to die associated with the act, then it can be considered an actual suicide attempt. There does not have to be any injury or harm, just the potential for injury or harm. Even if an individual denies intent/wish to die, it may be inferred clinically from the behavior or circumstances. Also, if someone denies intent to die, but they thought that what they did could be lethal, intent may be inferred.

Personality disorders were assessed with the Structured Clinical Interview for DSM-IV personality disorders (SCID II) [29], which includes a self-report survey of 119 items and a subsequent semi-structured interview, administered by the clinician. Each item provides a dichotomous yes/no answer (yes if the symptom is present, no if the symptom is not present). The interrater reliability and internal consistency are adequate [30].

For a dimensional assessment of psychopathology, all individuals were assessed with the Child Behavior Checklist (CBCL) [31] a 118-item scale, completed by parents, clustered in two broad-band scores, designated as Internalizing Problems and Externalizing Problems, a Total Problem Score, and with 8 different syndromes scales (Withdrawal, Somatic complaints, Anxiety/depression, Social problems, Thought problems, Attention problems, Rule-breaking behavior, Aggressive behavior). For each item, responses are recorded on a Likert scale: 0 = Not True, 1 = Somewhat or Sometimes True, 2 = Very True or Often True. The total problems scale has excellent test–retest reliability (r = 0.93) and fair internal consistency (a = 0.68), as well as excellent internal consistency, test–retest reliability, and crossinformant agreement for DSM-oriented scales [32]. We assessed also a CBCL Dysregulation Profile (CBCL-DP), based on the sum of t-scores of the three CBCL subscales, Anxiety/depression, Attention problems, and Aggressive behaviour which is an index of Emotional Dysregulation [33]. Moreover, all the patients received the Youth Self Report (YSR) [30], including 112 items, with the same possible responses and the same eight subscales of the CBCL, clustered in Externalizing or Internalizing Problems.

Patients completed a self-report measure of depressive symptomatology, the Children's Depression Inventory (CDI) [34], including 27 items, with the following subscales: Negative Mood, Interpersonal Problems, Ineffectiveness, Anhedonia and Negative Self Esteem. Patients rate themselves based on how they feel and think in the last two weeks, with each statement being identified with a rating from 0 to 2. The CDI was translated into Italian, and normative data for the Italian CDI were collected [35].

Anxiety symptoms were assessed with the Multidimensional Anxiety Scale for Children (MASC) [36] including 39 items, with four subscales: Physical Symptoms, Harm Avoidance, Social Anxiety and Separation/Panic. Patients are asked to rate their own behavior on a 4-point scale: 0-Never true about me, 1-Rarely true about me, 2-Sometimes true about me, 3-Often true about me. Studies using the MASC have reported high retest reliability [37], favorable divergent and convergent validity [38], and good internal reliability within the four subscales [39].

The study conformed to Declaration of Helsinki; the Ethics Committee of the Hospital approved the study (Identification Code 2014/0001507).

4. Statistical Analyses

Descriptive analyses were used to describe demographic and clinical characteristics of the whole sample. Chi-square analyses were performed on categorical variables, and two-ways ANOVA controlling for gender on continuous variables, taking into account that there were notable gender differences between the clinical groups and the control group.

Regarding the comparisons between three groups, a post hoc Bonferroni correction was applied for the quantitative variables, while for dichotomous variables we used z test. p values were based on two-tailed tests with $\alpha = 0.05$.

As samples size is limited, the analysis is prone to Type II Error, so Partial Eta Squared had to be calculated (and highlighted only for significant values).

To elaborate on the research question, a regression model is used to identify whether the predictors of suicidality might differ in each group: to analyze associations between suicidality, depression symptoms and biosocial values, univariate (simple) logistic regression were performed (overall percentage >70) and then a multivariate multiple logistic regression was performed in order to evidence risk factors for suicide (overall percentage >70).

5. Results

The three groups, SASIB, NSSIB and CB, did not differ according to mean age (14.8 ± 1.9 years, 15.0 ± 1.6 years, and 14.5 ± 1.9 years, respectively, F = 0.633, df = 2, $p = 0.533$). As regards gender ratio, there was a prevalence of females in the SASIB (F/M 22/8) and NSSIB (F/M 29/6) groups, while there was a slight prevalence of males in the CB (F/M 12/18) ($\chi^2 = 14.25$, df = 2, $p = 0.001$). Based on the WISC-IV scores, the three groups did not differ according to the full scale IQ, the Verbal Comprehension Index, the Perceptual Reasoning Index, the Working Memory Index and the Processing Speed Index.

About the frequency of the BD types, there was a clear prevalence of BD II than BD I in the three groups (SASIB BD I/BD II 7/23, NSSIB BD I/BD II 4/31, CB BD I/BD II 6/24), and differences among groups were not statistically significant ($\chi^2 = 1.69$, df = 2, $p = 0.429$).

Regarding psychiatric comorbidities, according to the K-SADS-PL and the SCID II, borderline personality disorder was significantly more frequent in the SASIB (21 [70%]) and NSSIB (23 [65.7%]) groups, compared to the CB (7 [23.3%]) (χ^2 = 16.36, df = 2, p = 0.000). Attention deficit hyperactivity disorder (ADHD) was significantly more frequent in the CB group (17 [56.7%]) than in the SASIB (2 [6.7%]) and NSSIB (5 [14.3%]) (χ^2 = 23.4, df = 2, p = 0.000). Eating disorders (seven [23.3%] in the SASIB group, four [11.4%] in the NSSIB and 0 [0%] in the CB) were significantly prevalent in the SASIB group than in the CB. According to the type of eating disorders, in the SASIB group there were three subjects with anorexia nervosa restrictive type, three subjects with anorexia nervosa binge/purging type and one subject with binge eating disorder; in the NSSIB group there were one subject with bulimia nervosa, one subject with anorexia nervosa restrictive type and two subjects with binge eating disorder. All the other categorical diagnoses, including Learning disabilities (χ^2 = 3.35, df = 2, p = 0.188), autism spectrum disorder (χ^2 = 3.41, df = 2, p = 0.182), conduct disorder (χ^2 = 4.09, df = 2, p = 0.130), oppositional defiant disorder (χ^2 = 2.5, df = 2, p = 0.287), anxiety disorders (χ^2 = 1.5, df = 2, p = 0.472), psychotic symptoms (χ^2 = 2.35, df = 2, p = 0.309), obsessive compulsive disorder (χ^2 = 4.02, df = 2, p = 0.134), substance use disorder (χ^2 = 0.38, df = 2, p = 0.829) and sleep disorders (χ^2 = 2.4, df = 2, p = 0.301) did not differ between groups.

When clinical severity (CGI-S) and functional impairment (C-GAS) were considered, patients in the SASIB group presented greater clinical severity (CGI-S score 6.2 ± 0.5) than patients in the NSSIB (CGI-S score 4.9 ± 0.5) and CB (CGI-S score 5.2 ± 0.6) (F = 46.49, df = 2, p < 0.001). Patients in the SASIB group also showed greater functional impairment (C-GAS score 32.8 ± 6.1) than patients in the NSSIB (C-GAS score 44.6 ± 7.8) and CB (C-GAS score 41 ± 8.6) (F = 20.24, df = 2, p < 0.001) with a high significance maintained with Bonferroni correction. By correcting this analysis for gender, the statistic power is maintained (partial eta squared 0.307).

There were no statistically significant differences among groups according to the presence of familial psychiatric disorders, familial attempted or completed suicides, and familial mood disorders. Similarly, groups did not differ according to the history of adverse childhood experiences (ACE), parental separation/divorce and family mourning.

Conversely, the presence of bullying was significantly higher in the SASIB group (21 [70%]) than in the NSSIB (10 [30.3%]) (two unknown) and the CB (eight [27.6%]) (one unknown) (χ^2 = 15.92, df = 4, p = 0.003). The presence of second-generation immigration (10 [33.3%] in the SASIB group, five [14.3%] in the NSSIB and two [6.7%] in the CB) was significantly higher in the SASIB group than in the CB (χ^2 = 15.92, df = 4, p = 0.003). Comparing the three groups according to the total number of adverse childhood experiences, the SASIB group presented a significantly higher total number of adverse childhood experiences (4.1 ± 1.52) than the NSSIB (2.65 ± 1.37) and the CB (1.86 ± 1.27) (F = 19.8, df = 2, p = 0.000). For CBCL the results are listed in Table 1.

Emotional dysregulation (based on comparison in the CBCL Dysregulation Profile) did not differ among groups, and it was over-represented in all three groups, affecting 89.3% of individuals in the SASIB group, 82.9% in the NSSIB and 86.2% in the CB (Partial Eta Squared 0.019). For the YSR results are listed in Table 2.

According to the CDI the results are listed in Table 3.

Table 1. Two-way ANOVA corrected by gender: Comparison between the three groups according to the Child Behavior Checklist (CBCL) (parent reports).

	SASIB (n = 28) (Mean ± SD)	NSSIB (n = 35) (Mean ± SD)	CB (n = 29) (Mean ± SD)	Two Ways Anova (F;df)	p	Partial Eta Squared	Bonferroni-Holm (Multiple Comparisons)
Internalizing problems	71.43 ± 7.188	71.54 ± 6.688	69.45 ± 6.328	(0.917;2)	ns		
Externalizing problems	64.21 ± 8.085	69.46 ± 8.326	70.38 ± 8.205	Group (4.724;2)	0.049 *	0.068	SASIB/NSSIB 0.035 * SASIB/CB 0.014 *
Total problems	68.61 ± 6.332	72.06 ± 6.721	70.59 ± 6.625	(2.142;2)	ns		
Anxious/depressed	75.14 ± 11.437	70.80 ± 10.975	68.76 ± 8.357	(0.817;2)	ns		
Withdrawn/depressed	74.00 ± 11.576	71.06 ± 11.008	6.21 ± 9.522	(1.441;2)	ns		
Somatic complaints	61.68 ± 8.944	67.17 ± 9.919	64.07 ± 8.031	(2.910;2)	ns		
Social problems	64.39 ± 6.849	65.46 ± 8.326	64.07 ± 7.473	(0.294;2)	ns		
Thought problems	70.79 ± 6.839	69.71 ± 7.775	66.66 ± 9.401	(2.044;2)	ns		
Attention problems	63.61 ± 9.589	68.80 ± 12.388	66.93 ± 10.330	(1.762;2)	ns		
Rule-breaking behavior	63.39 ± 7.752	68.20 ± 10.070	68.62 ± 8.621	(3.271;2)	0.043 *	0.071	
Aggressive behavior	65.14 ± 9.411	69.69 ± 11.287	71.90 ± 10.001	(0.944;2)	ns		

Legend: SASIB = Suicidal attempt or suicidal ideation bipolar; NSSIB = Nonsuicidal self-injury bipolar; CB = Controls bipolar; ns = not significant; * = $p < 0.05$.

Table 2. Two-way ANOVA corrected by gender: Comparison between the three groups according to the Youth Self Report (YSR).

	SASIB (n = 30) (Mean ± SD)	NSSIB (n = 33) (Mean ± SD)	CB (n = 26) (Mean ± SD)	Two Ways Anova (F;df)	p	Partial Eta Squared	Bonferroni-Holm (Multiple Comparisons)
Internalizing problems	71.37 ± 7.188	69.33 ± 6.688	60.38 ± 6.328	Group (5.864;2)	0.004 **	0.124	SASIB/CB 0.001 *** NSSIB/CB 0.008 **
Externalizing problems	59.97 ± 8.126	64.18 ± 8.133	65.81 ± 9.896	(3.465;2)	ns		
Total problems	67.33 ± 9.960	68.91 ± 7.966	64.08 ± 8.207	(2.255;2)	ns		
Anxious/depressed	73.47 ± 14.680	70.30 ± 10.953	62.12 ± 10.328	Group (5.296;2) Gender × Group (3.710;2)	0.007 ** 0.029	0.113 0.082	SASIB/CB 0.002 ** NSSIB/CB 0.029 *
WWithdrawn/depressed	72.43 ± 15.593	68.18 ± 10.984	61.88 ± 11.660	(4.683;2)	ns		
Somatic complaints	64.27 ± 11.341	64.55 ± 10.016	57.58 ± 9.390	Group (4.050;2) Gender × Group (3.687;2)	0.015 * 0.029 *	0.096 0.082	SASIB/CB 0.042 ** NSSIB/CB 0.027 *
Social problems	65.47 ± 11.575	63.73 ± 10.260	58.15 ± 8.748	(3.761;2)	ns		
Thought problems	67.33 ± 10.880	67.39 ± 11.233	60.35 ± 7.440	Group (3.312;2)	0.041 *	0.074	SASIB/CB 0.036 * NSSIB/CB 0.029 *
Attention problems	64.30 ± 9.642	68.18 ± 10.135	64.08 ± 9.082	(1.766;2)	ns		
Rule-breaking behavior	59.47 ± 8.212	62.18 ± 8.060	64.58 ± 10.207	Gender × Group (3.884;2)	0.024 *	0.086	
Aggressive behavior	59.87 ± 6.776	64.24 ± 8.832	65.73 ± 9.332	Group (3.263;2)	0.043 *	0.073	SASIB/CB 0.034 *

Legend: SASIB = Suicidal attempt or suicidal ideation bipolar; NSSIB = Nonsuicidal self-injury bipolar; CB = Controls bipolar; ns = not significant; * = $p < 0.05$; ** = $p < 0.005$; *** = $p < 0.001$.

Table 3. Two-way ANOVA corrected by gender: Comparison between the three groups according to the Children's Depression Inventory (CDI).

	SASIB (n = 30) (Mean ± SD)	NSSIB (n = 17) (Mean ± SD)	CB (n = 28) (Mean ± SD)	Two Ways Anova (F;df)	p	Partial Eta Squared	Bonferroni-Holm (Multiple Comparisons)
Total	73.17 ± 18.084	65.71 ± 15.430	55.50 ± 10.479	Gender (11.112;1) Group (5.046;2)	<0.001 *** 0.009 **	0.139 0.128	SASIB/CB 0.000 ***
Negative mood	67.53 ± 16.258	61.53 ± 13.342	51.75 ± 11.610	Gender (3.854;1) Group (5.302;2)	0.054 * 0.007 **	0.053 0.133	SASIB/CB 0.000 ***
Interpersonal problems	65.13 ± 17,290	64.06 ± 9.915	55.79 ± 11.262	Gender (4.610;1)	0.035 *	0.063	SASIB/CB 0.029 *
Ineffectiveness	65.87 ± 13.718	63.12 ± 9.980	55.07 ± 10.760	Gender (7.161;1)	0.009 **	0.094	SASIB/CB 0.002 **
Anhedonia	63.30 ± 13.298	56.35 ± 13.1	52.04 ± 8.905	Gender (5.410;1) Group (3.469;2)	0.023 * 0.037 *	0.073 0.091	SASIB/CB 0.001 ***
Negative self esteem	72.63 ± 18.011	67.35 ± 17.755	57.54 ± 10.868	Gender (12.650;1)	<0.001 ***	0.155	SASIB/CB 0.000 ***

Legend: SASIB = Suicidal attempt or suicidal ideation bipolar; NSSIB = Nonsuicidal self-injury bipolar; CB = Controls bipolar; ns = not significant; * = $p < 0.05$; ** = $p < 0.005$; *** = $p < 0.001$.

Finally, regarding anxiety symptoms according to the MASC the results are listed in Table 4.

Table 4. Two-way ANOVA corrected by gender: Comparison between the three groups according to the Multidimensional Anxiety Scale for Children (MASC).

	SASIB (n = 27) (Mean ± SD)	NSSIB (n = 18) (Mean ± SD)	CB (n = 24) (Mean ± SD)	Two Ways Anova (F;df)	p	Partial Eta Squared	Bonferroni-Holm (Multiple Comparisons)
Total	60.59 ± 13.776	52.39 ± 13.426	49.50 ± 14.179	Gender × Group (3.449;2)	0.038 *	0.099	SASIB/CB 0.013 *
Tense/restless	61.78 ± 12.744	59.28 ± 13.141	55.38 ± 12.427	(1.616;2)	ns		
Somatic/autonomic	57.33 ± 14.085	54.61 ± 12.733	51.79 ± 9.991	Gender × Group (3.708;2)	0.030 *	0.105	
Total physical symptoms	60.89 ± 12.816	57.61 ± 13.465	53.96 ± 10.980	Gender × Group (3.185;2)	0.048 *	0.092	
Perfectionism	42.63 ± 10.525	40.22 ± 12.591	39.29 ± 10.564	(0.612;2)	ns		
Anxious coping	45.56 ± 10.610	36.50 ± 12.075	41.50 ± 9.943	Gender × Group (3.818;2)	ns		
Total harm avoidance	43.48 ± 10.067	36.61 ± 12.103	38.71 ± 9.603	(2.614;2)	ns		
Humiliation/rejection	63.15 ± 13.601	54.00 ± 12.485	52.63 ± 12.576	(4.881;2)	ns		
Performance fears	64.70 ± 13.044	58.56 ± 14.076	51.00 ± 13.062	Group (4.651;2)	0.013 *	0.129	SASIB/CB 0.001 ***
Total social anxiety	65.00 ± 14.563	56.61 ± 12.705	52.25 ± 11.509	Group (3.614;2)	0.033 *	0.103	SASIB/CB 0.002 **
Separation/panic	55.89 ± 14.750	50.78 ± 10.664	52.08 ± 11.938	(1.004;2)	ns		SASIB/NSSIB 0.021 *
ADI (Anxiety disorder index)	56.96 ± 12.936	46.33 ± 14.471	45.67 ± 10.320	Group (4.120;2)	0.021 *	0.116	SASIB/CB 0.006 **

Legend: SASIB = Suicidal attempt or suicidal ideation bipolar; NSSIB = Nonsuicidal self-injury bipolar; CB = Controls bipolar; ns = not significant; * = $p < 0.05$; ** = $p < 0.005$; *** = $p < 0.001$.

Univariate logistic regression was performed on the clinical group by taking each significative item of two ways ANOVA as dependent variable (considering an overall percentage of 70 or above). The data analysis highlighted an explanatory power for factors linked to mood (YSR internalizing, CDI total score, CDI Ineffectiveness, CDI negative self-esteem) linked to anxiety dimensions (MASC total social anxiety, anxiety dimension index), linked to global functioning assessment (CGAS) and linked to biosocial factors (total ESI number); the results are listed in Table 5.

Table 5. Univariate Logistic Regression.

	Overall%	B	Exp (B)	df	Sig	95% CI for Exp (B) Lower	95% CI for Exp (B) Upper
CBCL externalizing	ns						
CBCL rule breaking	ns						
YSR Internalizing	70.8	0.044	1.045	1	0.030 *	1.004	1.087
YSR anxious depressed	ns						
YSR somatic complaints	ns						
YSR Thought problems	ns						
YSR Rule breaking	ns						
YSR Aggression	ns						
CDI total	73.3	0.055	1.056	1	0.001 ***	1.022	1.091
CDI negative mood	ns						
CDI Interpersonal problems	ns						
CDI ineffectiveness	70.7	0.052	1.053	1	0.012 *	1.011	1.097
CDI Anhedonia	ns						
CDI negative self esteem	70.7	0.044	1.045	1	0.006 *	1.013	1.078
MASC Total	ns						
MASC performance fears	ns						
MASC total social anxiety	72.5	0.062	1.064	1	0.003 **	1.022	1.108
MASC Anxiety Disorder Index	71	0.071	1.074	1	0.002 **	1.026	1.123
CGAS	70.5	−0.187	0.829	1	0.000 ***	0.763	0.901
Total number of Adverse Childhood Events	78.5	0.898	2.454	1	0.000 ***	1.623	3.712

Legend: CBCL: Child Behavior Checklist; YSR: Youth Self Report; CDI: Children Depression Inventory; MASC: Multidimensional Anxiety Scale for Children; CGAS: Children Global Assessment Scale; ns = not significant; * = $p < 0.05$; ** = $p < 0.005$; *** = $p < 0.001$.

A multiple logistic regression was conducted analysing the power of predicting suicide, finding Total ESI number, CGAS and CDI total score, taking together in the same block, account for 85% explanatory risk factor for suicide, as showed in Table 6.

Table 6. Multiple Logistic Regression.

	Overall %	B	df	Sig.	Exp(B)	95% CI per EXP(B)	
						Lower	Upper
ACE_TOT	85.1	1.156	1	0.001 **	3.178	1.637	6.167
CGAS		−0.237	1	0.000 **	0.789	0.691	0.901
CDI_tot		0.052	1	0.040 *	1.054	1.002	1.108
constant		1.047	1	0.683	2.850		

Legend: ACE_TOT: Total number of Adverse Childhood Events; CGAS: Children Global Assessment Scale; CDI: Children Depression Inventory; ns = not significant; * = $p < 0.05$; ** = $p < 0.001$.

6. Discussion

The aim of this study was to compare in a consecutive sample of bipolar adolescents referred to an emergency psychiatric unit those with suicidality but not NSSI, those with NSSIs but without suicidality, and those without the two conditions.

The three groups did not differ in age, while there was a significantly larger proportion of females in the SASIB and NSSIB groups. Females prevalence in the NSSIB group is consistent with all the available studies including both clinical and non-clinical samples [40].

Regarding the gender differences in the suicidal group, our finding is consistent with prior studies, which showed that in adolescents suicide rates are higher in males than females, while suicide attempts are more common in females [41] This phenomenon, known as the "gender paradox", can be explained by several reasons, including the use of more lethal means in males, such as firearms and hanging methods [42], while drug poisoning is more frequent in females [43]. Another reason is the greater suicidal intentionality presented by males than females, regardless of the suicidal method [43]. Lastly, the higher rates of suicide deaths among male adolescents may be associated with a higher prevalence of externalizing disorders (with more impulsive behaviors), while females show more frequently internalizing disorders [44].

The greater presence of second-generation immigrants in the SASIB group compared to the CB is confirmed by a recent review, suggesting a higher risk of suicidal behaviour in migrant populations and ethnic minorities than in native populations [45] Risk factors among migrants and ethnic minorities are language barriers, separation from family, lack of information on the health care system, poor socio-economic status, acculturative stress, social exclusion and discrimination [45].

The significant role of bullying in the SASIB group is supported by our findings. Consistently, a longitudinal study showed that frequent exposure to bullying by peers during childhood increased the risk of deliberate self-harm at the age of 12 [46]. Moreover, this association was independent of potential confounding selection effects of maltreatment by an adult, family environmental risk factors, early behavioural and emotional problems and low IQ [46].

We found a greater prevalence of borderline personality disorder in the SASIB and NSSIB groups than in the CB. The impaired sense of identity and of interpersonal relationships, as well as the higher sensitivity to adverse life events, all core features of borderline personality disorder, can explain its association with suicidality and NSSI.

Interestingly, we also found a greater prevalence of eating disorders in the SASIB group than in the CB, as previously reported [47] In particular, suicidal behavior has been linked to bulimia nervosa and anorexia nervosa binge/purging type, where impulsivity is a central feature [48]. This finding highlights the importance of a close monitoring of specific features (sense of guilt, dysmorphophobia, perfectionism and low motivation for change) which may be more related to the development of self-injurious thoughts and behaviors.

The prevalence of ADHD in the CB group can be related to the gender differences between the groups, being males significantly more represented in CB group than SASIB and NSSI groups. Boys are indeed more than twice as likely as girls to receive a diagnosis of ADHD and a significantly higher comorbidity of ADHD in bipolar rather than non-bipolar boys is well documented [49]. Nevertheless, it is important to underline that the role of ADHD in promoting self-injurious behavior has been described particularly in depressed subjects, while suicidality in ADHD-bipolar subjects is more likely linked to bipolar disorder itself.

Comparing the three groups according to the CBCL (parent report), individuals in the CB group showed the highest levels of externalizing problems, and individuals in the NSSIB group greater externalizing problems than those in the SASIB. Rule breaking appears to be significant but lost its significance when corrected with Bonferroni post hoc analysis.

Regarding the YSR (self-report), individuals in the SASIB and NSSIB groups presented significantly higher scores on the internalizing problems, so we can hypothesize that subjective internalizing symptoms might be associated to a higher likelihood of engaging in self-harm. Neither Anxious/depressed nor Withdrawn/depressed symptoms differ between the SASIB and NSSIB groups. Anxious/depressed symptoms do differ between SASIB and CB, and NSSIB and CB with a portion of significance which is due to gender influence (significance to Gender×Group influence). In line with our results, Muehlenkamp and Gutierrez [50] found comparable levels of anxious and depressive symptoms between adolescents with NSSI and adolescents with previous suicide attempts.

The finding of greater somatic problems in the SASIB and NSSIB groups than in the CB, slightly influenced by Gender×Group effect, reflects Idenford's [51] finding of a strong correlation between somatic compliants, NSSIB and the gateway toward suicide attempts: Idenford sustained that individuals who had complained of somatic disorders in the 12 months before an episode of self-injury were also at a higher risk of suicide; so the authors concluded that it is important to check for a possible self-injuring or suicidal risk in adolescents who access healthcare for somatic symptoms.

The finding of greater thought problems in the SASIB and NSSIB groups than in the CB underlines the importance of dysfunctional thinking (obsessive thinking, psychotic thinking, ruminative thinking) in suicidality and NSSI.

Interestingly, in the SASIB and NSSIB groups internalizing problems are reported by adolescents, but not by parents. Failure in the family to recognize these symptoms might increase the subjective suffering of adolescents and their perception of lack of familial support, leading to suicidal ideation, NSSI or suicide attempts. It should be emphasized that, in our sample, the SASIB and NSSIB groups are mainly characterized by internalizing problems, while the CB group shows a prevalence of externalizing problems. This finding might be partly explained by gender differences between groups, as we know that females are more prone to show internalizing disorders, while males present a higher prevalence of externalizing disorders.

Emotional dysrgulation (ED) is defined as a poor ability to manage emotional responses or to keep them within an acceptable range of typical emotional reactions. Interestingly, ED profiles shown by CBCL was highly represented both in CB and SASIB/NSSI groups, indicating ED as a core feature of BD itself, regardless of the association with suicidality and self-injurious behaviours [52]. This finding is widely confirmed by literature, reporting ED as a transdiagnostic trait, identified in multiple disorders such as ADHD, BD and BPD [53].

Comparing the three groups according to the CDI, the total score and all the subscales scores were significantly higher in the SASIB group than in the CB, with a noticeable gender effect weighting on the significance. In line with our results, prior work has shown that adolescents with NSSI did not significantly differ from adolescents with suicide attempt in depressive symptoms [14,50]. Furthermore, some authors [54] found significantly greater depressive symptoms in bipolar adolescents engaged in suicide attempts compared to bipolar adolescents without previous suicide attempts.

Finally, comparing the three groups according to the MASC, the total score, performance fears, total social anxiety scores and anxiety disorder index score, were significantly higher in the SASIB group compared to the CB while anxiety disorder index was also significantly higher in SASIB than in NSSIB. In line with our results, a recent study has found that comorbid anxiety increases the risk of suicidal behaviors in bipolar adolescents by 46% and, after controlling for demographic confounders and psychiatric comorbidities, the risk of association with suicidal behaviors remained statistically significant and increased by 35% [55]. In our study, anxiety disorders represent a frequent comorbidity in all three groups, but higher anxiety symptoms seem to be associated with suicidal ideation and behavior.

The analysis of results for univariate and multiple logistic regression highlights a strong predictivity for mood variables (in particular CDI total score), global functioning and adverse childhood experiences (ACE), finding that total ACE number, CGAS and CDI total score together in the same block account for 85% explanatory risk factor for suicide. These findings confirm recent assumptions that comorbid anxiety disorders and childhood maltreatment have worse outcomes of BP with increased severity and suicidal attempts [55].

Our naturalistic study presents several methodological limitations, namely the small sample size. Furthermore, the cross-sectional design of the study does not allow for firm conclusions about possible mechanisms affecting the transition from NSSI to severe suicidal ideation or attempts, as only a longitudinal, perspective design may consent an exploration of risk factors in this transition, supporting or not the continuum model between the two conditions.

In summary, in our sample of bipolar adolescents, suicidality and NSSI are both associated with female sex, borderline personality disorder and self-reported internalizing disorders, anxiety/depression and thought disorders. The NSSIs are specifically associated with somatic problems, reflecting a preferential use of the body for the manifestation of psychic distress. Severe suicidal ideation and suicide attempts are associated with adverse childhood experiences, immigration, bullying, eating disorders, lower externalizing disorders, depressive feelings, performance and social anxiety with a sense of rejection and humiliation. Lower CGAS, presence of adverse childhood experiences and higher CDI total scores, strongly predict attempting suicide. These aspects may represent possible risk factors and targets for early diagnosis, specific prevention and treatment, both in the general population and in clinical samples of bipolar adolescents, engaged or not in self-harm.

7. Conclusions

The clinical implications in clinical practice may be relevant. In at risk populations, such as adolescents with BD, the exploration of factors associated with suicidality, compared to those associated to NSSI, may help not only to focus intervention on specific targets, but also to prevent acute anticonservative behaviors. Indeed, at-risk adolescents often act impulsively suicidal or self-harm behaviors, without previous explicit communications, on the basis of contingent environmental factors and/or momentary internal experiences. These dynamic properties of suicidal risk account for a "fluid vulnerability" [56], with temporal fluctuation (acute dimension of risk), which may be crucial in the management and prevention of real suicidal behaviors. In these patients, environmental safety and support are fundamental in order to prevent the triggering of an acute suicidal crisis, sometimes without previous active suicidal ideation. Suicidal ideation, in fact, is not followed in the next two years by suicidal behavior in more than 92% of individuals [57]. In addition, the correlation between the anticonservative intent and the lethality of a suicidal attempt is weak in adolescents [58]. In bipolar adolescents with high suicidal risk, a specific attention to contingent and biosocial factors (namely adverse childhood experiences) implies a careful prevention of contact with potential lethal means, parental supervision of medications, avoid social isolation, and, above all, monitor possible triggers of negative emotions, such as acute anxiety, humiliation, bullying, victimization, exclusion from peers, with possible cumulative effect., with global functioning that strongly modifies individual resilience of adolescent patients.

In these at-risk patients, when the conditions explored in our study are present, learning training and exercise of coping skills for adolescents and their parents may reduce the impact of negative contingent factors, and support specific skills. Among these interventions, multimodal adapted program to adolescents of the Dialectical Behavioral Therapy (DBT) includes a multi-family group skill training setting, in the DBT-A [59] specifically aimed at reducing suicide attempts, self-injurious over time and the resort itself to hospitalization for suicidality [60]. The implementation of this clinical perspective (diagnostic and therapeutic) in mental health professionals, especially in a psychiatric Emergency Hospital Care Unit for adolescents, represents a desirable goal for improving the quality and effectiveness of the clinical practice, with the structuring and implementation of differentiated therapeutic paths and ad hoc organizational models for populations of adolescents at high suicidal risk, together with their families.

Author Contributions: Conceptualization: G.M., I.L., A.M., D.F., U.M., S.B., F.L., M.M. Methodology G.D., F.L.; Writing—original draft preparation G.M., I.L., M.M., A.M., S.B. All authors have read and agreed to the published version of the manuscript.

Funding: This research was funded by the Italian Ministry of the Health RC2019 and 5 × 1000 founds.

Institutional Review Board Statement: The study was conducted according to the guidelines of the Declaration of Helsinki, and approved by the Ethics Committee of Hospital Meyer, Florence Italy, protocol code 0001507, 2014.

Informed Consent Statement: Informed consent was obtained from all subjects involved in the study.

Data Availability Statement: The data presented in this study are available on request from the corresponding author. The data are not publicly available due to privacy.

Conflicts of Interest: Masi was in advisory boards for Angelini, received grants from Lundbeck and Humana, and was speaker for Angelini, FB Health, Janssen, Lundbeck, and Otsuka. The other authors report no other conflicts of interest.

References

1. World Health Organization. *Preventing Suicide: A Global Imperative*; WHO Press: Luxembourg, 2014.
2. Hawton, K.; Saunders, K.E.A.; O'Connor, R.C. Self-Harm and suicide in adolescents. *Lancet* **2012**, *379*, 2373–2382. [CrossRef]
3. American Psychiatric Association. *Diagnostic and Statistical Manual of Mental Disorders (DSM-5)*; American Psychiatric Association: Philadelphia, PA, USA, 2013.
4. Walsh, B. *Treating Self-Injury: A Practical Guide*; Guilford Press: New York, NY, USA, 2006.
5. Muehlenkamp, J.J.; Kerr, P.L. Untangling a complex web: How non-suicidal self-injury and suicide attempts differ. *Prev. Res.* **2010**, *17*, 8–10.
6. Klonsky, E.D.; May, A.M.; Glenn, C. The relationship between nonsuicidal self-injury and attempet suicide: Converging evidence from four samples. *J. Abnorm. Psychol.* **2013**, *122*, 231–237. [CrossRef] [PubMed]
7. Kapur, N.; Cooper, J.; O'Connor, R.C.; Hawton, K. Non-suicidal self-injury v. attempted suicide: New diagnosis or false dichotomy? *Br. J. Psychiatry* **2013**, *202*, 326–328. [CrossRef] [PubMed]
8. Scott, L.N.; Pilkonis, P.A.; Hipwell, A.E.; Keenan, K.; Stepp, S.D. Non-suicidal self-injury and suicidal ideation as predictors of suicide attempts in adolescent girls: A multi-wave prospective study. *Compr. Psychiatry* **2015**, *58*, 1–10. [CrossRef]
9. Nock, M.K.; Joiner, T.E., Jr.; Gordon, K.H.; Lloyd-Richardson, E.; Prinstein, M.J. Non-suicidal self injury among adolescents: Diagnostic correlates and relation to suicide attempts. *Psychiatry Res.* **2006**, *144*, 65–72. [CrossRef]
10. Muehlenkamp, J.J.; Kerr, P.L.; Bradley, A.R.; Adams, L.M. Abuse subtypes and nonsuicidal self injury: Preliminary evidence of complex emotion regulation patterns. *J. Nerv. Ment. Dis.* **2010**, *198*, 258–263. [CrossRef]
11. Lynam, D.R.; Miller, J.D.; Miller, D.J.; Bornovalova, M.A.; Lejuez, C.W. Testing the relations between impulsivity-related traits, suicidality, and nonsuicidal self-injury: A test of the incremental validity of the UPSS Model. *Personality Disord.* **2011**, *2*, 151–160. [CrossRef]
12. Connor, J.J.; Rueter, M.A. Parent–child relationships as a systems of support or risk for adolescent suicidality. *J. Fam. Psychol.* **2006**, *20*, 143–155. [CrossRef]

13. Muehlenkamp, J.J.; Ertelt, T.W.; Miller, A.L.; Claes, L. Borderline personality symptoms differentiate non-suicidal and suicidal self-injury in ethnically diverse adolescent outpatients. *J. Child Psychol. Psychiatry* **2011**, *52*, 148–155. [CrossRef]
14. Asarnow, J.R.; Porta, G.; Spirito, A.; Emslie, G.; Clarke, G.; Wagner, K.D.; Vitiello, B.; Keller, M.; Birmaher, B.; McCracken, J.; et al. Suicide Attempts and Nonsuicidal Self-Injury in the Treatment of Resistant Depression in Adolescents: Findings from the TORDIA Study. *J. Am. Acad. Child Adolesc. Psychiatry* **2011**, *50*, 772–781. [CrossRef]
15. Dougherty, D.M.; Mathias, C.W.; Marsh-Richard, D.M.; Prevette, K.N.; Dawes, M.A.; Hatzis, E.S.; Palmes, G.; Nouvion, S.O. Impulsivity and clinical symptoms among adolescents with non-suicidal self-injury with or without attempted suicide. *Psychiatry Res.* **2009**, *169*, 22–27. [CrossRef]
16. Guertin, T.; Lloyd-Richardson, E.; Spirito, A.; Donaldson, D.; Boergers, J. Self-mutilative behavior in adolescents who attempt suicide by overdose. *J. Am. Acad. Child Adolesc. Psychiatry* **2001**, *39*, 470–480. [CrossRef]
17. Claes, L.; Muehlenkamp, J.; Vandereycken, W.; Hamelinck, L.; Martens, H.; Claes, S. Comparison of non-suicidal self-injurious behavior and suicide attempts in patients admitted to a psychiatric crisis unit. *Personal. Individ. Differ.* **2010**, *48*, 83–87. [CrossRef]
18. Jacobson, C.M.; Muehlenkamp, J.J.; Miller, A.L.; Turner, J.B. Psychiatric impairment among adolescents engaging in different types of deliberate self-harm. *J. Child Psychol.* **2008**, *37*, 363–375. [CrossRef] [PubMed]
19. Csorba, J.; Dinya, E.; Plener, P.; Nagy, E.; Páli, E. Clinical diagnoses, characteristics of risk behaviour, differences between suicidal and non-suicidal subgroups of Hungarian adolescent outpatients practising self-injury. *Eur. Child Adolesc. Psychiatry* **2009**, *18*, 309–320. [CrossRef]
20. Baetens, I.; Claes, L.; Muehlenkamp, J.; Grietens, H.; Onghena, P. Non-suicidal and suicidal self-injurious behavior among Flemish adolescents: A web-survey. *Arch. Suicide Res.* **2011**, *15*, 56–67. [CrossRef]
21. Baldessarini, R.J.; Tondo, L. Suicide risk and treatments for patients with bipolar disorder. *JAMA* **2003**, *290*, 1517–1519. [CrossRef] [PubMed]
22. Pavuluri, M.; Birmaher, B.; Naylor, M. Pediatric bipolar disorder: A review of the past 10 years. *J. Am. Acad. Child Adolesc. Psychiatry* **2005**, *44*, 846–871. [CrossRef]
23. Gore, F.; Bloem, P.; Patton, G.; Ferguson, J.; Joseph, V.; Coffey, C.; Sawyer, S. Global burden of disease in young people aged 10–24 years: A systematic analysis. *Lancet* **2011**, *377*, 2093–2102. [CrossRef]
24. Wechsler, D. *The Wechsler Intelligence Scale for Children*, 4th ed.; Pearson: London, UK, 2003.
25. Kaufman, J.; Birmaher, B.; Brent, D.; Rao, U.; Flynn, C.; Moreci, P.; Williamson, D.; Ryan, N. Schedule for Affective Disorders and Schizophrenia for School-Age Children-Present and Lifetime Version (K-SADS-PL): Initial reliability and validity data. *J. Am. Acad. Child Adolesc. Psychiatry* **1997**, *36*, 980–988. [CrossRef] [PubMed]
26. Posner, K.; Brown, G.K.; Stanley, B.; Brent, D.A.; Yershova, K.V.; Oquendo, M.A.; Currier, G.W.; Melvin, G.A.; Greenhill, L.; Shen, S.; et al. The Columbia–Suicide Severity Rating Scale: Initial Validity and Internal Consistency Findings From Three Multisite Studies With Adolescents and Adults. *Am. J. Psychiatry* **2011**, *168*, 1266–1277. [CrossRef] [PubMed]
27. Guy, W. *ECDEU Assessment Manual for Psychopharmacology, Revised*; US Department of Health, Education and Welfare: Rockville, MD, USA, 1976.
28. Shaffer, D.; Gould, M.S.; Brasic, J.; Ambrosini, P.; Fisher, P.; Bird, H.; Aluwahlia, S. A children's Global Assessment Scale (CGAS). *Arch. Gen. Psychiatry* **1983**, *40*, 1228–1231. [CrossRef] [PubMed]
29. First, M.B.; Gibbon, M.; Spitzer, R.L.; Benjamin, L.S.; Williams, J.B. *Structured Clinical Interview Interview for DSM-IV® Axis II Personality Disorders SCID-II*; American Psychiatric Publications: Washington, DC, USA, 1997.
30. Maffei, C.; Fossati, A.; Agostoni, I.; Barraco, A.; Bagnato, M.; Deborah, D.; Petrachi, M. Interrater reliability and internal consistency of the Structured Clinical Interview for DSM–IV Axis-II Personality Disorder (SCID–II) Version 2.0. *J. Pers. Disord.* **1997**, *11*, 279–284. [CrossRef]
31. Achenbach, T.; Rescorla, L. *Manual for the ASEBA School-Age Forms & Profiles*; University of Vermont: Burlington, VT, USA, 2001.
32. Achenbach, T.M.; Dumenci, L.; Rescorla, L.A. DSM-oriented and empirically based approaches to constructing scales from the same item pools. *J. Clin. Child Adolesc. Psychol.* **2003**, *32*, 328–340. [CrossRef]
33. Deutz, M.H.; Geeraerts, S.B.; van Baar, A.L.; Deković, M.; Prinzie, P. The Dysregulation Profile in middle childhood and adolescence across reporters: Factor structure, measurement invariance, and links with self-harm and suicidal ideation. *Eur. Child Adolesc. Psychiatry* **2016**, *25*, 431–442. [CrossRef]
34. Kovacs, M. *Children's Depression Inventory: Manual (p. Q8)*; Multi-Health Systems: North Tonawanda, NY, USA, 1992.
35. Camuffo, M.C.R.; Lucarelli, R.; Mayer, M. *Children's Depression Inventory, Italian Version*; Giunti OS: Firenze, Italy, 2006.
36. March, J.S.; Parker, J.D.; Sullivan, K.; Stallings, P.; Conners, C.K. The Multidimensional Anxiety Scale for Children (MASC): Factor structure, reliability, and validity. *J. Am. Acad. Child Adolesc. Psychiatry* **1997**, *36*, 554–565. [CrossRef]
37. March, J.S.; Sullivan, K.; Parker, J. Test-retest reliability of the multidimensional anxiety scale for children. *J. Anxiety Disord.* **1999**, *13*, 349–358. [CrossRef]
38. Baldwin, J.S.; Dadds, M.R. Reliability and validity of parent and child versions of the Multidimensional Anxiety Scale for Children in community samples. *J. Am. Acad. Child Adolesc. Psychiatry* **2007**, *46*, 252–260. [CrossRef] [PubMed]
39. Dierker, L.C.; Albano, A.M.; Clarke, G.N.; Heimberg, R.G.; Kendall, P.C.; Merikangas, K.R.; Lewinsohn, P.M.; Offord, D.R.; Kessler, R.; Kupfer, D.J. Screening for Anxiety and Depression in Early Adolescence. *J. Am. Acad. Child Adolesc. Psychiatry* **2001**, *40*, 929–936. [CrossRef]

40. Barrocas, A.L.; Giletta, M.; Hankin, B.L.; Prinstein, M.J.; Abela, J.R. Nonsuicidal self-injury in adolescence: Longitudinal course, trajectories, and intrapersonal predictors. *J. Abnorm. Child Psychol.* **2015**, *43*, 369–380. [CrossRef] [PubMed]
41. Freeman, A.; Mergl, R.; Kohls, E.; Székely, A.; Gusmao, R.; Arensman, E.; Koburger, N.; Hegerl, U.; Rummel-Kluge, C. A cross-national study on gender differences in suicide intent. *BMC Psychiatry* **2017**, *17*, 234. [CrossRef] [PubMed]
42. Rhodes, A.E.; Lu, H.; Skinner, R. Time trends in medically serious suicide-related behaviours in boys and girls. *Can. J. Psychiatry* **2014**, *59*, 556–560. [CrossRef] [PubMed]
43. Mergl, R.; Koburger, N.; Heinrichs, K.; Székely, A.; Tóth, M.D.; Coyne, J.; Quintão, S.; Arensman, E.; Coffey, C.; Maxwell, M.; et al. What are reasons for the large gender differences in the lethality of suicidal acts? An epidemiological analysis in four European countries. *PLoS ONE* **2015**, *10*, e0129062. [CrossRef]
44. Kaess, M.; Parzer, P.; Haffner, J.; Steen, R.; Roos, J.; Klett, M.; Brunner, R.; Resch, F. Explaining gender differences in non-fatal suicidal behaviour among adolescents: A population-based study. *BMC Public Health* **2011**, *11*, 597. [CrossRef]
45. Forte, A.; Trobia, F.; Gualtieri, F.; Lamis, D.A.; Cardamone, G.; Giallonardo, V.; Fiorillo, A.; Girardi, P.; Pompili, M. Suicide Risk among Immigrants and Ethnic Minorities: A Literature Overview. *Int. J. Environ. Res. Public Health* **2018**, *15*, 1438. [CrossRef]
46. Fisher, H.L.; Moffitt, T.E.; Houts, R.M.; Belsky, D.W.; Arseneault, L.; Caspi, A. Bullying victimisation and risk of self harm in early adolescence: Longitudinal cohort study. *BMJ* **2012**, *344*, e2683. [CrossRef]
47. Miotto, P.; De Coppi, M.; Frezza, M.; Preti, A. Eating disorders and suicide risk factors in adolescents: An Italian community-based study. *J. Nerv. Ment. Dis.* **2003**, *191*, 437–443. [CrossRef]
48. Corcos, M.; Taieb, O.; Benoit-Lamy, S.; Paterniti, S.; Jeammet, P.; Flament, M.F. Suicide attempts in women with bulimia nervosa: Frequency and characteristics. *Acta Psychiatr. Scand.* **2002**, *106*, 381–386. [CrossRef]
49. Masi, G.; Perugi, G.; Toni, C.; Millepiedi, S.; Mucci, M.; Bertini, N.; Pfanner, C. Attention-deficit hyperactivity disorder–bipolar comorbidity in children and adolescents. *Bipolar Disord.* **2006**, *8*, 373–381. [CrossRef]
50. Muehlenkamp, J.J.; Gutierrez, P.M. An investigation of differences between self-injurious behavior and suicide attempts in a sample of adolescents. *Suicide Life Threat. Behav.* **2004**, *34*, 12–23. [CrossRef] [PubMed]
51. Idenfors, H.; Strömsten, L.M.J.; Renberg, E.S. Are non-psychiatric hospitalisations before self-harm associated with an increased risk for suicide among young people? *J. Psychosom. Res.* **2019**, *120*, 96–101. [CrossRef] [PubMed]
52. Kweon, K.; Lee, H.J.; Park, K.J.; Joo, Y.; Kim, H.W. Child behavior checklist profiles in adolescents with bipolar and depressive disorders. *Compr. Psychiatry* **2016**, *70*, 152–158. [CrossRef] [PubMed]
53. Masi, G.; Muratori, P.; Manfredi, A.; Pisano, S.; Milone, A. Child behaviour checklist emotional dysregulation profiles in youth with disruptive behaviour disorders: Clinical correlates and treatment implications. *Psychiatry Res.* **2015**, *225*, 191–196. [CrossRef]
54. Francisco, A.P.; Motta, G.L.C.L.; Zortea, F.; Mugnol, F.E.; Acosta, J.; Kohmann, A.M.; Brun, J.B.; Souza, A.C.M.L.; Ramos, B.R.; Bogie, B.J.; et al. Lower estimated intelligence quotient is associated with suicide attempts in pediatric bipolar disorder. *J. Affect. Disord.* **2020**, *261*, 103–109. [CrossRef]
55. Amuk, O.C.; Patel, R.S. Comorbid anxiety increases suicidal risk in bipolar depression: Analysis of 9720 adolescent inpatients. *Behav. Sci.* **2020**, *10*, 108. [CrossRef]
56. Bryan, C.J.; Butner, J.E.; May, A.M.; Rugo, K.F.; Harris, J.A.; Oakey, D.N.; Rozek, D.C.; Bryan, A.O. Nonlinear change processes and the emergence of suicidal behavior: A conceptual model based on the fluid vulnerability theory of suicide. *New Ideas Psychol.* **2020**, *57*, 100758. [CrossRef]
57. Have, M.T.; De Graaf, R.; Van Dorsselaer, S.; Verdurmen, J.; Van't Land, H.; Vollebergh, W.; Beekman, A. Incidence and course of suicidal ideation and suicide attempts in the general population. *Can. J. Psychiatry* **2009**, *54*, 824–833. [CrossRef]
58. Rimkeviciene, J.; De Leo, D. Impulsive suicide attempts: A systematic literature review of definitions, characteristics and risk factors. *J. Affect. Disord.* **2015**, *171*, 93–104. [CrossRef]
59. Rathus, J.H.; Miller, A.L. *DBT Skills Manual for Adolescents*; Guilford Publications: New York, NY, USA, 2014.
60. Asarnow, J.R.; Mehlum, L. Practitioner Review: Treatment for suicidal and self-harming adolescents–advances in suicide prevention care. *J. Child Psychol. Psychiatry* **2019**, *60*, 1046–1054. [CrossRef]

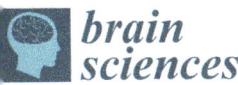

Article

Forgiveness in the Modulation of Responsibility in a Sample of Italian Adolescents with a Tendency towards Conduct or Obsessive–Compulsive Problems

Carlo Buonanno [1,*], Enrico Iuliano [1,2], Giuseppe Grossi [1,2], Francesco Mancini [1,3], Emiliana Stendardo [1], Fabrizia Tudisco [1] and Barbara Pizzini [1,4,*]

1. School of Cognitive Psychotherapy srl, 00162 Roma, Italy; iulianoenrico@libero.it (E.I.); g.grossi@hotmail.it (G.G.); mancini@apc.it (F.M.); stendardoe@gmail.com (E.S.); fabrizia-tudisco@virgilio.it (F.T.)
2. InMovement Center, 04022 Fondi, Italy
3. Department of Human Sciences, University of Studies Guglielmo Marconi, 00193 Roma, Italy
4. Department of Psychology, University of Campania "Luigi Vanvitelli", 81100 Caserta, Italy
* Correspondence: buonanno@apc.it (C.B.); barbarapizzini.17@gmail.com (B.P.)

Citation: Buonanno, C.; Iuliano, E.; Grossi, G.; Mancini, F.; Stendardo, E.; Tudisco, F.; Pizzini, B. Forgiveness in the Modulation of Responsibility in a Sample of Italian Adolescents with a Tendency towards Conduct or Obsessive–Compulsive Problems. *Brain Sci.* **2021**, *11*, 1333. https://doi.org/10.3390/brainsci11101333

Academic Editor: Suresh Sundram

Received: 21 September 2021
Accepted: 6 October 2021
Published: 9 October 2021

Publisher's Note: MDPI stays neutral with regard to jurisdictional claims in published maps and institutional affiliations.

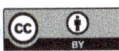

Copyright: © 2021 by the authors. Licensee MDPI, Basel, Switzerland. This article is an open access article distributed under the terms and conditions of the Creative Commons Attribution (CC BY) license (https:// creativecommons.org/licenses/by/ 4.0/).

Abstract: Although obsessive–compulsive disorder (OCD) and the conduct disorders (CD) express a contrasting symptomatology, they could represent different answers to a common matrix about morality. In the literature, some theoretical models describe people with OCD as individuals who experience high levels of responsibility and guilt. On the other hand, adolescents with a CD are described as if they do not feel guilty at all or consider anti-social purposes as more important than existing moral purposes. The aims of this study were to investigate the role of forgiveness in responsibility and guilt levels and to test whether this putative relation was influenced by tendencies towards obsessive–compulsive problems (OCP) or conduct problems (CP). In total, 231 adolescents aged between 16 and 18 years were self-assessed using a Youth Self-Report, Child Responsibility Attitudes Questionnaire, Heartland Forgiveness Scale, and Test Of Self-Conscious Affect. The results show that self-forgiveness predicted responsibility levels, while guilt was predicted by self-forgiveness and situation-forgiveness. Moreover, mediation analyses revealed that the effects of OCP on responsibility and guilt were mediated by self-forgiveness and situation-forgiveness. Regarding CP, no mediated effects were found. In conclusion, lower proneness to forgive increases responsibility and guilt, and this is particularly evident in subjects with higher levels of OCP.

Keywords: forgiveness; responsibility; guilt; obsessive-compulsive problems; conduct problems; adolescence

1. Introduction

Morality can be defined as a set of prescriptive norms concerning others' welfare, rights, fairness, and justice [1,2]. It refers to the way people choose to live their lives according to a set of principles that lead their decisions about what is right or wrong, good or evil. Theoretical constructs of morality can be considered as consisting of three main dimensions: a pure cognitive aspect regarding moral reasoning (e.g., a specific type of reasoning, by which moral principles provide the grounds for moral judgments) [3]; moral behaviours (e.g., expression of behaviours that benefit society) [4]; and moral emotions (e.g., shame, guilt, sympathy, and empathy) [5].

Seeds of morality emerge early in children with typical trajectories of development. Young children (i.e., 2–3 years old) spontaneously engage in prosocial behaviours and, conversely, want to avoid antisocial behaviour [6,7]. Regarding moral reasoning, from preschool age onwards, children show an ability to recognise and protest injustice or harmful behaviour [8–11], suggesting that children grasp concepts of harm and unfairness. Regarding moral emotions, Frick et al. [12] argued that, while in early childhood it may be difficult to distinguish between moral emotions, they become more differentiated over development, with guilt becoming more specifically related to prosocial behaviour [13]. Therefore, as children become adolescents, they able to integrate cognitive, emotional, and behavioural aspects of their morality by applying their moral judgments and emotions to social situations while they coordinate competing concerns in different contexts [14].

Among moral emotions, guilt is the one more strongly associated with morality (especially with prosocial behaviours). It is believed that it influences human behaviour, particularly when transgressions that violate social prescriptions happen. Indeed, guilt has been defined as thoughts and feelings of distress associated with transgressions [15–17]. Moreover, in the field of social psychology, guilt is considered an adaptive emotion able to improve social relationships through the development of an empathic concern for the well-being of others [18–20].

Always adopting an interpersonal view of guilt, some authors [21] relate the moral emotion of guilt with the perceived sense of personal responsibility by sustaining that guilt is a moral emotion composed of five factors (including distress and beliefs about responsibility) interacting with each other. In this view, the magnitude of guilt is proportional to the relative importance of each factor, namely, to perceived responsibility.

Responsibility can be described as the belief that a person possesses a pivotal power to provoke or prevent crucial negative consequences of their behaviour [22]. Results have shown that a perceived sense of responsibility is mediated by guilt, even if the contrary is not true [23]. This result highlights that those differences in guilt, although strongly influenced by responsibility, cannot be accounted for entirely in terms of responsibility [24,25].

Therefore, considering all the above, adolescents are called upon to find the right balance between social and personal demands on moral issues. Obstacles to this balance can lead to symptom spectra, such as obsessive–compulsive disorder on one hand or conduct disorders on the other.

In obsessive–compulsive disorder (OCD), a strong sensitivity to guilt is considered a crucial element, particularly in cognitive-behavioural models [22,25–28]. Excessive responsibility (also called 'inflated responsibility') has been suggested as a central cognitive variable associated with this disorder [22,26,29–32]. In this view, obsessions and compulsive behaviours take place in order to avoid situations that can trigger guilt, namely, to avoid the perception of being responsible for the occurrence of negative events [33]. These possible negative outcomes are perceived as essential to prevent. They may be actual, i.e., having consequences in the real world, and/or at a moral level [34]. Results from numerous studies using questionnaires [35] or experimental manipulations [36] suggest that obsessive symptoms are aimed at preventing, reducing, or neutralising the possibility of being guilty and responsible [37], sustaining evidence for such a link between responsibility and obsessive–compulsive symptoms. In OCD, an excessive engagement to deontological morality is present [28,38,39], which leads in turn to hyper-prudential checking behaviours. Control of thought processes and obsessive doubts are useful to avoid deontological guilt and a sense of responsibility [28]. In OC patients, the possibility of being guilty is evaluated by itself as a catastrophe, and it is represented as something unforgivable and unbearable [28,40]. On the other hand, the feeling of guilt can work as a signal of a possible looming threat ('If I feel guilty, the event I have to prevent will occur') [41]. According to the Diagnostic and Statistical Manual of Mental Disorders (DSM-5), it is possible to make a diagnosis of OCD even in children and, moreover, the early-onset of obsessive–compulsive disorder is one of the more common mental illnesses of children and adolescents, with a prevalence of 1% to 3% [42]. Furthermore, clinical manifestations of OCD in adolescents are very similar to those observed in adults [42,43].

On the opposite side of an imaginary morality continuum seems to be the conduct disorder (CD) diagnosis, which results in aggressive and antisocial behaviours. In fact, some authors consider it as the outcome of a total lack of morality. Recent studies have shown that guilt has the role of inhibiting antisocial behaviour [44–47] and plays a central role in predicting a high level of antisocial conduct. Diffusion of responsibility [48], a phenomenon in which people, when in a group, feel less responsible for the negative outcome of their behaviour compared to a situation in which they act alone, has been found to be the primary reason for increased antisocial and aggressive behaviours. Numerous studies have reported that, in people with problematic conduct, a fearless temperament, marked by behavioural disinhibition, prepares for a lack of moral reasoning that does not allow these patients to gain an internal system of rules [49,50]. These results seem to show that the total absence of guilt and empathy combine to predict very high levels of antisocial behaviours, proactive aggression, and school bullying [51,52]. As previously noted, empathy and guilt are considered moral emotions because they help to encourage prosocial behaviours [53]. Adolescents with CD are described as not feeling guilty [12]. Normally, developing children will increasingly internalise moral attributions and judgments [54]. However, this process of internalisation will be hindered if the negative arousal associated with guilt is attenuated due to the child's temperament [12]. An opposite view about patients with a CD diagnosis posits that they feel guilty but consider anti-social purposes, such as dominance for example [55], as more important compared to moral purposes [56]. It could be plausible that these patients do have an internal system of moral rules but that they are considered at the same level as conventional ones [57]. Thus, the outcome of aggressive behaviours is a mechanism of moral disengagement [58] that acts by leading the deontological guilt to decrease. In line with this view, it might be assumed that patients with CD feel guilty, but this emotion is assessed as something from which to defend themselves. The lack of credit to morality also depends on the limited importance of moral goals compared to the high relevance of antisocial goals, including dominance, for example [55]. In this view, moral lack can occur not because of a patient's lack of empathy or their fearless temperament, but because patients diagnosed with CD do not picture the moral consequences of the pain they can induce in others [56]. Namely, they may not anticipate the feeling of guilt or excess responsibility that would result from hurting others. Finally, clinical experience highlights how some beliefs in CD children ('Authorities and their rules are unreliable and arbitrary'; 'Nobody really cares about me'; 'Since I have suffered, then the world is in credit to me') induce the child to renounce affiliation with healthy peer groups [59] and to consider subordination to authority as useless and dangerous [60].

Therefore, in our opinion, although OCD and CD express a different symptomatology in adolescents, they could represent different answers to a common matrix about morality. In both diagnoses, an excessive sense of responsibility seems to be something that is unacceptable. In OC diagnosis, the patient feels guilty, and the sense of responsibility is hard to accept; the patient has to reassure themselves to not feel guilty and is not forgiving until a solution is found. In CD patients, the adolescent at first feels guilty and then tries to defend themselves by acting with anger to the authorities, who are considered unfair [61], by showing themselves to be someone who does not care about other people's feelings, pain, and suffering.

Self-forgiveness and interpersonal forgiveness could represent a variable that determines the shift into a disorder or into the other. Our hypothesis is that this variable, i.e., the ability to forgive, might modulate different behavioural outcomes.

Forgiveness has been shown to be an effective aspect in regulation of negative emotions [62–64]. It has been defined as 'a willingness to abandon one's right to resentment, negative judgement, and indifferent behaviour towards one who has unjustly hurt us' [65]. When people forgive, there is a reduction in angry and resentful emotions, thoughts and behaviours, and an increase in positive and benevolent ones towards the offending person [66]. It has also been reported that promoting forgiveness increases anger control and reduces trait anger and anger expressions [67,68]. The forgiving inclination may act as a protective factor against the detrimental effects of dysfunctional behaviours triggered by anger. Most of the literature, in studying forgiveness, often refers to the willingness to forgive others when a wrongdoing has been done. In fact, although the recent literature has paid remarkable attention to the role of forgiveness in interpersonal relationships, less effort has been put into studying self-forgiveness. In the psychological literature, self-forgiveness has been defined as 'a willingness to abandon self-resentment in the face of one's own acknowledged objective wrong, while fostering compassion, generosity, and love toward oneself' [65] (p. 115). Some research on the topic found that being unable to forgive oneself is associated with lower self-esteem and life satisfaction and higher neuroticism, depression, anxiety, and hostility [69–72]. In addition, Thompson and colleagues [69] introduced another dimension of forgiveness, namely, situation-forgiveness, defined as the willingness to forgive situations beyond anyone's control (e.g., an illness or natural disaster).

Considering the abovementioned literature, in the present study performed on a non-clinical adolescent sample, the role of forgiveness in responsibility and guilt levels was investigated. We additionally tested whether this putative relation was influenced by tendencies towards obsessive–compulsive problems (OCP) or conduct problems (CP), i.e., whether forgiveness mediated the effect of OCD or CD symptoms on guilt and responsibility.

2. Materials and Methods

The study was conducted according to the guidelines of the Declaration of Helsinki and approved by the Ethics Committee of the Italian Association of Cognitive Psychotherapy (Associazione di Psicoterapia Cognitiva, APC) (protocol code: 3/2021; date of approval: 28 April 2021). Informed consent was obtained from all subjects involved in the study. For participants aged under 18 years, informed consent was signed by both parents. Participants did not receive any incentive for participating in the study. All research procedures conformed to the Declaration of Helsinki for Human Subjects or its later Amendments.

2.1. Participants

Participants were 261 Italian students (52.3% F) attending year III, IV, or V of five different secondary schools in southern Italy. Participants were aged between 16 to 18 years (M = 17.37; SD = 0.84). Thirty subjects were excluded from the final sample due to incomplete tests. The final size of the sample was 231 subjects (110 M; 121 F). Subjects were naïve to the objectives and the predictions of the study.

2.2. Procedure

Participants were administered a booklet in the pencil and paper version, including all measures reported in the following 'Questionnaire measures' section. Administration of the questionnaires took place in the participants' classroom during regular class hours under researcher supervision. Students were instructed to work alone and not to talk to each other while completing the questionnaires. The order of the presentation of the instruments was randomised.

2.3. Questionnaire Measures

2.3.1. Personal Information Form

Participants first completed the folder in an anonymous way: they were asked to generate a personal code (given by the first letter of their mother's name + their date of birth + exact number of their brothers and sisters) and to copy it on each sheet of the questionnaire set. Participants were then asked to indicate information about their gender, age, and school level.

2.3.2. Symptomatic Tendencies

The Youth Self-Report (YSR) [73,74] is a 112-item self-report questionnaire that evaluates adolescents' behaviours during the recent 6 months by using a three-point Likert scale (from 0 never true to 2 sometimes true). Through the sum of different items, it is possible to calculate for each participant a total problem score, two summary scores (internalising and externalising problems), and syndrome scales based on DSM (Diagnostic and Statistical Manual, APA) syndromes. In the present study, the Obsessive–compulsive Scale (YSR-OCS) and Conduct Problems Scale (YSR-CPS) were used.

2.3.3. Forgiveness

The Heartland Forgiveness Scale (HFS) [65,75] is an 18-item self-report questionnaire that measures the person's dispositional forgiveness (Total HFS), forgiveness of the self (Self-forgiveness), forgiveness of a particular situation (Situation-forgiveness), and forgiveness of the others (Others-forgiveness).

2.3.4. Responsibility

The Child Responsibility Attitude Scale (CRAS) is a self-report measure which has been adapted from the adult Responsibility Attitude Scale (RAS) [76]. The CRAS is a measure of general responsibility attitudes and consists of 20 items that ask the child to rate a series of statements on a seven-point Likert scale. Higher levels on this scale mean a lower responsibility attitude. Since the Italian version of the CRAS is not yet available, for the present study, a version independently translated by two professional interpreters was used.

2.3.5. Guilt

The Test of Self-Conscious Affect (TOSCA-A) [77] is a scenario-based measure of characteristic guilt-proneness and shame-proneness. The original scale consists of 15 scenarios, generated from adult participants' descriptions of personal experiences of guilt, shame, and pride, followed by potential responses reflecting different affective tendencies. Respondents rate each response on a five-point Likert scale indicating how likely they would be to react in the manner described (1 = not likely, 5 = very likely). Ratings are summed across scenarios to obtain indices of guilt-proneness, shame-proneness, externalisation of blame, detachment/unconcern, alpha pride (i.e., pride in self), and beta pride (i.e., pride in behaviour). Since the Italian version of the TOSCA-A is not yet available, for the present study, a version independently translated by two professional interpreters was used.

2.4. Statistical Analyses

Data analyses were carried out using IBM SPSS, version 18. The α level was set at $p < 0.05$. For the assessment of normality, the Kolmogorov-Smirnov (K-S) test was used.

At first, to analyse the relationship between variables taken into account in the study, Pearson correlation coefficients were calculated. Then, a hierarchical regression analysis was conducted in which it was determined which variable, among three types of forgiveness (independent variables; IV), significantly predicted responsibility levels. Another hierarchical regression analysis was conducted to test the effect of the same IV on guilt levels. With the aim of testing a mediation model in which the putative effect of OCP or CP scales on responsibility levels was mediated by dimensions of forgiveness, two mediation analyses (one for each tendency scale) were performed using the bootstrap method. The last two mediational analyses were then conducted with the aim of investigating whether the two tendency scales (OCP or CP) influenced guilt levels and whether this effect was mediated by forgiveness.

3. Results

Mean and standard deviations of all measures taken into account as part of the study are reported in Table 1.

Correlational analysis revealed no significant relations among two problematic tendencies and age. CP levels were negatively related to guilt levels to a significant degree, and no significant correlations were found with three types of forgiveness and responsibility. Conversely, higher levels of OCP were found to be negatively related to self-forgiveness and situation-forgiveness and positively related to responsibility levels. No significant correlation was found between OCP and guilt. See Table 2 for the correlational analysis results.

Table 1. Means and standard deviations of all measures taken into account as part of the study.

	Mean	Std. Deviation
YSR_OCS	5,33	3450
YSR_CPS	2,77	3113
HFS_TOT	82,43	15,503
Self-forgiveness	29,09	6208
Others-forgiveness	26,79	6520
Situation-forgiveness	26,65	6884
Responsibility (CRAS)	68,87	14,465
Guilty (TOSCA)	53,61	7846

Note. YSR_OCS = Obsessive–compulsive Scale; YSR-CPS = Conduct Problems Scale; HFS_TOT = Heartland Forgiveness Scale total score.

Table 2. Correlations among the study variables.

	1.	2.	3.	4.	5.	6.	7.
1. Self-forgiveness	-	0.208 **	0.571 **	−0.145 *	413 **	−0.487 **	−0.075
2. Others-forgiveness		-	0.419 **	0.158 *	0.017	0.029	−0.122
3. Situation-forgiveness			-	0.081	0.216 **	−0.259 **	−0.111
4. Guilt				-	−0.266 **	0.106	−0.185 **
5. Responsibility					-	−0.324 **	0.066
6. OCP						-	0.231
7. CP							-

Note. $p < 0.05$ *; $p < 0.01$ **.

The first regression analysis showed that age (B = −2.304; β = − 0.134; t = −2.179; $p = 0.030$) and self-forgiveness (B = 0.938; β = 0.403; t = 6.704; $p = 0.000$) significantly predicted responsibility levels, explaining almost 20% of the total of variance (R^2adj = 0.177; F_{3227} = 17.488; $p = 0.000$). The results revealed in detail that higher levels of self-forgiveness, along with younger age, predicted lower levels of perceived responsibility. The second regression analysis revealed that self-forgiveness (B = −0.347; β = −0.275; t = −3.509; $p = 0.001$) and situation-forgiveness (B = 0.214; β = 0.188; t = 2.229; $p = 0.001$) significantly predicted guilt levels. Specifically, lower levels of self-forgiveness and higher levels of situation-forgiveness predicted higher levels of guilt (R^2adj = 0.067; F_{3225} = 14.315; $p = 0.001$).

The mediation analyses were carried out using the PROCESS 3.1 macro for SPSS [78]. It employs a bootstrapping method for estimating indirect effects; 95% bias-corrected confidence intervals were calculated through 5000 bootstrap samples. From the variety of models proposed by the program, representative of different conceptual models, Model 4 was tested because it considers the effect of IV on the DV through mediators. Specifically, further mediational analyses were conducted that considered the regression results, namely, by not considering others-forgiveness in models in which the DV was guilt and not considering situation-forgiveness and others-forgiveness in models in which the DV was responsibility.

Mediational analysis tested the model in which OCP was inserted as the IV and guilt as the DV; self-forgiveness and situation-forgiveness were settled as putative mediators, revealing that OCP does not exert significant direct and total effects on guilt levels, but rather has an indirect effect through the occurrence of both self-forgiveness and situation-forgiveness (Table 3). A suppression effect [79] was probably revealed: namely, a non-significant total effect of the IV on the DV due to the opposite in sign direct and indirect effects of the IV on the DV. Specifically, higher OCP led both self- and situation-forgiveness to decrease, which in turn led guilt levels to increase (self-forgiveness) and to decrease (situation-forgiveness). This resulted in a positive indirect effect exerted by self-forgiveness, by increasing guilt, and a negative indirect effect through situation-forgiveness, by decreasing guilt (Figure 1).

Table 3. Results of the mediation analysis (Model 4) testing the effects of obsessive–compulsive problems (IV) on guilt (DV) through self-forgiveness and situation-forgiveness (mediators).

Model Summary	R-Sq	F		p	
	0.062	4.996		0.002	
Model	B	t	p		CI
Constant	55.493	16.602	<0.001		[48.906; 62.079]
Obsessive–compulsive Problems	−0.090	0.538	0.591		[−0.240; 0.420]
Self-forgiveness	−0.333	−3.046	0.003		[−0.549; −0.118]
Situation-forgiveness	0.275	3.082	0.002		[0.099; 0.451]
	Total Effects of IV on DV (R-Sq = 0.011; F = 2.579; p = 0.110)				
	Effect	t	p		CI
Constant	52.327	55.186	<0.001		[50.459; 54.195]
Obsessive–compulsive Problems	0.240	1.606	0.110		[−0.055; 0.535]
	Significant Relative Indirect Effect of IV on DV Through Mediators				
Mediators	Effect			CI	
Self-forgiveness	0.292			[0.095; 0.519]	
Situation-forgiveness	−0.142			[−0.271; −0.050]	

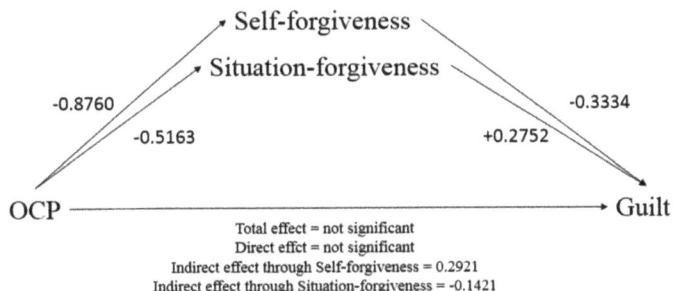

Figure 1. Mediation model tested: Obsessive–compulsive Problems (IV) on Guilt (DV) through Self-forgiveness and Situation-forgiveness (Mediators). Numbers reported are coefficient (B) of the effect represented. Coefficients are presented in Table 3.

The same mediational analysis, with the same DV and putative mediators, was then carried out, replacing OCP with CP. The results showed no effects of CP on either self- or situation-forgiveness. Higher CP levels led guilt to decrease, but no indirect effects were revealed (Table 4).

Two further mediational analyses were conducted to test mediation models in which the effect of OCP or CP on responsibility was mediated by self-forgiveness. The first analysis revealed that higher OCP led responsibility levels to increase both directly and indirectly through self-forgiveness. That is, higher OCP levels led self-forgiveness to decrease, which in turn led responsibility scores to decrease: the multiplication of these effects gave a positive indirect effect such that higher OCP levels led responsibility to increase through the mediation of self-forgiveness (Table 5 and Figure 2).

Table 4. Results of the mediation analysis (Model 4) testing the effects of conduct problems (IV) on guilt (DV) through self-forgiveness and situation-forgiveness (mediators).

Model Summary	R-Sq	F		p	
	0.093	7.778		<0.001	
Model	B	t	p		CI
Constant	58.612	22.765	<0.001		[53.539; 63.686]
Conduct Problems	−0.457	−2.851	0.004		[−0.773; −0.141]
Self-forgiveness	−0.363	−3.728	<0.001		[−0.556; −0.171]
Situation-forgiveness	0.256	2.904	0.004		[0.082; 0.429]
	Total Effects of IV on DV (R-Sq = 0.034; F = 8.072; p = 0.005):				
	Effect	t	p		CI
Constant	54.897	80.510	<0.001		[53.553; 56.240]
Conduct Problems	−0.465	−2.841	0.005		[−0.788; −0.143]

Table 5. Results of the mediation analysis (Model 4) testing the effects of obsessive–compulsive problems (IV) on responsibility (DV) through self-forgiveness (mediator).

Model Summary	R-Sq	F		p	
	0.191	26.821		<0.001	
Model	B	t	p		CI
Constant	49.767	8.896	<0.001		[38.744; 60.790]
Obsessive–compulsive Problems	−0.674	−2.357	0.019		[−1.238; −0.111]
Self-forgiveness	0.780	4.910	<0.001		[0.467; 1.094]
	Total Effects of IV on DV (R-Sq = 0.105; F = 26.825; p = 0.000)				
	Effect	t	p		CI
Constant	76.111	45.761	<0.001		[72.833; 79.388]
Obsessive–compulsive problems	−1.358	−5.180	<0.001		[−1.874; −0.841]
	Significant Relative Indirect Effect of IV on DV Through Mediator				
Mediator	Effect			CI	
Self-forgiveness	−0.684			[−1.013; −0.386]	

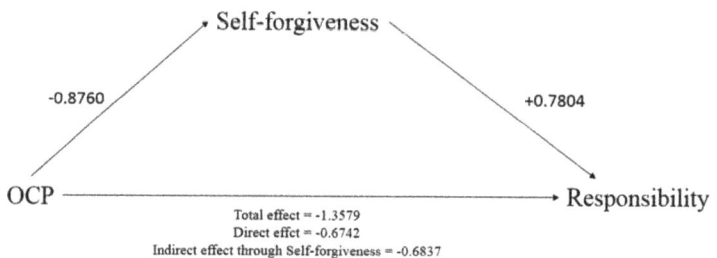

Figure 2. Mediation model tested: Obsessive–compulsive Problems (IV) on Responsibility (DV) through Self-forgiveness (Mediator). Numbers reported are coefficient (B) of the effect represented. Coefficients are presented in Table 5.

The second mediational analysis was carried out assuming that the effect of CP on responsibility levels was mediated by self-forgiveness, but this analysis actually showed no significant effects (either direct or indirect) of the IV on the DV (Table 6).

Table 6. Results of the mediation analysis (Model 4) testing the effects Conduct problems (IV) on Responsibility (DV) through Self-forgiveness (mediator).

Model Summary	R-Sq	F		p	
	0.180	25.077		<0.001	
Model	B	t		p	CI
Constant	39.102	9.107		<0.001	[30.642; 47.563]
Conduct Problems	0.456	1.632		0.104	[−0.095; 1.007]
Self-forgiveness	0.980	6.995		<0.001	[0.704; 1.256]
	Total Effects of IV on DV (R-Sq = 0.004; F = 1.014; p = 0.315)				
	Effect	t		p	CI
Constant	68.018	53.295		<0.001	[65.504; 70.533]
Conduct Problems	0.309	1.007		0.315	[−0.295; 0.912]
	Significant Relative Indirect Effect of IV on DV Through Mediator				
Mediator	Effect	CI			
Self-forgiveness	−0.148	[−0.399; 0.098]			

4. Discussion

The aim of the present study was to investigate the role of forgiveness in the modulation of guilt and responsibility in a non-clinical sample of adolescents. Specifically, in the present study, the role of forgiveness was investigated in regard to responsibility and guilt levels, and we tested whether this putative relation was influenced by tendencies towards OCP or CP, i.e., whether specific dimensions of forgiveness mediate the effect of OCD or CD symptoms on guilt and responsibility.

Regarding the role of guilt in the two problematic trends (i.e., OCP and CP), our results confirmed the hypothesis that high levels of OCP are strongly related with high sensitivity to guilt [22,26–28], confirming that in OCD, the control of thought processes and obsessive doubt seem to be useful tools to avoid an ethical sense of guilt [28]. However, in relation to the absence of a correlation found between the OCP and TOSCA-A scores, we believe that this data may be due to the inability of the latter tool to grasp two different types of guilt, i.e., deontological and altruistic [56]. Our results also demonstrated that adolescents with a tendency towards CD actually feel guilty, in contrast to the position of Frick (2014), but less than adolescents without this problematic tendency, supporting alternative hypotheses for which they first feel guilty but develop processes that lead them to consider antisocial purposes as more important compared to moral purposes [56]; alternatively, they have an internal system of moral rules, but these rules are considered at the same level as conventional ones [57]. Regarding responsibility, our results confirmed only its role in the OCP tendency, whilst no effect was observed in CP. While these results support the idea that excessive responsibility is a central cognitive variable associated with OCP [22,26,29–32], they also suggest that, in adolescents with a tendency towards CP, no different levels of responsibility are observed compared to adolescents without this tendency. Taken together, our results regarding guilt and responsibility levels in adolescents with tendencies towards OCP or CP seem to confirm our hypothesis that although OCD and CD express a different symptomatology in adolescence, they could represent different answers to a common matrix about morality. Further research considering clinical samples are needed in order to better delineate these trajectories in diagnosed patients.

Regarding the role of forgiveness in levels of responsibility and experienced guilt, our results revealed that self-forgiveness has an important role in modulating levels of a sense of responsibility, while either self-forgiveness or situation-forgiveness play a crucial role in guilt levels. In both regression analyses, the R^2 values were not very high, with a very low coefficient in the regression that had guilt as the DV; this was probably because few putative predictors were inserted in the model. Indeed, guilt and responsibility are very complex constructs in which many variables (see, for example, social context and external models of emotion regulation) not considered in the present study have a modulating role. Therefore, further research considering a wider set of putative predictors is needed in order to improve our comprehension of the relationship between self-forgiveness, guilt, and responsibility. Moreover, mediation analyses revealed that two types of forgiveness (i.e., self- and situation-forgiveness) mediated the effect of OCP tendency on guilt levels. Furthermore, self-forgiveness mediated the role of OCP on responsibility levels. Regarding the effect of CP on guilt, this was not mediated by forgiveness. No effects of CP on responsibility levels were revealed. Thus, our results confirmed the need to include self-forgiveness in future models of forgiveness [72,80,81] for both theoretical and clinical implications. Moreover, the results of the present study highlight for the first time how the relation between self-forgiveness, guilt, and responsibility could lead to pathological outcomes, such as OCD. In fact, although our study was performed on a non-clinical sample, as Mancini and colleagues [43] stated, there is a 'connection between normal and pathological obsessions and thus a similarity in the cognitive processes involved', suggesting that non-clinical and clinical samples may differ more in degree than in kind [82]. In other words, in adolescents with higher levels of OCP, an increase in guilt and responsibility is considered to be something unacceptable and something to defend oneself against; these adolescents do not forgive themselves until they find a solution. The relationship between an inflated sense of responsibility and guilt and low proneness to self-forgiveness could be considered a vicious cycle underlying OCD. The present results seem to support its necessity in OCD: as stated by Barcaccia, Tenore, and Mancini [83], 'besides the already available treatments, it would be advantageous to design protocols aimed [. . .] at developing a more general compassionate and forgiving stance towards oneself' [84,85].

On the contrary, adolescents with higher CP levels experience guilt, albeit less than the rest of the sample and even if it is not affected by the degree of forgiveness. This result could be in line with a hypothesis in which CD patients at first feel guilty and then try to defend themselves by appearing to be someone who does not care about other people's feelings, pain, and suffering.

Finally, forgiveness of the situation, namely, the willingness to forgive situations beyond anyone's control (for example, an illness or a natural disaster), was also a significant predictor of the level of guilt in our results, confirming the importance of considering it in further conceptual models. More specifically, our results showed that adolescents who experienced higher levels of forgiveness of the situation experienced more guilt. This seems to represent a process whereby people who are faced with internal or external events (for example, an illness) are called upon to decide whether or not they have personal responsibility for that situation. When they attribute responsibility to themselves, then the situation (external or internal) is 'discharged'.

5. Limitations and Strengths

Although this study was the first to investigate an important issue, i.e., the role of forgiveness in guilt and responsibility in tendencies towards OCP and/or CP, some limitations need to be acknowledged. First of all, the results of the study are based on self-reported measures, which, especially in the clinical field, could represent a problem in terms of the generalisability of the results. Adolescents could, in fact, not be fully aware of how their thoughts or behaviours could represent a problematic issue in terms of pathology. The second limitation might be in not having considered clinical samples composed of OCP and CP diagnosed groups, which could have clarified the role of forgiveness in guilt and responsibility when the presence OCD and CD symptoms is problematic. Finally, the TOSCA-A was found to be a tool unable to grasp two different types of guilt, i.e., deontological and the altruistic. This probably affected the results regarding guilt. Further investigations should include instruments more able to make this very relevant distinction.

6. Conclusions

In conclusion, the results of the present study show that a lower proneness to forgiveness increases responsibility and guilt and that this is particularly evident in subjects with higher levels of OCP. The present study is the first to highlight the important role of forgiveness in experiencing guilt and responsibility, particularly in adolescents with a higher presence of OC traits. Moreover, it initially evidenced the role of the interplay between these variables in a shift along the potential symptom spectrum (see OCP).

Author Contributions: Conceptualization, C.B., F.M. and B.P.; methodology, E.I. and B.P.; formal analysis, B.P.; investigation, G.G., F.T. and E.S.; data curation, G.G., F.T. and E.S.; writing—original draft preparation, B.P.; writing—review and editing, C.B.; supervision, F.M.; project administration, C.B., G.G. and F.M.; funding acquisition, F.M. All authors have read and agreed to the published version of the manuscript.

Funding: This research was funded by Scuola di Psicoterapia Cognitiva srl.

Institutional Review Board Statement: The study was conducted according to the guidelines of the Declaration of Helsinki, and approved by the Ethics Committee of the Italian Association of Cognitive Psychotherapy (Associazione di Psicoterapia Cognitiva, APC) (protocol code: 3/2021; date of approval: 28/04/2021).

Informed Consent Statement: Informed consent was obtained from all subjects involved in the study. For participants aged under 18 years, informed consent was signed by both parents.

Data Availability Statement: The data presented in this study are available upon request of the corresponding author. The data is not publicly available because it was collected on a sample of minors.

Conflicts of Interest: The authors declare no conflict of interest. The funders had no role in the design of the study; in the collection, analyses, or interpretation of data; in the writing of the manuscript; or in the decision to publish the results.

References

1. Killen, M.; Rutland, A. *Children and Social Exclusion: Morality, Prejudice, and Group Identity*; Wiley-Blackwell: New York, NY, USA, 2011.
2. Dahl, A.; Killen, M. Moral Reasoning: Theory and Research in Developmental Science. In *Stevens' Handbook of Experimental Psychology and Cognitive Neuroscience*, 4th ed.; Wixted, J.T., Ghetti, S., Eds.; Wiley: New York, NY, USA, 2018; pp. 323–353.
3. Kohlberg, L. The Development of Children's Orientations Toward a Moral Order. *Hum. Dev.* **1963**, *6*, 11–33. [CrossRef]
4. Eisenberg, N.; Fabes, R.A. Prosocial development. In *Handbook of Child Psychology, Social, Emotional, And Personality Development*, 5th ed.; Damon, W., Eisenberg, N., Eds.; Wiley: New York, NY, USA, 1998; Volume 3, pp. 701–778.
5. Tangney, J.P.; Dearing, R.L. *Shame and Guilt*; Guilford Press: New York, NY, USA, 2002.
6. Thompson, R.A.; Meyer, S.; McGinley, M. Understanding values in relationship: The development of conscience. In *Handbook of Moral Development*; Killen, M., Smetana, J., Eds.; Erlbaum: Mahwah, NJ, USA, 2006; pp. 267–297.
7. Warneken, F.; Tomasello, M. The roots of human altruism. *Br. J. Psychol.* **2009**, *100*, 455–471. [CrossRef] [PubMed]
8. Smetana, J.G. The development of autonomy in adolescence: A social domain theory view. In *The Meaning and Role of Autonomy in Adolescent Development: Towards Conceptual Clarity*; Soenens, B., Vansteenkiste, M., Van Petegem, S., Eds.; Routledge: New York, NY, USA, 2018; pp. 53–73.
9. Hepach, R.; Vaish, A.; Tomasello, M. Young Children Are Intrinsically Motivated to See Others Helped. *Psychol. Sci.* **2012**, *23*, 967–972. [CrossRef]
10. Vaish, A.; Missana, M.; Tomasello, M. Three-year-old children intervene in third-party moral transgressions. *Br. J. Dev. Psychol.* **2011**, *29*, 124–130. [CrossRef]
11. Davidson, P.; Turiel, E.; Black, A. The effect of stimulus familiarity on the use of criteria and justifications in children's social reasoning. *Br. J. Dev. Psychol.* **1983**, *1*, 49–65. [CrossRef]
12. Frick, P.J.; Ray, J.V.; Thornton, L.C.; Kahn, R.E. Annual Research Review: A developmental psychopathology approach to understanding callous-unemotional traits in children and adolescents with serious conduct problems. *J. Child Psychol. Psychiatry* **2013**, *55*, 532–548. [CrossRef] [PubMed]
13. Tangney, J.P.; Wagner, P.; Gramzow, R. Proneness to shame, proneness to guilt, and psychopathology. *J. Abnorm. Psychol.* **1992**, *101*, 469–478. [CrossRef]
14. Killen, M.; Smetana, J.G. Origins and development of morality. In *Handbook of Child Psychology and Developmental Science*, 7th ed.; Lamb, M., Ed.; Wiley-Blackwell: New York, NY, USA, 2015; pp. 701–749.

15. Baker, E.; Baibazarova, E.; Ktistaki, G.; Shelton, K.H.; van Goozen, S.H.M. Development of fear and guilt in young children: Stability over time and relations with psychopathology. *Dev. Psychopathol.* **2012**, *24*, 833–845. [CrossRef]
16. Kochanska, G.; Gross, J.N.; Lin, M.; Nichols, K.E. Guilt in young children: Development, determinants and its relation with a broader system of standards. *Child Dev.* **2002**, *73*, 461–482. [CrossRef]
17. Zahn-Waxler, C.; Kochanska, G.; Krupnick, J.; Mcknew, D. Patterns of guilt in children of depressed and well mothers. *Dev. Psy.* **1990**, *26*, 51–59. [CrossRef]
18. Hoffman, M.L. Development of prosocial motivation: Empathy and guilt. In *The Development of Prosocial Behavior*; Eisenberg, N., Ed.; Academic Press: New York, NY, USA, 1982; pp. 281–313.
19. Hoffman, M.L. Varieties of empathy-based guilt. In *Guilt and Children*; Bybee, J., Ed.; Academic Press: San Diego, CA, USA, 1998; pp. 91–112.
20. Baumeister, R.F.; Stillwell, A.M.; Heatherton, T.F. Guilt: An interpersonal approach. *Psychol. Bull.* **1994**, *115*, 243–267. [CrossRef]
21. Kubany, E.S.; Watson, S.B. Guilt: Elaboration of a multidimensional model. *Psychol. Rec.* **2003**, *53*, 51–90.
22. Salkovskis, P.M.; Richards, C.H.; Forrester, E. The relationship between obsessional problems and intrusive thoughts. *Behav. Cogn. Psychother.* **1995**, *23*, 281–299. [CrossRef]
23. Berndsen, M.; Manstead, A.S.R. On the Relationship between Responsibility and Guilt: Antecedent Appraisal or Elaborated Appraisal Eur. *J. Soc. Psychol.* **2007**, *37*, 774–792. [CrossRef]
24. Baumeister, R.F.; Stillwell, A.M.; Heatherton, T.F. Personal narratives about guilt: Role in action control and interpersonal relationships. *Basic Appl. Soc. Psychol.* **1995**, *17*, 173–198. [CrossRef]
25. Frijda, N.H. Mood, Emotion Episodes, and Emotions. In *Handbook of Emotions*; Lewis, M., Haviland, J.M., Eds.; Guilford Press: New York, NY, USA, 1993; pp. 381–403.
26. Rachman, S. Obsessions, responsibility and guilt. *Behav. Res. Ther.* **1993**, *31*, 149–154. [CrossRef]
27. Mancini, F.; Gangemi, A. Fear of Guilt from Behaving Irresponsibly in Obsessive-Compulsive Disorder. *J. Behav. Exp. Psychiat.* **2004**, *35*, 109–120. [CrossRef]
28. Mancini, F. *La Mente Ossessiva*; Raffaello Cortina Editore: Milano, Italy, 2016.
29. Salkovskis, P.M. Cognitive-behavioural factors and the persistence of intrusive thoughts in obsessional problems. *Behav. Res. Ther.* **1989**, *27*, 677–682. [CrossRef]
30. Mancini, F.; Gangemi, A. The Role of Responsibility and Fear of Guilt in Hypothesis-Testing. *J. Behav. Ther. Exp. Psychiat.* **2006**, *37*, 333–346. [CrossRef]
31. Mancini, F.; Gangemi, A. Responsibility, guilt and decision under risk. *Psychol. Rep.* **2003**, *93*, 1077–1079. [CrossRef]
32. Mancini, F.; Gragnani, A.; D'Olimpio, F. The Connection between Disgust and Obsessions and Compulsions In a non-clinical Sample. *Pers. Ind. Diff.* **2001**, *31*, 1171–1178. [CrossRef]
33. Miceli, M. How to make someone feel guilty: Strategies of guilt inducement and their goals. *J. Theory Soc. Behav.* **1992**, *22*, 81–104. [CrossRef]
34. Salkovskis, P.M. *The Cognitive Approach to Anxiety: Threat Beliefs, Safety-Seeking Behavior, and the Special Case of Health Anxiety and Obsessions*; Guilford Press: New York, NY, USA, 1996; pp. 48–74.
35. Rheaume, J.; Freeston, M.H.; Dugas, M.J.; Letarte, H.; Ladouceur, R. Perfectionism, Responsibility and Obsessive-Compulsive Symptoms. *Behav. Res. Ther.* **1995**, *33*, 785–794. [CrossRef]
36. Ladouceur, R.; Rhéaume, J.; Freeston, M.H.; Aublet, F.; Jean, K.; Lachance, S.; Langlois, F.; de Pokomandy-Morin, K. Experimental manipulations of responsibility: An analogue test for models of obsessive-compulsive disorder. *Behav. Res. Ther.* **1995**, *33*, 937–946. [CrossRef]
37. Shapiro, L.J.; Stewart, E.S. Pathological guilt: A persistent yet overlooked treatment factor in obsessive-compulsive disorder. *Ann. Clin. Psychiatry* **2011**, *23*, 63–70.
38. Giacomantonio, M.; Salvati, M.; Mancini, F. Am I Guilty or Not? Deontological Guilt, Uncertainty and Checking Behavior. *Appl. Cogn. Psychol.* **2019**, *33*, 1279–1287. [CrossRef]
39. Mancini, F.; Gangemi, A. Obsessive patients and their guilt. *Psychopathol. Rev.* **2017**, *7*, 155–168. [CrossRef]
40. Enholt, K.A.; Salkovskis, P.M.; Rimes, K.A. Obsessive-Compulsive Disorder, Anxiety Disorders and Self-Esteem: An Exploratory Study. *Behav. Res. Ther.* **1999**, *37*, 771–781. [CrossRef]
41. Mancini, F. Current Targets in Obsessive-Compulsive Patients. *Psicoterapia Cognitiva e Comportamentale* **2010**, *15*, 353–363.
42. Walitza, S.; Melfsen, S.; Jans, T.; Zellmann, H.; Wewetzer, C.; Warnke, A.; Taub, E. Obsessive-compulsive disorder in children and adolescents. *Dtsch. Arztebl. Int.* **2011**, *108*, 173–179. [CrossRef]
43. Mancini, F.; Corsani, I.; Episcopo, A. Il ruolo della responsabilità nel disturbo ossessivo-compulsivo. *Psicoter. Cogn. Comport.* **1999**, *5*, 15–30.
44. Arsenio, W. Moral emotion attributions and aggression. In *Handbook of Moral Development*; Killen, M., Smetana, J., Eds.; Lawrence Erlbaum: Mahwah, NJ, USA, 2014; pp. 235–255.
45. Kochanska, G.; Barry, R.A.; Jiménez, N.B.; Hollatz, A.L.; Woodard, J. Guilt and effortful control: Two mechanisms that prevent disruptive developmental trajectories. *J. Pers. Soc. Psychol.* **2009**, *97*, 322–333. [CrossRef]
46. Menesini, E.; Camodeca, M. Shame and guilt as behaviour regulators: Relationships with bullying, victimization and prosocial behaviour. *Br. J. Dev. Psychol.* **2008**, *26*, 183–196. [CrossRef]

47. Malti, T.; Ongley, S.F. The development of moral emotions and moral reasoning. In *Handbook of Moral Development*; Psychology Press: Hove, UK, 2014; pp. 163–183.
48. Dana, J.; Weber, R.A.; Kuang, J.X. Exploiting moral wiggle room: Experiments demonstrating an illusory preference for fairness. *Econ. Theory* **2006**, *33*, 67–80. [CrossRef]
49. Lykken, D.T. *The Antisocial Personalities*; Lawrence Erlbaum Associates Inc.: Mahwah, NJ, USA, 1995.
50. Quay, H.C. The psychobiology of undersocialized aggressive conduct disorder: A theoretical perspective. *Dev. Psychopathol.* **1993**, *5*, 165–180. [CrossRef]
51. Frick, P.; White, S.F. Research review: The importance of callous-unemotional traits for developmental models of aggressive and antisocial behavior. *J. Child Psychol. Psychiatry* **2008**, *49*, 359–375. [CrossRef]
52. Van Noorden, T.H.; Haselager, G.J.; Cillessen, A.H.; Bukowski, W.M. Empathy and involvement in bullying in children and adolescents: A systematic review. *J. Youth Adolesc* **2014**, *44*, 637–657. [CrossRef]
53. Roose, A.; Bijttebier, P.; Decoene, S.; Claes, L.; Frick, P. Assessing the affective features of psychopathy in adolescence: A further validation of the inventory of callous and unemotional traits. *Assessment* **2010**, *17*, 44–57. [CrossRef]
54. Nunner-Winkler, G. Development of moral motivation from childhood to early adulthood. *J. Moral Ed.* **2007**, *36*, 399–414. [CrossRef]
55. Lochman, J.E.; Coie, J.D.; Underwood, M.K.; Terry, R. Effectiveness of a social relations intervention program for aggressive and nonaggressive, rejected children. *J. Consult. Clin Psychol.* **1993**, *61*, 1053–1058. [CrossRef]
56. Mancini, F. I sensi di colpa altruistico e deontologico. *Cogn. Clin.* **2008**, *5*, 123–144.
57. Hauser, M.D. *Moral Minds: How Nature Designed Our Universal Sense of Right and Wrong*; Harper Collins: New York, NY, USA, 2006.
58. Bandura, A. Moral disengagement in the perpetration of inhumanities. *Personal. Soc. Psychol. Rev.* **1999**, *3*, 193–209. [CrossRef] [PubMed]
59. Mancini, F.; Capo, R.; Colle, L. La moralità nel disturbo antisociale di personalità. *Cogn. Clin.* **2009**, *6*, 161–177.
60. Buonanno, C.; Capo, R.; Romano, G.; Di Giunta, L.; Isola, L. Caratteristiche genitoriali e stili di paenting associati ai disturbi esternalizzanti in età evolutiva. *Psichiatr. Psicoter.* **2010**, *29*, 176–188.
61. Robins, L. Conduct disorder. *J. Child Psychol. Psychiatry* **1991**, *32*, 193–212. [CrossRef] [PubMed]
62. Worthington, E.L.; Scherer, M. Forgiveness is an emotion-focused coping strategy that can reduce health risks and promote health resilience: Theory, review, and hypotheses. *Psychol. Health* **2004**, *19*, 385–405. [CrossRef]
63. Barcaccia, B.; Milioni, M.; Pallini, S.; Vecchio, G.M. Resentment or forgiveness? *The assessment of forgivingness in Italian adolescents*. *Child Indic. Res.* **2018**, *11*, 1407–1423. [CrossRef]
64. Barcaccia, B.; Pallini, S.; Pozza, A.; Milioni, M.; Baiocco, R.; Mancini, F.; Vecchio, G.M. Forgiving Adolescents: Far from Depression, Close to Well-Being. *Front. Psychol.* **2019**, *10*, 1725. [CrossRef]
65. Enright, R.D.; Freedman, S.; Rique, J. Exploring forgiveness. In *The Psychology of Interpersonal Forgiveness*; Enright, R.D., North, J., Eds.; University of Wisconsin Press: Madison, WI, USA, 1998; pp. 46–62.
66. Wade, N.G.; Hoyt, W.T.; Kidwell, J.E.M.; Worthington, E.L., Jr. Efficacy of psychotherapeutic interventions to promote forgiveness: A meta-analysis. *J. Consult. Clin. Psychol.* **2014**, *82*, 154–170. [CrossRef]
67. Wilkowski, B.M.; Robinson, M.D. The anatomy of anger: An integrative cognitive model of trait anger and reactive aggression. *J. Personal.* **2010**, *78*, 9–38. [CrossRef]
68. Akhtar, S.; Barlow, J. Forgiveness Therapy for the Promotion of Mental Well-Being: A Systematic Review and Meta-Analysis. *Trauma Violence Abuse* **2018**, *19*, 107–122. [CrossRef] [PubMed]
69. Thompson, L.Y.; Snyder, C.R.; Hoffman, L.; Michael, S.T.; Rasmussen, H.N.; Billings, L.S.; Heinze, L.; Neufeld, J.E.; Shorey, H.S.; Roberts, J.C.; et al. Dispositional Forgiveness of Self, Others, and Situations. *J. Pers.* **2005**, *73*, 313–360. [CrossRef] [PubMed]
70. Maltby, J.; Macaskill, A.; Day, L. Failure to forgive self and others: A replication and extension of the relationship between forgiveness, personality, social desirability and general health. *Personal. Individ. Differ.* **2001**, *30*, 881–885. [CrossRef]
71. Mauger, P.A.; Perry, J.E.; Freeman, T.; Grove, D.C. The measurement of forgiveness: Preliminary research. *J. Psychol. Christ.* **1992**, *11*, 170–180.
72. Wohl, M.J.A.; DeShea, L.; Wahkinney, R.L. Looking within: The state forgiveness scale. *Can. J. Behav. Sci.* **2008**, *40*, 1–10. [CrossRef]
73. Achenbach, T.M.; Rescorla, L.A. *Manual for the ASEBA School-Age Forms and Profiles*; University of Vermont Research Center for Children, Youth, & Families: Burlington, VT, USA, 2011.
74. Achenbach, T.M.; Edelbrock, C. *Manual for the Child Behavior Checklist*; University of Vermont Department of Psychiatry: Burlington, VT, USA, 1991.
75. Consoli, S.; Rossi, A.; Thompson, L.Y.; Volpi, C.; Mannarini, S.; Castelnuovo, G.; Molinari, E. Assessing Psychometric Properties of the Italian Version of the Heartland Forgiveness Scale. *Front. Psychol.* **2020**, *11*, 3360. [CrossRef]
76. Salkovskis, P.M.; Wroe, A.L.; Gledhill, A.; Morrison, N.; Forrester, E.; Richards, C.; Reynolds, M.; Thorpe, S. Responsibility attitudes and interpretations are characteristic of obsessive compulsive disorder. *Behav. Res. Ther.* **2000**, *38*, 347–372.
77. Tangney, J.P.; Wagner, P.E.; Gavlas, J.; Gramzow, R. *The Test of Self-Conscious Affect for Adolescents (TOSCA-A)*; George Mason University: Fairfax, VA, USA, 1991.
78. Hayes, A.F. Partial, conditional, and moderated moderated mediation: Quantification, inference, and interpretation. *Commun. Monogr.* **2017**, *85*, 4–40. [CrossRef]

79. MacKinnon, D.P.; Krull, J.L.; Lockwood, C.M. Equivalence of the Mediation, Confounding and Suppression Effect. *Prev. Sci.* **2000**, *1*, 173–181. [CrossRef]
80. Hall, J.H.; Finchman, F.D. Self-forgiveness: The stepchild of forgiveness research. *J. Soc. Clin. Psychol.* **2005**, *24*, 621–637. [CrossRef]
81. Jacinto, G.A.; Edwards, B.L. Therapeutic stages of forgiveness and self-forgiveness. *J. Hum. Behav. Soc. Environ.* **2011**, *21*, 423–437. [CrossRef]
82. Clark, D.A.; Purdon, C.L. The assessment of unwanted intrusive thoughts: A review and critique of the literature. *Behav. Res. Ther.* **1995**, *33*, 967–976. [CrossRef]
83. Barcaccia, B.; Tenore, K.; Mancini, F. Early Childhood Experiences Shaping Vulnerability to Obsessive-Compulsive Disorder. *Clin. Neuropsychiatry* **2015**, *12*, 141–147.
84. Mancini, F.; Saliani, A. Senso di colpa deontologico e perdono di sé nel disturbo ossessivo-compulsivo. In *Teoria e Clinica del Perdono*; Barcaccia, B., Mancini, F., Eds.; Raffaello Cortina Editore: Milano, Italy, 2013; pp. 131–144.
85. Petrocchi, N.; Barcaccia, B.; Couyoumdjian, A. Il Perdono di Sè: Analisi del Costrutto e Possibili Applicazoni Cliniche. In *Teoria e Clinica del Perdono*; Barcaccia, B., Mancini, F., Eds.; Raffaello Cortina Editore: Milano, Italy, 2013; pp. 146–185.

MDPI
St. Alban-Anlage 66
4052 Basel
Switzerland
Tel. +41 61 683 77 34
Fax +41 61 302 89 18
www.mdpi.com

Brain Sciences Editorial Office
E-mail: brainsci@mdpi.com
www.mdpi.com/journal/brainsci

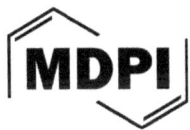

www.ingramcontent.com/pod-product-compliance
Lightning Source LLC
LaVergne TN
LVHW070737100526
838202LV00013B/1255